610.76

Score Hi

on the AT

Score Higher on the UKCAT

The expert guide from Kaplan, with over 1000 questions and a mock online test

SECOND EDITION

Brian Holmes
Kaplan Test Prep

Dr Marianna Parker
Kaplan Test Prep

Dr Katie Hunt
Kaplan Test Prep

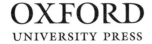

OXFORD
UNIVERSITY PRESS

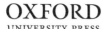

OXFORD
UNIVERSITY PRESS

Great Clarendon Street, Oxford, OX2 6DP,
United Kingdom

Oxford University Press is a department of the University of Oxford.
It furthers the University's objective of excellence in research, scholarship,
and education by publishing worldwide. Oxford is a registered trade mark of
Oxford University Press in the UK and in certain other countries

© Kaplan Test Prep, 2014

The moral rights of the authors have been asserted

First Edition published in 2012
Second Edition published in 2014

Impression: 1

Published in the United States of America by Oxford University Press
198 Madison Avenue, New York, NY 10016, United States of America

British Library Cataloguing in Publication Data
Data available

Library of Congress Control Number: 2014934231

ISBN 978-0-19-870431-7

Printed in Great Britain by
Clays Ltd, St Ives plc

Preface

One test stands between you and a place at the medical school of your dreams: the UKCAT.

No matter how strongly you perform in your GCSEs and A-levels, you are likely to find the UKCAT incredibly challenging. Most students who apply to study medicine get top results in their other exams, and are used to surpassing any academic challenge they have encountered. Such students make up virtually the entire UKCAT cohort, and so the UKCAT is designed to differentiate among this cohort of highly capable and resourceful students.

Most UKCAT test-takers do very little to prepare for the exam, and each year countless students find that Test Day comes as a rude surprise. They have never sat an exam that they were unable to finish, or in which they were unable to understand fully the nature of the questions being asked. Sadly, these students are unable to get a place studying medicine because of their poor UKCAT results, and must wait another year before taking the test again. At Kaplan, we have helped hundreds of students in this situation over the past few years, and they always tell us the same thing: they wish someone had told them they could prepare for the UKCAT.

Despite what you may have heard, the UKCAT is very much a test you can prepare for, and here's why: the UKCAT is a standardised test, meaning it asks the same types of questions in the same format in each section, regardless of the particular version of the test you may encounter on Test Day. Because the test is standardised, you can prepare for the specific question types, and build your confidence and score by practising for speed and accuracy—ideally with full-length mock tests in proper UKCAT format—before you sit the actual UKCAT. This book includes two full-length Kaplan UKCAT mock tests, a Diagnostic Test that will orient you to the format and challenges of the UKCAT, and a final Mock Test to complete your preparation, as you put the Kaplan top tips learnt in this book fully into practice.

This book includes Kaplan's top tips for building a higher score on each section of the UKCAT, and distils the basics of Kaplan's comprehensive UKCAT course into a self-study programme. We developed the top tips at Kaplan by working with dozens of UKCAT teachers and helping thousands of students prepare for the UKCAT since its inception in 2006. Our Kaplan top tips have a proven track record, in that they can be learnt and practised so that they become 'second nature' by Test Day, and are genuinely helpful for most students to improve their timing and their score.

We know that getting into medical school is a challenging endeavour, and we have written this book to help you navigate the challenges of the UKCAT. By learning and practising the Kaplan top tips, we hope you will achieve a score that will 'make the cut', so you can pursue your dream of becoming a doctor.

Study smart—and think success!

Brian Holmes
Dr Marianna Parker
Dr Katie Hunt

Contents

About the authors

Brian Holmes

Brian is the Academic Director at Kaplan Test Prep International and the head writer for Kaplan's UKCAT and BMAT courses. He scored a 3250 on the UKCAT. Before relocating to London in 2006, Brian lectured in drama, classics and film at Cornell University and the University of California, Los Angeles. He graduated *summa cum laude* from Tulane University with a Bachelor of Arts in English and Greek and Latin, and earned a master's degree in theater arts from UCLA.

Dr Marianna Parker MBBS, BSc

Marianna earned a Chemistry BSc from the Massachusetts Institute of Technology and a medical degree from St George's University of London, where she was nominated for the University of London Gold Medal. As a successful applicant to both UK and US universities, she has extensive personal experience with admissions tests. She is currently training as a paediatrician at Massachusetts General Hospital in Boston.

Dr Katie Hunt MA (Cantab) MBBS

Katie studied Pre-Clinical Medicine and Developmental Biology at the University of Cambridge and then completed her medical degree at King's College London School of Medicine, graduating with Distinction. She has always enjoyed teaching and training, with experience both abroad and in the UK. Katie has taught UKCAT and BMAT courses for Kaplan since 2007, including as lead UKCAT teacher. She is a Paediatric Trainee in London, currently working at St Thomas' Hospital, and also has a keen interest in medical education.

About Kaplan Test Prep

Kaplan Test Prep (**www.kaptest.co.uk**) has offered test preparation courses in the UK since 1993. Kaplan has been the leading provider of preparation for the UKCAT and BMAT since the tests were first introduced, and currently offers classroom-based and online courses and tutoring, in addition to this book.

First established in the United States in 1938, Kaplan Test Prep is the world leader in test preparation, offering preparation for more than 90 standardised tests, including entrance exams for UK and US universities, as well as some professional licensure exams. Kaplan Test Prep's course materials are updated on a regular basis so that Kaplan students have the most current and helpful test prep available.

Visit Kaplan Test Prep's website at **www.kaptest.co.uk/ukcattest** to access the free, full-length Kaplan UKCAT Mock Online Test, which we recommend that you complete after working through the practice questions and mock tests in this book.

Score Higher on the UKCAT: test updates and mock online test

The key to achieving a high score in the UKCAT is to become familiar with the style of questions and practise these to develop your technique. It is also very important to practise answering the questions within the timing of the real exam. Once you have finished working through the book you can undertake Kaplan's Mock Online Test. You will also want to check the test updates in our Online Resource Centre in the year you sit the UKCAT, to ensure you are aware of any test changes in that year.

Test Updates

Test updates are freely available to readers of this book, but are password protected. To access the test updates, simply visit the online resource centre at **www.oxfordtextbooks.co.uk/orc/kaplan_ukcat2e/** and enter the following username and password:

> *Username*: kaplan

> *Password*: medicalschool

Annual changes to the UK Clinical Aptitude Test by the exam provider are usually announced in April and July, and we will announce any updates on the Online Resource Centre soon thereafter.

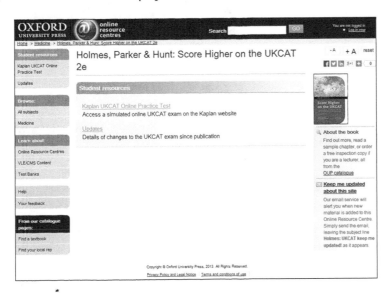

Mock Online Test

This is freely available at **www.kaptest.co.uk/ukcattest**

The Kaplan Mock Online Test looks and functions exactly like the real UKCAT exam so on Test Day you will be familiar with its layout and navigation. The test is automatically timed to mirror the official UKCAT so you can practise getting your timing just right.

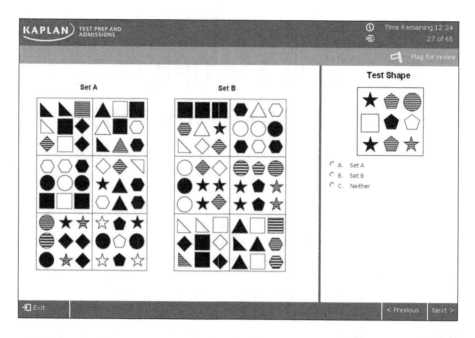

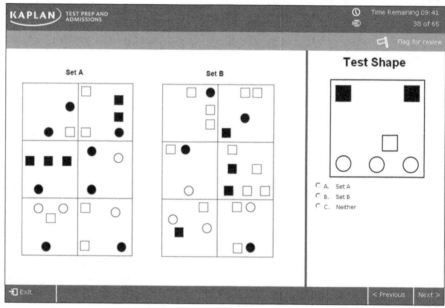

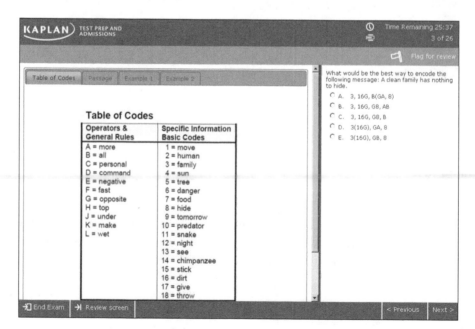

Assessing the UKCAT

Doctors cannot help patients get better without first completing an assessment, to ensure that they fully understand the issues and symptoms their patients are presenting. It is essential to adopt the same mindset when preparing for the UK Clinical Aptitude Test (UKCAT), which serves a very different purpose than any other exam you have taken, and presents very different challenges than you are likely to have encountered on any previous exam.

As part of your initial assessment of the UKCAT, you will complete the Kaplan UKCAT Diagnostic Test (Chapter 2), which will help you to understand the issues with question format and timing in each section. First, let's take a few minutes to consider the fundamental logic of the UKCAT.

Why sit the UKCAT?

The basic reason to sit the UKCAT is that it is required for admission to 26 medical and dental programmes in the UK. The 26 universities that require the UKCAT for medical and dental admissions are known as the UKCAT Consortium, the test-maker responsible for the UKCAT since its inception in 2006. Most universities in the UKCAT Consortium require the UKCAT for undergraduate admissions, though a few require the exam for postgraduate admissions. Check the test-maker's website (www.ukcat.ac.uk) for a current and complete list.

NB A few UK universities, including Oxford and Cambridge, require a different exam called the BMAT (www.bmat.org.uk) for medical admissions. Depending on which universities you plan to apply to, you may have to sit both the UKCAT and the BMAT.

How important is the UKCAT?

There is a further reason that the UKCAT is an essential part of the medical and dental admissions process: most programmes that require the UKCAT will use your results to determine which applicants are invited to interview. The most common approach is to set a 'cut-off' score: applicants with UKCAT results above the cut-off are invited to interview; those with UKCAT results below the cut-off are not. In this sense, then, your UKCAT result will likely be 'make or break' for getting into a medical or dental programme.

Most programmes that use a cut-off score are rather discreet about the fact that they do so, and as a result it can be difficult to find out exactly where they draw the line between scores that get invited to interview and scores that are out of luck. Anecdotal evidence from many students who have been through the admissions process recently reveals that the cut-off score is usually right around the average mark on the UKCAT, which is currently a total score of 2643, or an average of 660 in each section. To ensure that you score higher than the cut-off score, you will want to try and score above average on the UKCAT. The good news is that it is very possible to do so, but you will need to invest time in learning Kaplan's top tips and putting them into practice. In order to secure a medical or dental interview, it is essential to prepare for the UKCAT, and to do your absolute best to get the highest score possible on Test Day.

What does the UKCAT test?

The UKCAT is not a test of content that you studied at GCSE or A-level, and it has been designed with a very different format and timing than those exams. As such, the UKCAT will require a very different approach. The UKCAT consists of five sections, each of which tests your ability to provide the most correct answers in a very short time.

Here is a brief overview of the task, number of questions and timing in each section.

Verbal Reasoning: You must assess statements by finding relevant information and making inferences from a reading passage. You must answer 44 items in 21 minutes.

Quantitative Reasoning: You must find relevant data and complete basic calculations (most involve arithmetic, algebra and/or geometry). You must answer 36 questions in 22 minutes.

Abstract Reasoning: You must find patterns or progressions in sets of shapes, and match new shapes to existing patterns and progressions. You must answer 55 items in 13 minutes.

Decision Analysis: You must evaluate the logical meaning of messages using a table of codes. You must answer 28 questions in 33 minutes.

Situational Judgement: You must determine the most pressing issues in a clinical or educational scenario, and evaluate a series of possible responses to the scenario. You must answer 71 items in 26 minutes.

As you can see, the UKCAT will not require you to use any content that you learnt in school, with the exception of a few basic formulae (e.g. those involving percentage, mean, speed and geometry) in the Quantitative Reasoning section. Most of the work required to answer correctly in most sections is particular to the types of questions on the UKCAT. Thus, you will need to learn the workings of the various question types, so you can improve your speed and accuracy at answering individual questions and in working through each section.

Timing is also a significant challenge on the UKCAT. You have about a minute to answer each Decision Analysis question, and 30 seconds or less to answer each question in the other four sections. This timing is much quicker than you will likely have experienced on any exam you have sat previously. It is very common for students to be unable to finish one or more sections of the first UKCAT test paper they sit, so don't be alarmed if this happens to you on the Kaplan UKCAT Diagnostic Test. Just be glad that you are not one of the many unlucky students each year who have the experience of being unable to finish whilst sitting the actual UKCAT. Sitting the realistic practice tests in this book will be essential in preparing yourself for the timing and 'endurance' factors of answering 234 questions in 2 hours on Test Day. You can obtain a further practice test free of charge at www.kaptest.co.uk/ukcattest. Each additional practice test you sit will enable you to improve your timing, give you more opportunity to practise Kaplan's top tips and allow you to make mistakes. Remember: any mistake you make whilst practising for the UKCAT is one you can avoid on Test Day.

The test-taking format is a further challenge in that the UKCAT is taken on a computer at a testing centre. You can find a complete list of UKCAT testing centres on the UKCAT website, along with a tutorial and demonstration of the test-taking interface. The UKCAT Consortium also provides two full-length practice tests in the computerised interface, which are available for free on the UKCAT website. You are strongly advised to work through these tests, but you should do so after completing the chapters in this book. Don't worry if you have worked through the official computerised practice tests already. If you haven't, you will get more out of them once you have learnt Kaplan's top tips and completed the paper-based practice tests in this book. It is essential that you become familiar with the exact appearance and functions in the test-taking interface. These include the option to move back and forth between questions, to flag questions for review and to review questions (whether flagged, unanswered or all questions) at the end of a section. The computerised interface also includes an onscreen calculator, which you will want to practise using so you can be prepared for Quantitative Reasoning.

How is the UKCAT scored?

The first four sections of the UKCAT are each scored from 300 to 900. According to the test-maker, most people who sit the UKCAT score between 500 and 700 in each section. Scores above 700 in any section are considered difficult to achieve, and very impressive indeed. According to data provided by the UKCAT Consortium, the average score is just above or below 600 in each section.

Your results are tabulated by the computer, and you will be given a printout when you leave the testing room. Don't lose this printout, as there is a charge to obtain a replacement copy. Your results are automatically sent to the universities you select on your UCAS form; for this reason, you must sit the UKCAT in the year when you are applying for admission. Scores do not carry over from one year to another, and you can sit the UKCAT only once per year.

Although the scores are scaled from 300 to 900, the actual scoring is very simple. You get a mark for each correct answer. There is no negative marking, so you do not lose any marks for incorrect answers. You do not gain or lose any marks for questions that are left unanswered. Leaving many questions unanswered in one or more sections is the most common mistake made by UKCAT test-takers on Test Day. Doing so virtually ensures that you will score well below the average in at least one section, which will make it difficult to pass the cut-off score required for interview.

Situational Judgement scores are given from Band 1 to Band 4 (highest to lowest), depending how many of your answers match those determined by the panel of medical experts. You get full marks for choosing the correct answer, and partial marks for choosing an answer that is close to the correct answer. The exact details of the partial marking have not been disclosed by the UKCAT Consortium, but this means that you have a good chance of getting some marks for each Situational Judgement question, so long as you mark an answer.

How do you get top scores?

The first tip, if perhaps a somewhat obvious one, is to mark an answer for every question. You may not be comfortable with marking answers for questions you have not actually attempted. However, it is possible that you may find yourself running out of time as you get to the end of one or more sections, despite your best efforts in preparing for the UKCAT, as the timing is so tight. If you have a few questions you are unable to work out properly, it is better to mark an answer and gain a chance of picking up the marks than to leave them blank and have 0% chance of picking up the mark.

Verbal Reasoning and Abstract Reasoning questions have three or four answer choices. Situational Judgement questions have four answer choices. Quantitative Reasoning and Decision Analysis questions have five answer choices. Consider the odds of guessing correctly when guessing blindly—as compared to guessing strategically—in the following table.

Number of answer choices	Odds of correctly guessing blindly	Odds of correctly guessing strategically, after eliminating 1 answer	Odds of correctly guessing strategically, after eliminating 2 answers
3	33%	50%	100%
4	25%	33%	50%
5	20%	25%	33%

When you can eliminate one or more answer choices, guessing strategically gives you a much stronger chance of answering correctly and picking up the mark. The odds of guessing blindly are not bad, particularly when there are only three answer choices. Still, you should only guess blindly if you are running out of time and at risk of leaving questions unanswered.

You can minimise blind guessing by following the next tip: maximise your marks with question triage. Since you have so little time to answer each question, the UKCAT can challenge you by presenting you with a few questions in each section that take far longer than the average timing per question to answer properly. For instance, you might see a few questions in the Quantitative section that would take 2 or more minutes to solve using straightforward maths, rather than the 30 seconds allotted. If you take the time to answer one such question by doing the straightforward maths, and spending 90 seconds more than you have, then you will effectively have ensured that you are unable to answer 3 questions later in the section. Unless you were on the final Quantitative set, you could be sure that there would be at least 3 more questions that you could reasonably answer in 30 seconds each. Answering those 3 questions would earn you 3 more marks, whereas answering the one long question picks up only a single mark. Since there are fairly few questions in each section that are meant to be very time-consuming, you must triage these questions. Rather than following the usual timing, spend no more than 10 seconds on one that appears to be very time-consuming. Make a strategic or blind guess, mark an answer, flag the question for review and move on. You will need to practise for triage—and to build up your confidence in deploying triage as a test-taking strategy—but students who do so usually score well above 700 in most (if not all) sections of the UKCAT.

The reason for this has to do with the exact correspondence of the number of correct answers in each section to the scaled scores from 300 to 900. Based on extensive feedback from students who have sat the UKCAT, we have prepared a scoring table which you can find at the end of the two practice tests in this book (on p. 72 and p. 280). If you check the scoring table, you will notice that you can score 700 or above by answering approximately three-quarters of the questions in a section correctly. A score of 700 in a section would place you in the top 10% of UKCAT test-takers—a phenomenal achievement, and one you can attain without answering all the questions in a section correctly.

All the questions in the UKCAT have been written for a certain objective level of difficulty. If you think of question difficulty as a continuum from easy to medium to hard, most questions will be in the 'medium' range on the continuum, with a few towards the extremes of 'easy' and 'hard'. Time-consuming questions (i.e. those that take more than the allotted time per question to answer) are always objectively at the 'hard' end of the difficulty continuum, and the test cannot give you very many of these in any one section. Triage can thus help you maximise your marks in each section, by spending the time allotted on the easy and medium questions, which should certainly account for at least three-quarters of the total. Maximising your marks on these questions will be essential to earning a high score.

The final tip for getting a top score on the UKCAT is to make the most of this book. Learn the test formats and tips for each section. Practise for strategy as well as pacing. This book is loaded with Kaplan timed practice sets, which will allow you to practise triage, while also deploying Kaplan's top tips and ensuring that you answer every question before time is up. Review the worked answers for every question you attempt while practising, so you can ensure that you are getting the right answers for the right reasons, and in the fastest time possible.

When you are ready to begin your UKCAT preparation, set aside a couple of hours and sit the Kaplan UKCAT Diagnostic Test in Chapter 2. Be sure to review all the worked answers soon after the test—ideally the same day, or the next day. Many UKCAT test-takers never sit a full-length practice test, so you will have a huge advantage over the competition after finishing the next chapter.

2

Kaplan UKCAT Diagnostic Test

You have 2 hours to complete the Kaplan UKCAT Diagnostic Test. You will need the following items:

- This book.
- A pen or pencil to record your answers.
- Scrap paper for any written calculations and notations.
- A timer (such as one on your watch, mobile or computer).
- A calculator.

Time each section strictly, so you can practise under test-like conditions.

On Test Day, you will have an additional minute to read the directions for each section. That minute cannot be used to answer test questions, so it has not been included here. Time yourself using the timings given once you turn each instructions page and start work on each section.

Answer the questions as quickly and accurately as possible. There is no negative marking, so you are strongly encouraged to mark an answer for every question in each section.

Pace yourself so you can attempt all the items in each section.

Record your answers on a sheet of paper, and check them against the explanations in Appendix B once you finish.

NB You cannot write on the test paper on Test Day, because the test is taken on a computer. So be careful not to get into the habit of writing on the practice questions in this book. Make any notations, eliminations, etc., entirely on scrap paper, and not directly on the questions themselves.

Your score on Test Day corresponds to the number of questions you answer correctly. You can find your equivalent score on the scoring table at the end of the test.

Section 1: Verbal Reasoning (21 Minutes)

This section contains 11 passages, each of which is followed by four items. Some passages in this section will be followed by four statements. Your task is to decide whether each statement logically flows from the information presented in the passage. You have three answer choices for each statement:

True: The information in the statement is stated explicitly in the passage or is a valid inference.

False: The information in the statement contradicts what is stated in the passage.

Can't tell: There is not enough information to determine whether the statement is True or False.

Some passages in this section will be followed by four questions; each question will have four answer choices. Choose the best answer, based on the passage.

Answer all 44 items in Section 1, selecting one of the possible answers and circling the letter corresponding to the appropriate answer in your test book.

When you are finished with this section, you may use any remaining time to review your work in this section only. Once you proceed to the next section, you may not return to this section.

You will have 21 minutes to answer the questions. It is in your best interest to select an answer for every item as there is no penalty for wrong answers.

Set your timer for 21 minutes, turn the page and begin the section.

Recent research has demonstrated that all of today's polar bears are descended from prehistoric (and long since extinct) brown bears that lived in Ireland. Female brown bears of this very ancient species interbred with a similarly prehistoric species of polar bear during the last Ice Age, which ultimately wiped out the earlier, non-hybrid polar bears. Scientists were able to prove that today's polar bears maintain a direct hereditary line to the prehistoric brown bears of Ireland using mitochondrial DNA. An offspring's mitochondrial DNA is identical to its mother's, and can be used to trace maternal ancestry back through the generations. Bones and teeth from about a dozen female brown bears that lived in Ireland 100 to 380 centuries ago—during the last Ice Age—match the mitochondrial DNA found in polar bears today.

Polar bears and brown bears are usually known to favour very different behaviours and climates. Polar bears eat a diet composed exclusively of meat and fish, and excel at swimming and hunting prey in the cold, icy seas that are their required habitat. Brown bears live in the forest and eat a diet that includes carnivorous options, along with plants and berries.

Of course, Ireland is far too warm for polar bears today, though its climate would have cooled considerably during the Ice Age, bringing the prehistoric polar bears into contact with the ancient brown bears that would join them in creating the polar bear as we know it today.

1. Which of these statements about brown bears cannot be true?
   A. They are known to eat plants and berries.
   — B. They eat only meat and fish.
   C. They favour a habitat with trees.
   D. They prefer a habitat that is not watery or icy.

2. The ancestry of polar bears has been traced to prehistoric brown bears in Ireland because the two types of bears have:
   A. identical mitochondria.
   — B. the same mitochondrial DNA.
   C. mothers with similar traits.
   D. an unbroken chain of paternal genes.

3. In the last Ice Age, it must be true that:
   A. Iceland's climate cooled.
   B. Ireland's climate warmed up.
   C. Iceland's climate warmed up.
   __ D. Ireland's climate cooled.

4. The author would be most likely to agree with which of the following assertions?
   — A. Some bears survived the Ice Age.
   B. Mating between species is a common occurrence.
   C. No bears survived the Ice Age.
   D. There are no examples of successful mating between species.

Sarah Bernhardt was a French stage and early film actress, known in her day as 'the most famous actress the world has ever known'. She was educated at the French Conservatoire, the Government-sponsored school of acting at that time, from the age of 13, and made her debut as a member of the French national theatre company Comédie-Française in 1862. Bernhardt did not really become recognised, though, until 1868, when she performed the role of Anna Danby in Alexandre Dumas' play *Kean* at the Odéon Theatre in Paris.

Bernhardt's fame grew further in the 1870s, and she enjoyed a decades-long career as an actress across Europe and the Americas. Among her most famous roles were Zanetto in the verse play *Le Passant* by François Coppée, which she played by special request before Napoleon III, and the title role in Voltaire's *Zaire*, performed after her return to the Comédie-Française in 1872. Bernhardt was also well known off-stage for her strange habits and complicated personality. The novelist Alexandre Dumas, son of the author Alexandre Dumas (who wrote *Kean*) and author himself of *The Three Musketeers*, described Bernhardt as a notorious liar, and she was widely rumoured to sleep every night in a coffin, rather than a bed. Little is known about her biography or early life; her birth certificate was lost in a fire when she was young, and she fabricated new birth records in order to prove citizenship for the French Légion d'honneur. Even though her past is largely inscrutable, her work has been immortalised on screen, in art and in photographs; her image appears in a number of paintings by the famous Art Nouveau painter and decorative artist Alphonse Mucha. She was a pioneer in film, playing Hamlet in the short film *Le Duel d'Hamlet* in 1900 and starring in eight motion pictures and two biographical films. Today, she is best remembered as a serious dramatic actress, for the work that earned her the nickname 'The Divine Sarah' in the late nineteenth and early twentieth century.

5. All of these statements regarding Sarah Bernhardt's career are true except:
   A. She never appeared in films.
   B. She played the role of Hamlet.
   C. Her career spanned two centuries.
   D. Her career spanned multiple continents.

6. An unusual fact about the novelist who wrote *The Three Musketeers* is that:
   A. his father was also a novelist.
   B. he and his father were not actually French.
   C. he and his father had the same name.
   D. his father was France's best-known actor.

7. The author suggests that Sarah Bernhardt's personal history:
   A. was entirely fabricated.
   B. was based in unfounded rumours that she was a vampire.
   C. is more or less unknowable.
   D. is irrelevant to her reputation.

8. According to the passage, in the 19th century the French government:
   A. fully funded the French national theatre.
   B. invested heavily in early films.
   C. supported the work of Art Nouveau painters.
   D. subsidised a theatre training scheme.

The Town and Country Planning Act, passed in 1947, established the national system of town planning and development still in use across the UK today. The act outlined laws governing ownership, construction and development of property across the UK, administered on the local level by 421 Local Planning Authorities. The system is plan-led, meaning that all development of properties in the UK must begin with a development plan, public consultation and planning permission.

Over time, the Town and Country Planning Act has become a particularly effective vehicle through which the Government has been able to achieve its objectives for climate control, reduction of carbon emissions and housing access, among other initiatives. In addition, the act makes provisions for the protection and maintenance of listed buildings, those that carry architectural or historical interest. Owners of such structures can be required by law to keep these buildings in good repair, and must receive listed building consent before they are able to make any alterations that would affect the structure's character or appearance.

Fifty-nine years after its institution, the Town and Country Planning Act was revised, and the Development Plan formerly required by the law was replaced by the Local Development Framework. The change was designed to increase community and public involvement and also to help promote such government initiatives as energy-efficient transportation, highway safety, housing supply and natural preservation. Today, planning applications must also include a Design and Access statement, which describes the proposed design and the process by which it was determined, the extent of public engagement and the ways in which the proposed development adheres to the relevant principles of good design. The Design and Access statement is one way in which the government creates planning policies with an eye to broad public interests, rather than the private interests or profitability of a single individual or corporation.

9. It must be true that the Town and Country Planning Act:

   A. has not changed fundamentally since it became law.
   B. was revised in 2006.
   C. no longer requires a Local Development Framework.
   D. applies only in England and Wales.

10. According to the passage, which of these assertions must be false?

    A. Listed buildings can be refurbished.
    B. Listed buildings have some architectural or historical relevance.
    C. Listed buildings can never be repaired.
    D. Listed buildings cannot be altered without consent.

11. A planning application in the UK today must include:

    A. some evidence of engagement with the public.
    B. a Development Plan.
    C. consent of the local council.
    D. a study of projected impact on local roads.

12. The author would most likely agree that town planning:

    A. cannot impact the housing supply.
    B. can reduce carbon emissions.
    C. cannot improve highway safety.
    D. should only apply to publicly owned property.

All testimony taken by the commission must be transcribed in the language in which it is given. The possible languages for testimony to the commission are English, French, Arabic or a tribal language.

All testimony must also be summarised in either English or French. Summaries of testimony may be prepared in the field, or at the commission's head office in Strasbourg. Due to a lack of translators who speak both Arabic and French in the field, all testimony transcribed in Arabic can only be summarised into French at the head office. No one at head office speaks the tribal languages, so all testimony taken and transcribed in a tribal language must be summarised in English or French by translators working in the field.

All summarised testimonies will be translated into the alternate language (English or French), before being indexed with all other summaries in the same language. The alternate translation of summaries and indexing of summaries must be completed at head office.

13. No one at head office translates Arabic.

    A. True
    B. False
    C. Can't tell

14. A testimony may be taken, transcribed and initially summarised entirely in English.

    A. True
    B. False
    C. Can't tell

15. Testimony taken in a tribal language must be transcribed in French.

    A. True
    B. False
    C. Can't tell

16. Summaries of testimony taken in Arabic must be completed in Strasbourg.

    A. True
    B. False
    C. Can't tell

In 2008, UK Culture Secretary Andy Burnham initiated a process that reviewed the standing and worth of the UK's World Heritage Sites. The committee review followed a request by UNESCO for represented countries to slow their nominations and produce a statement of their intention to give priority to land and sea habitats in need of protection. Though UNESCO was founded to catalogue, name and preserve sites of both cultural and natural importance to humanity across the world, the vast majority of currently designated World Heritage Sites are cultural landmarks.

Founded in November 1945, the United Nations Educational, Scientific, and Cultural Organization (UNESCO) has listed a total of 911 sites, of which 704 are sites of outstanding cultural importance. The sites span 151 countries, but countries in Europe are far better represented than those in most other continents. There are 28 identified World Heritage Sites in the UK and its overseas territories: 17 in England; 4 in Scotland; 3 in Wales; and 1 each in Northern Ireland, Bermuda, the Pitcairn Islands and St Helena. Only seven nations have a greater number of identified World Heritage Sites.

Burnham's interest in reviewing the value of the UK's sites was more than just a charitable gesture to those countries currently underrepresented, though. The cost of World Heritage Sites has been on the rise for a number of years. As part of its commitment to the United Nations Educational, Scientific and Cultural Organization, the UK contributes £130,000 per year to the preservation of sites in developing countries, and £150,000 per year to maintain the UK's sites. In addition, the cost of application to UNESCO has risen to around £400,000. In the wake of the financial crisis, Burnham's inquiry into the value of these sites reflected the ongoing challenges of balancing the budget and investing in sites of national and international importance.

17. What proportion of the World Heritage Sites in the UK and its overseas territories are in England, Scotland or Wales?

    A. 79%

    B. 86%

    C. 90%

    D. 100%

18. The UK's total annual cost of preserving World Heritage Sites in the UK and developing countries is:

    A. £130,000

    B. £150,000

    C. £280,000

    D. £680,000

19. The author would most likely agree that UNESCO's priority is recognising more

    A. World Heritage Sites in Europe.

    B. sites of cultural and national importance.

    C. cultural sites located south of the Equator.

    D. ecosystems, including marine ecosystems, that are at risk.

20. Which of these statements must be false?

    A. Most of the World Heritage Sites are cultural landmarks.

    B. Some of the World Heritage Sites are ecological areas.

    C. Some of the World Heritage Sites are cultural landmarks.

    D. None of the World Heritage Sites are ecological areas.

The last few winters in the UK have proven especially harsh. Each winter seems to bring several major snowfalls of 5 to 8 inches in 24 hours; most of the UK is not equipped for such 'blizzards'. Only a few local authorities in England have snow ploughs, as gritting lorries are usually sufficient for snowfalls of 3 inches or less. Unfortunately, gritting salt is not effective during snowfalls with larger accumulations, with the consequence that thousands of schools have had to shut, sometimes for a week or even longer, until the snow has melted, because there is no other way of clearing the roads and pavements.

Many people have suggested that the UK must plan better and invest in appropriate winter equipment, so the country does not continue to stop working and travelling whenever there is more than a few inches of snow. Some countries with very harsh winters, such as Norway and Sweden, view road safety as a shared responsibility of all drivers (rather than purely a matter of state spending), and require all cars and lorries to switch to studded tyres during fixed dates each winter. Other countries that experience frequent blizzards in winter, such as the USA and Canada, invest in mechanised equipment that can clear airport runways quickly, dig out snow that has settled around planes parked at boarding gates and 'de-ice' planes so they are safe to fly in the harshest of winter conditions. Sadly, there is no such equipment at major British airports such as Heathrow, where a blizzard in December 2010 required hundreds of planes that were parked at passenger gates as the snow fell to be dug out by hand, resulting in severe flight delays for five days and costing the airlines and the British economy to lose tens of millions of pounds.

21. The author would least likely agree with which of these assertions?
    A. Snowfall of 5 inches in 24 hours is not, strictly speaking, a blizzard.
    B. Winters in the UK have been much snowier in the last few years.
    C. Snowfall of 5 inches in 24 hours constitutes a blizzard.
    D. The UK experienced a blizzard in 2010.

22. Gritting salt works best when:
    A. applied to roads before snow falls.
    B. used in combination with studded tyres.
    C. supplied from North America or Scandinavia.
    D. fewer than 3 inches of snow accumulates.

23. The passage suggests that Heathrow does not have:
    A. any of the equipment found at American airports.
    B. all the same equipment as Canadian airports.
    C. a plan to deal with passengers in a blizzard.
    D. a method of clearing snow from parked planes.

24. The most severe consequence of heavy snow in the UK mentioned in the passage is that:
    A. children missed a day of school.
    B. pavements were especially slippery.
    C. financial losses in the tens of millions were incurred.
    D. Heathrow had to hire American de-icing equipment.

Kathleen Mansfield Beauchamp Murry, better known by her pseudonym Katherine Mansfield, was born in 1888 in New Zealand. The daughter of a prominent banker, she moved to London in 1903 to attend Queen's College, where she trained as a professional cellist. She would go on to become one of the early twentieth-century's most significant short story writers, best known for writing in which she explored alienation, mental illness and disruption. Some of her short stories, such as *The Garden Party*, *The Daughters of the Late Colonel* and *The Fly*, continue to be taught in schools and universities today.

Though she lived for only 34 years, Mansfield had an active and tumultuous life. She was close to many important members of the literary community in London of her day, including notable writers like Virginia Woolf and D.H. Lawrence. She was engaged several times and, in 1909, married George Bowden, a singing teacher, whom she left just hours after their wedding. This hasty marriage and divorce particularly distressed her parents, who sent her away to a spa town in Germany later that year. Though a very difficult time in Mansfield's life, her time in Germany was enormously influential on her writing. It was here that she was introduced to the work of the late Russian playwright Anton Chekhov, who would become one of her most important literary inspirations.

Mansfield was incredibly prolific while she was in Germany. Returning to London the following January, she published more than a dozen short stories in A.R. Orage's socialist magazine *The New Age*, though she had managed to publish only one story and one poem in the previous fifteen months she'd spent living in London. Her time in Germany also set the foundation for the first published collection of her stories, *In a German Pension*. The collection was well received by critics in the UK and inspired her to submit a short story, *The Woman at the Store*, to John Middleton Murry's magazine *Rhythm*. The two would marry in London in 1918, a year after Mansfield was diagnosed with tuberculosis. Though Mansfield sought treatment abroad in her later years, her illness prevented her from ever returning to her home in New Zealand. She died in 1922 in France, while seeking treatment.

25. Chekhov lived in Germany for a time.

    A. True

    B. False

    C. Can't tell

26. Of all the arts, Mansfield achieved greatest recognition for her accomplishments in music.

    A. True

    B. False

    C. Can't tell

27. Mansfield was a prominent socialist.

    A. True

    B. False

    C. Can't tell

28. Virginia Woolf lived in London in the early 1900s.

    A. True

    B. False

    C. Can't tell

As schoolchildren, we all learned that the circumference of a circle is equal to the radius multiplied by two, multiplied by the mathematical constant pi. Pi has always been defined as the ratio of a circle's circumference to its diameter, without controversy—until now. A dissenting group of mathematicians and scientists are advocating that pi be replaced with tau, a new maths constant defined as the ratio of a circle's circumference to its radius, or approximately 6.28, exactly double the value of pi.

Proponents of tau fault pi for mistakenly making a circle's diameter more important than its radius. Because all other calculations involving circles (and circle-based solids, such as spheres and cylinders) are based on the radius, solving for these values using the diameter and pi almost always involves an extra factor of 2, which must be divided out; such calculations would be easier with tau, according to its supporters. The one exception, which opponents of tau are quick to point out, is the area of a circle, which equals pi times radius squared. Tau would have to be divided by 2 for equations involving a circle's area (including the area of a sector of a circle and of the base of a cylinder), which is proof of tau's uselessness to its opponents. Tau's supporters, meanwhile, would argue that the vast majority of circle-based calculations in real-life applications, such as engineering, computing and science, do not involve area, so pi continues to require unnecessary factors of 2 in most (if not nearly all) cases beyond the maths classroom.

29. The author would most likely agree that most teachers and scientists prefer:
    A. a vote by mathematicians on whether to replace pi with tau.
    B. an international conference on the future of maths.
    C. replacing pi with tau for circle-based calculations.
    D. continuing to use pi for circle-based calculations.

30. Traditionally, pi has been understood as:
    A. the proportion of circumference to diameter.
    B. the only essential measurement of a circle.
    C. the most critical mathematical constant.
    D. a subject of controversy among mathematicians.

31. Proponents of tau would agree that pi unnecessarily involves a factor of 2 in calculations by all of these professionals except:
    A. teachers
    B. scientists
    C. engineers
    D. computer programmers

32. A circle's radius does not relate in any direct way to:
    A. its area.
    B. the height of a cylinder.
    C. its circumference.
    D. the area of the base of a cylinder.

The British Film Academy, now known as the British Academy of Film and Television Arts, was founded in 1947 to promote and reward great films, inspire future film-makers and benefit the public. Today, BAFTA is perhaps best known for its annual film awards ceremony, which is typically held in February, just before the Academy Awards (or the awards given by the Academy of Motion Picture Arts and Sciences, to give the Oscars their full, proper name) in Los Angeles. Like the Oscars, the BAFTA film awards are open to nominees of all nationalities, though some awards—Best British Film and Best Newcomer, for example—are reserved for British films and film-makers.

Like most other award-granting organisations in the film industry, BAFTA gives its film awards (known as Baftas) almost entirely to feature-length films. They require that all eligible films have had a UK theatrical release in a public UK cinema for at least one week in the last year. The members of the Academy, which has Prince William as its president, vote on most of these awards, but the Academy also makes special provision for one award to be voted on by the British public: the Rising Star Award, dedicated to the memory of legendary casting director Mary Selway, who passed away in 2004, recognises new talent in the acting industry. Nominees are selected by Bafta judges, but this is the only Bafta winner chosen entirely by the public, via text, online and phone voting. The first Rising Star Award was presented to James McAvoy in 2006 in recognition of his role in *Starter for Ten*, based on the novel by David Nicholls. That same year McAvoy also starred alongside Forest Whitaker in *The Last King of Scotland*.

33. BAFTA gives awards for television as well as film.
    A. True
    B. False
    C. Can't tell

34. Only Americans are eligible for Oscar nominations.
    A. True
    B. False
    C. Can't tell

35. The first BAFTA Rising Star Award was given in 2004.
    A. True
    B. False
    C. Can't tell

36. James McAvoy is a Bafta winner.
    A. True
    B. False
    C. Can't tell

Why do sixth-formers think they must celebrate the end of exams with an enormously expensive dance? We used to make do with a disco in the school hall; if we were lucky, the crisps weren't stale and someone in our year would have some quality cassettes for us all to pretend we weren't terribly interested in dancing to, whilst staring into our cordials with cool (but not overly cool) indifference.

Nowadays, the end of exams seems to almost always bring a hideously costly 'prom', in the full-on American style. Boys hire tuxedos and limousines, and girls simply *must* buy a formal dress—many girls (or, rather, their parents) spend hundreds of pounds on a frock to be worn only once, at an event that did not exist (in the UK, anyway) ten years ago. Add in the cost of catering, decorating and hiring a DJ (no one brings their own music to a prom), and a school could easily pay £10,000 or more, all in. There is something to be said for tradition, so I say, bring back the days of the sixth-form disco! Bigger isn't always better, but it's certainly more expensive.

37. Sixth-formers traditionally mark the end of exams by celebrating with food and music.

    A. True
    B. False
    C. Can't tell

38. American-style proms did not exist ten years ago.

    A. True
    B. False
    C. Can't tell

39. Most girls spend hundreds of pounds on a prom dress.

    A. True
    B. False
    C. Can't tell

40. Some schools spend £10,000 or more on a DJ.

    A. True
    B. False
    C. Can't tell

The Office for National Statistics has released data showing the length of people's commutes from home to work in London and in the rest of the UK. Forty-two per cent of people in the UK have a commute of 15 minutes or less; the figure is much lower in London (18%) than in the rest of the UK (46%). A further 33% of people in the UK have a commute of 16 to 30 minutes; again, the figure is lower in London (26%) than in the rest of the UK. A further 12% of the national population has a commute of 31 to 45 minutes; 20% of people in London have a commute of this length. Commutes of 46 to 60 minutes and commutes in excess of one hour are taken by 20% and 16% of the population of London, respectively.

A total of 71% of the UK's workers drive a car to get to work; however, the figure for workers in London who drive (35%) is less than half that for workers who commute by driving in the rest of the UK (76%). Only 9% of UK workers outside London use public transport to commute to work; in London, 20% travel to work by train, 18% commute by underground and 12% travel to work by bus.

41. A majority of people in London have a commute that is:
   A. 30 minutes or less.
   B. 45 minutes or less.
   C. between 16 and 45 minutes.
   D. longer than 45 minutes.

42. It must be true that the proportion of workers in the rest of the UK (outside London) that drive a car to work is nearest to:
   A. three-fifths.
   B. two-thirds.
   C. seven-tenths.
   D. three-quarters.

43. The author would least likely agree with the assertion that:
   A. there are negligible differences between commutes in London and the rest of the UK.
   B. commutes in London are not representative of those in the UK as a whole.
   C. there is some variation in the lengths of commutes in the UK.
   D. there is data about the means by which people in the UK travel to work.

44. Which of these conclusions must be false?
   A. Most people commute by public transport.
   B. Most people in the UK commute by public transport.
   C. Most people commute by car.
   D. Most people in the UK commute by car.

STOP. IF YOU FINISH BEFORE TIME IS UP, CHECK ANY QUESTIONS YOU HAVE MARKED FOR REVIEW. YOU MAY GO BACK TO QUESTIONS IN THIS SECTION ONLY.

This section contains 9 sets of data, each of which is followed by four questions. Each question will have five answer choices. Your task is to select the best option based on the data provided.

Answer all 36 questions in Section 2, selecting one of the possible answers and circling the letter corresponding to the appropriate answer in your test booklet.

When you are finished with this section, you may use any remaining time to review your work in this section only. Once you proceed to the next section, you may not return to this section.

You will have 22 minutes to answer the questions. It is in your best interest to select an answer for every item as there is no penalty for wrong answers.

You may use a calculator to answer the questions in this section. On Test Day, you will be provided with an onscreen calculator that can perform the four basic operations (addition, subtraction, multiplication and division) along with only a few extra features (percentage, reciprocal, square root and memory buttons). You should not use any functions beyond these on the calculator used for this Kaplan UKCAT Diagnostic Test.

Set your timer for 22 minutes, turn the page and begin the section.

The table below shows the crime rates for Lincoln, and for the UK as a whole, in 2005–2006.

[AQ1]

Offence	Total Locally	Per 1000 Population	
		Locally	Nationally
Robbery	73	0.84	1.85
Theft of a motor vehicle	283	3.27	4.04
Theft from a motor vehicle	789	9.12	9.56
Sexual offences	186	2.15	1.17
Violence against a person	2885	33.33	19.97
Burglary	552	6.38	5.67
TOTAL	4768		

	Local	National
Population	86,547	60,200,000
Households	37,000	24,900,000

1. What percentage of crimes committed locally were thefts of motor vehicles?
   - A. 6%
   - B. 9%
   - C. 14%
   - D. 17%
   - E. 25%

2. What was the rate of crimes per person in Lincoln in 2005–2006?
   - A. 1:22
   - B. 1:21
   - C. 1:20
   - D. 1:19
   - E. 1:18

3. Approximately how many crimes of violence against a person were committed nationally in 2005–2006?
   - A. 120,000
   - B. 160,000
   - C. 1.2 million
   - D. 1.4 million
   - E. 1.6 million

4. How many burglaries were recorded in Lincoln in 2006–2007, if the total number of burglaries increased by 10% from 2005–2006?
   - A. 582
   - B. 607
   - C. 624
   - D. 648
   - E. 652

Each year the University of Chalvey keeps a record of its visitors. Below is a chart showing which subject areas the different visitors came from in 2011.

Student visitors in the library by faculty in 2011 (%)

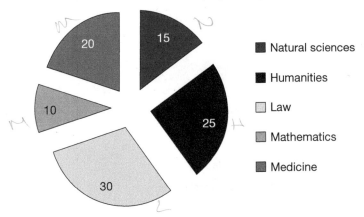

- Natural sciences
- Humanities
- Law
- Mathematics
- Medicine

The different segments of the chart indicate the percentages of students from the different faculties.

5. Which faculty had the fewest student visitors to the library in 2011?

    A. Humanities
    B. Law
    C. Mathematics
    D. Medicine
    E. Natural Sciences

6. If there were 800 student visitors from the Faculty of Medicine, how many students in total visited the library in 2011?

    A. 3,200
    B. 4,000
    C. 5,000
    E. 6,500
    F. 8,000

7. If there were 400 student visitors from the Faculty of Mathematics and 25% of all student visitors are first-year students, approximately how many first-year Law student visitors were there in 2011?

    A. 300
    B. 600
    C. 900
    D. 1,200
    E. 1,500

8. What percentage of total student visitors were not students in the Law or Humanities faculties?

    A. 35%
    B. 45%
    C. 55%
    D. 65%
    E. 75%

Omar is preparing for a raffle draw at a local charity event. He has made a list of prize items he purchased last week and their costs, which are the only prizes in the raffle.

Item	Price
Mountain Bike	£185
Tennis Racket	£45
MP3 Player	£75
Picnic Hamper	£32
Hair Dryer	£19

- Raffle tickets are priced at £1.50 each.
- Omar has set a sales target of 300 raffle tickets.
- The MP3 player and hairdryer are the only electrical prizes.

9. How much did Omar spend on the prizes?
   - A. £85
   - B. £115
   - C. £140
   - D. £356
   - E. £435

10. If Omar meets the sales target exactly, how much profit will Omar make on the raffle?
   - A. £77
   - B. £94
   - C. £114
   - D. £122
   - E. £144

11. This week, electrical products are on sale for 50% off. How much could Omar have saved if he bought the electrical prizes this week?
   - A. £9
   - B. £27
   - C. £47
   - D. £126
   - E. £309

12. How many raffle tickets must Omar sell to make a profit of £300?
   - A. 372
   - B. 437
   - C. 438
   - D. 512
   - E. 513

Russell and his friend Pauline decide to buy the total unshaded piece of land at £70 per square metre to use it as a shared vegetable patch. The unshaded piece of land, shown below, has a total area of 18 m². They plan to split the land into symmetrical vegetable patches of equal area.

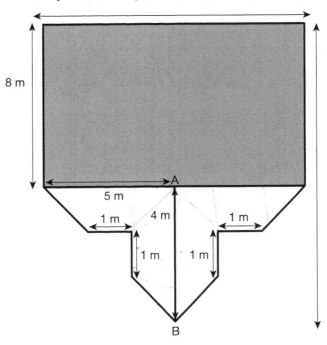

13. What is the total price that Russell and Pauline must pay for the unshaded land?

    A. £1040
    B. £1180
    C. £1260
    D. £1300
    E. £1420

14. After buying the land, they split the area equally with a 4 m fence (along line AB) to mark the borders of their respective vegetable patches. What is the area of Russell's vegetable patch, in cm²?

    A. 900 cm²
    B. 9,000 cm²
    C. 18,000 cm²
    D. 90,000 cm²
    E. 180,000 cm²

15. After a few months, Pauline decides to buy 30% of the shaded area to expand her vegetable patch, but the price of land has increased to £114 per square metre. How much will it cost her to buy the extra land?

    A. £2,394
    B. £2,736
    C. £3,468
    D. £5,700
    E. Can't tell

16. What is the total area of Pauline's vegetable patch in m², if Russell sells her half of his vegetable patch after she buys 30% of the shaded area?

    A. 28.5 m²
    B. 33 m²
    C. 37.5 m²
    D. 42 m²
    E. Can't tell

There are four different models that car manufacturer Royal produce. Below is a graph showing how many miles each of the cars can travel for every gallon of fuel used.

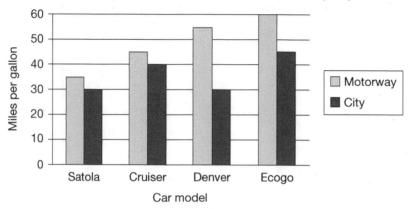

The fuel consumption of different cars manufactured by Royal cars

1 litre = 4.5 gallons

17. How many miles could you drive on a motorway on one gallon of fuel in the Denver car?
    A. 50
    B. 55
    C. 60
    D. 65
    E. 70

18. If fuel costs £1.10 a litre, approximately how much would a 30 mile city journey in a Satola cost?
    A. £1.10
    B. £2.20
    C. £3.65
    D. £4.50
    E. £4.95

19. Which of the models would be most economical for a journey that consists of 25 miles on the motorway and 5 miles in the city?
    A. Cruiser
    B. Denver
    C. Ecogo
    D. Satola
    E. Can't tell

20. How many gallons of fuel do you need if you wanted to travel 405 miles on the motorway in a Cruiser?
    A. 6
    B. 7
    C. 8
    D. 9
    E. 10

Peter wants to convert money for a series of holidays. The table below shows the currency conversions as they stood at the beginning of 2011.

	US dollar	Euro	Pound	Australian dollar	New Zealand dollar	Japanese yen
US $1 (1 US dollar)		0.71948	0.622205	0.98561	1.34644	81.9100
€1 (1 euro)	1.38990		0.86458	1.36990	1.87142	113.846
£1 (1 pound)	1.60760	1.16667		1.58447	2.16453	131.678

21. How much, to the nearest cent, will Peter receive if he converted £540 to US dollars?

    A. $802.10

    B. $840.16

    C. $868.10

    D. $890.41

    E. $914.04

22. Peter returns from his holidays with $38. How much of his original sum in US dollars did he spend?

    A. 46%

    B. 67%

    C. 76%

    D. 79%

    E. 96%

23. How many €2 coins are required to convert £108 into euros, if no other euro notes or coins are available?

    A. 63

    B. 84

    C. 92

    D. 126

    E. 141

24. What is the value of 1000 Japanese yen, in New Zealand dollars?

    A. NZ $14.60

    B. NZ $14.64

    C. NZ $16.40

    D. NZ $16.44

    E. Can't tell

Arabella has four horses: Dazzle, Truffles, Peppermint and Jack of Hearts. Her brother Leander has a horse, Galaxy, with an average trotting speed of 9.2 miles per hour. A riding trail starts at the edge of their estate, and extends a length of 11 miles through the neighbouring woodland.

25. Arabella rides Truffles at a trot for the full length of the riding trail, from one end to the other, in 1 hour, 14 minutes. What is his average trotting speed on the ride, in miles per hour?

   A. 7.8
   B. 8.1
   C. 8.9
   D. 9.2
   E. 9.6

26. Arabella rides Jack of Hearts at a canter from the start of the trail to the far end, and then all the way back to the start at a trot. She notes that his speed on the ride out (which he completed in 44 minutes) was twice his speed on the ride back. What was his average speed on the total ride?

   A. 7.5 mph
   B. 10 mph
   C. 12.5 mph
   D. 15 mph
   E. Can't tell

27. Arabella rides Dazzle and Peppermint the full length of the trail and then all the way back to its start, both at a trot, on consecutive days. Dazzle's average trotting speed was 1.4 mph faster than Peppermint's, and Dazzle completed the ride 23 minutes faster than Peppermint's time of 2 hours, 39 minutes. What was Peppermint's average trotting speed, in miles per hour?

   A. 6.9
   B. 7.6
   C. 7.9
   D. 8.3
   E. 9.7

28. Which horse has the fastest average trotting speed?

   A. Dazzle
   B. Galaxy
   C. Jack of Hearts
   D. Peppermint
   E. Truffles

The pie chart below shows the total number of hours Joe spent watching different genres of TV programmes as a proportion of his total viewing hours in two consecutive months, May (150 hours total) and June (234 hours total).

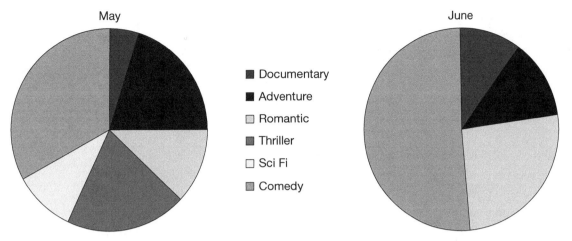

29. What proportion of Joe's TV viewing hours in May were comedies?
    A. ⅙
    B. ⅕
    C. ¼
    D. ⅓
    E. ½

30. How many hours did Joe spend watching romantic programmes in June?
    A. 28 hours
    B. 38 hours
    C. 45 hours
    D. 55 hours
    E. 60 hours

31. Documentaries and adventure programmes were what percentage of Joe's total viewing in May?
    A. 10%
    B. 20%
    C. 25%
    D. 30%
    E. 33%

32. What is the approximate percentage increase in hours spent watching comedy programmes from May to June?
    A. 70%
    B. 140%
    C. 180%
    D. 200%
    E. 240%

Five weeks of singles sales figures for five bands vying for the Christmas Number 1 chart position are shown below. Sales figures correspond to one single release per band. The Christmas Number 1 went to the group with the most sales in Week 3.

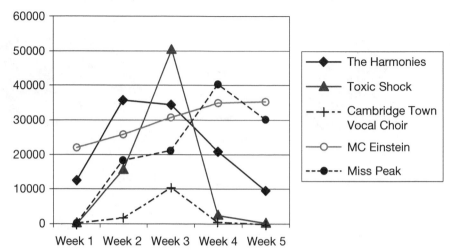

33. Which band saw the greatest percentage rise in sales from Week 2 to Week 3?
    A. Cambridge Town Vocal Choir
    B. The Harmonies
    C. MC Einstein
    D. Miss Peak
    E. Toxic Shock

34. In which week did the bands record the greatest total sales?
    A. Week 1
    B. Week 2
    C. Week 3
    D. Week 4
    E. Week 5

35. Which band saw the greatest decrease in sales from one week to the next?
    A. Cambridge Town Vocal Choir
    B. The Harmonies
    C. MC Einstein
    D. Miss Peak
    E. Toxic Shock

36. MC Einstein's Week 5 sales were what percentage of Week 5's total sales?
    A. 38%
    B. 41%
    C. 44%
    D. 47%
    E. 50%

STOP. IF YOU FINISH BEFORE TIME IS UP, CHECK ANY QUESTIONS YOU HAVE MARKED FOR REVIEW. YOU MAY GO BACK TO QUESTIONS IN THIS SECTION ONLY.

This section contains 55 questions, in one or two of the following question types:

- Type 1 questions will include a total of 5 test shapes, along with a Set A in which all the items are similar to each other and a Set B in which all the items are similar to each other. Your task is to determine in what way the shapes in each set are similar and to decide whether each test shape fits into Set A, Set B or neither set.

- Type 2 questions will include a progression of four boxes in a single row. Your task is to select the test shape that comes next in the progression.

- Type 3 questions will include a statement, with two boxes in the top row and two boxes in the bottom row. There is some progression from the first box to the second box in the top row, and the second box in the bottom row is blank. Your task is to select the test shape that fills the blank box, so that the progression in the bottom row is the same as the progression in the top row.

- Type 4 questions will include a Set A in which all the items are similar to each other and a Set B in which all the items are similar to each other. Your task is to choose the test shape that belongs to the set mentioned in the question.

Answer all 55 questions in Section 3, selecting one of the possible answers and circling the letter corresponding to the appropriate answer in your test booklet.

When you are finished with this section, you may use any remaining time to review your work in this section only. Once you proceed to the next section, you may not return to this section.

You will have 13 minutes to answer the questions. It is in your best interest to select an answer for every item as there is no penalty for wrong answers.

Set your timer for 13 minutes, turn the page and begin the section.

Set A   **Set B**

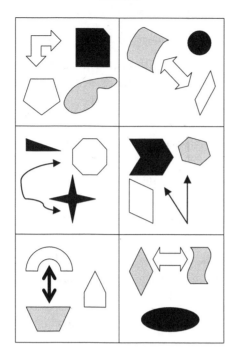   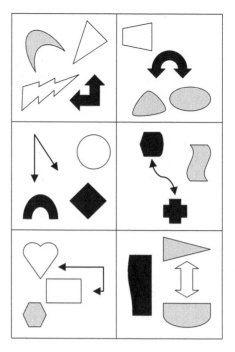

Test Shapes

1	2	3	4	5

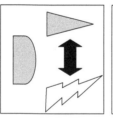 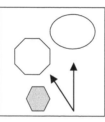 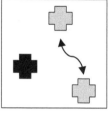

1	2	3	4	5
A. Set A	A. Set A	A. Set A	A. Set A	A. Set A
B. Set B	B. Set B	B. Set B	B. Set B	B. Set B
C. Neither	C. Neither	C. Neither	C. Neither	C. Neither

Set A   **Set B**

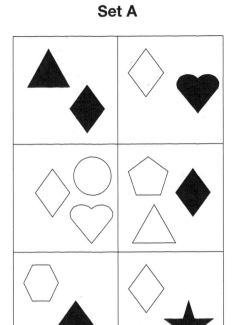
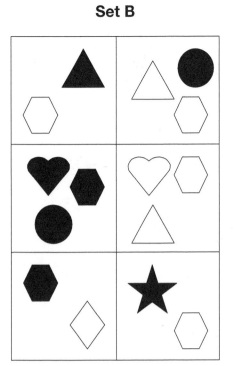

Test Shapes

6	7	8	9	10
		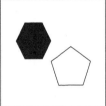	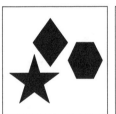	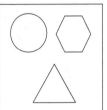

A. Set A	A. Set A	A. Set A	A. Set A	A. Set A
B. Set B	B. Set B	B. Set B	B. Set B	B. Set B
C. Neither	C. Neither	C. Neither	C. Neither	C. Neither

Set A

Set B

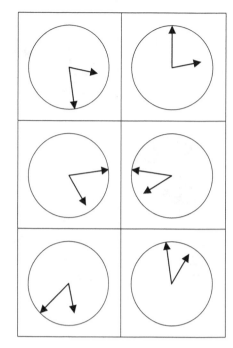

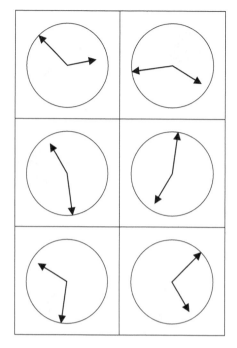

Test Shapes

11	12	13	14	15

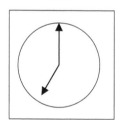
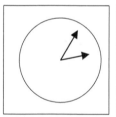
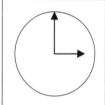
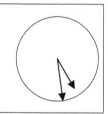
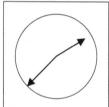

A. Set A
B. Set B
C. Neither

A. Set A
B. Set B
C. Neither

A. Set A
B. Set B
C. Neither

A. Set A
B. Set B
C. Neither

A. Set A
B. Set B
C. Neither

Set A   **Set B**

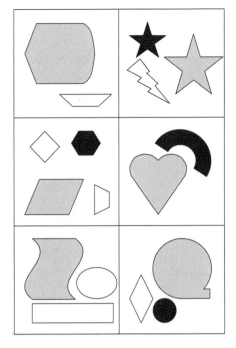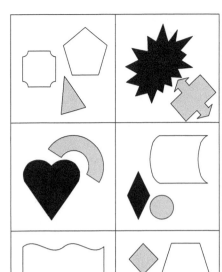

Test Shapes

16	17	18	19	20

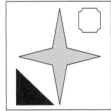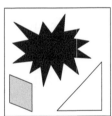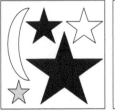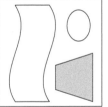

16	17	18	19	20
A. Set A	A. Set A	A. Set A	A. Set A	A. Set A
B. Set B	B. Set B	B. Set B	B. Set B	B. Set B
C. Neither	C. Neither	C. Neither	C. Neither	C. Neither

Set A   **Set B**

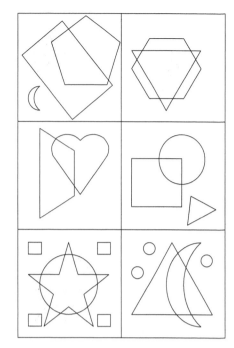   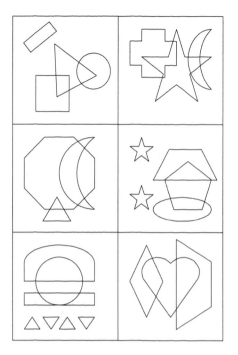

Test Shapes

21	22	23	24	25

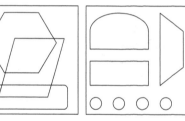 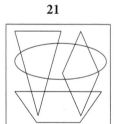   

A. Set A	A. Set A	A. Set A	A. Set A	A. Set A
B. Set B	B. Set B	B. Set B	B. Set B	B. Set B
C. Neither	C. Neither	C. Neither	C. Neither	C. Neither

Set A   **Set B**

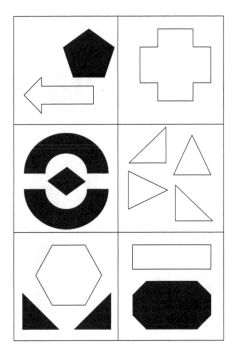
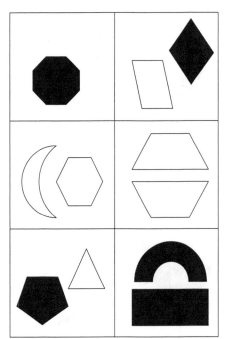

Test Shapes

26	27	28	29	30

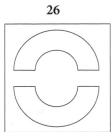 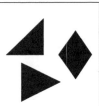 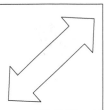 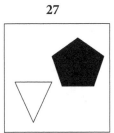 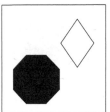

26	27	28	29	30
A. Set A	A. Set A	A. Set A	A. Set A	A. Set A
B. Set B	B. Set B	B. Set B	B. Set B	B. Set B
C. Neither	C. Neither	C. Neither	C. Neither	C. Neither

Set A **Set B**

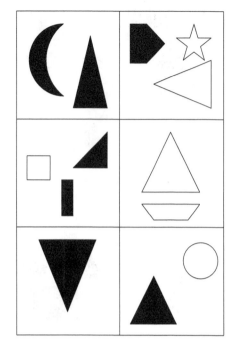 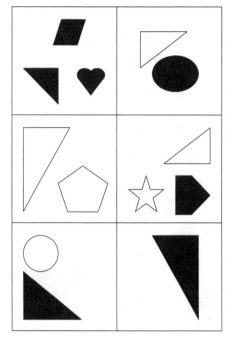

Test Shapes

31	32	33	34	35

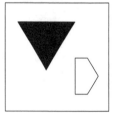 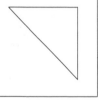 

- A. Set A
  B. Set B
  C. Neither

- A. Set A
  B. Set B
  C. Neither

A. Set A
- B. Set B
  C. Neither

- A. Set A
  B. Set B
  C. Neither

A. Set A
- B. Set B
  C. Neither

Set A

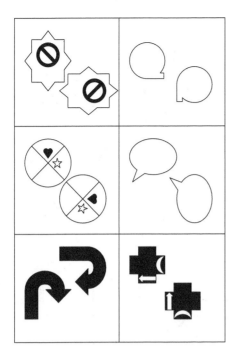

Set B

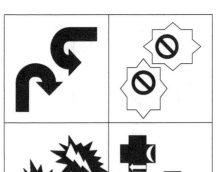
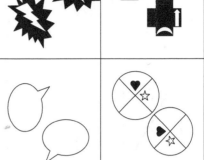

Test Shapes

36	37	38	39	40

A. Set A	A. Set A	A. Set A	A. Set A	A. Set A
B. Set B	B. Set B	B. Set B	B. Set B	B. Set B
C. Neither	C. Neither	C. Neither	C. Neither	C. Neither

Set A   **Set B**

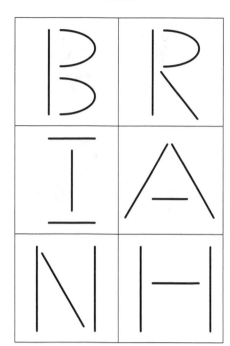 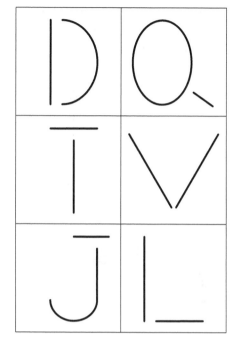

Test Shapes

41	42	43	44	45

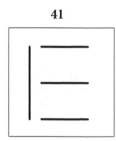 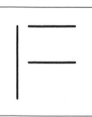 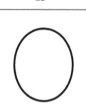 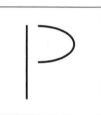 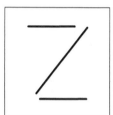

A. Set A	A. Set A	A. Set A	A. Set A	A. Set A
B. Set B	B. Set B	B. Set B	B. Set B	B. Set B
C. Neither	C. Neither	C. Neither	C. Neither	C. Neither

Set A

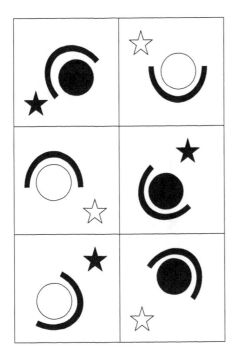

Set B

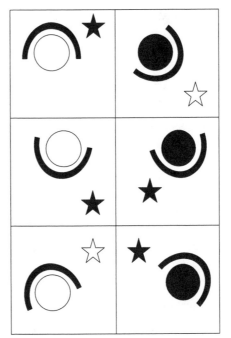

Test Shapes

46	47	48	49	50

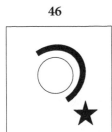 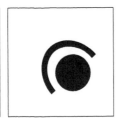 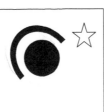  

46	47	48	49	50
A. Set A	A. Set A	A. Set A	A. Set A	A. Set A
B. Set B	B. Set B	B. Set B	B. Set B	B. Set B
C. Neither	C. Neither	C. Neither	C. Neither	C. Neither

Score Higher on the UKCAT

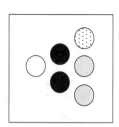 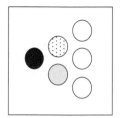 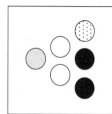 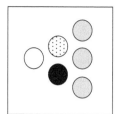

51. Which figure completes the series?

A

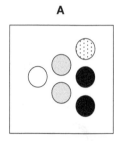

C

B

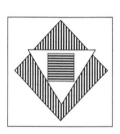 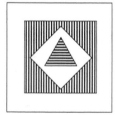 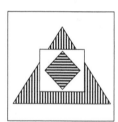 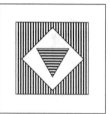

D

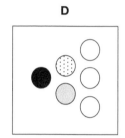

52. Which figure completes the series?

A

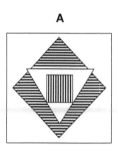

C

B

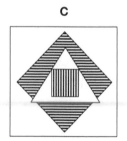 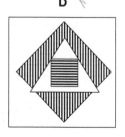

D

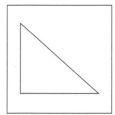
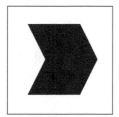
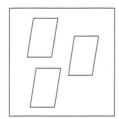
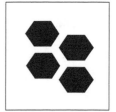

53. Which figure completes the series?

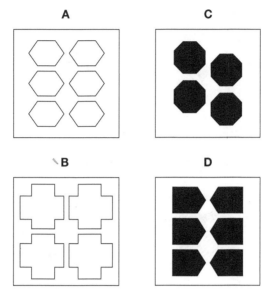

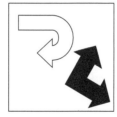
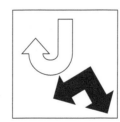
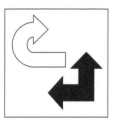

54. Which figure completes the series?

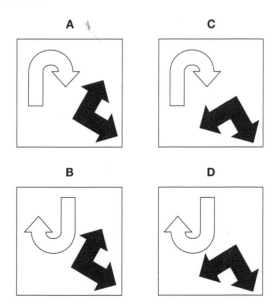

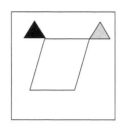 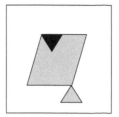 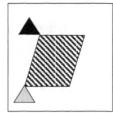 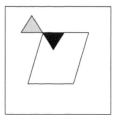

55. Which figure completes the series?

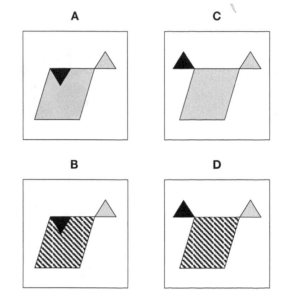

A   C

B   D

STOP. IF YOU FINISH BEFORE TIME IS UP, CHECK ANY QUESTIONS YOU HAVE
MARKED FOR REVIEW. YOU MAY GO BACK TO QUESTIONS IN THIS SECTION ONLY.

This section contains information relating to a scenario. Your task is to answer a number of questions based on your interpretation of the information provided. Additional information will be presented after you have completed some of the questions. This new information will apply to subsequent questions.

Answer all 28 questions in Section 4, selecting one of the possible answers and circling the letter corresponding to the appropriate answer in your test booklet. A few questions will require you to select two answers from the options given, as two correct answers must be chosen in order to answer such questions correctly.

When you are finished with this section, you may use any remaining time to review your work in this section only. Once you proceed to the next section, you may not return to this section.

You will have 33 minutes to answer the questions. It is in your best interest to select an answer for every item as there is no penalty for wrong answers.

Set your timer for 33 minutes, turn the page and begin the section.

Egyptology Code

You spend your summer holidays with a team of archaeologists who are preparing for their next big dig in the desert near Cairo. One afternoon, whilst exploring a previously discovered pyramid, you come across what appear to be a series of messages written in code by Egyptologists who visited the pyramid in an earlier era. A secret chamber in the pyramid includes a table of translations for the code, painted on the wall by some earlier proponents of Egyptology, and you study the table and the messages carefully with your torch, trying to determine the code's exact logical workings.

Some of the information will be strange or incomplete but all of the messages contain some logic. You will therefore need to make assessments based on the codes rather than what seems like the most predictable translation. Every code has a best answer that makes the most sense based on all the information presented, but remember that this test requires you to make judgements rather than simply apply logic and rules.

Table of Codes

Operators & General Rules	Specific Information Basic Codes
A = old	1 = Egypt
B = increase	2 = woman
C = pharaoh	3 = triangle
D = under	4 = build
E = command	5 = sand
F = past	6 = sun
G = negative	7 = temple
H = place	8 = river
J = god	9 = leave
K = kill	10 = sleep
L = big	11 = snake
M = opposite	12 = guard
	13 = perfume
	14 = jar
	15 = find
	16 = wash
	17 = camel
	18 = brain
	19 = wheat

Example 1

What is the best interpretation of the coded message: M2, F(M9), B17, 3H

    A. The man took the large camel to the pyramid. *(message has increase camel, not big camel)*

    B. The man took the camels to the pyramid. *(CORRECT)*

    C. The girl took the camels to the pyramid. *(girl is not the opposite of woman)*

    D. The man left the camels at the pyramid. *(omits opposite)*

    E. The man took the camels to the three-sided building. *(build is in the table, but not the message)*

Example 2

What is the best interpretation of the coded message: 7(6J), BA, (L5)H

    A. The temple of the sun is older than the desert. *(omits god)*

    B. The temple of the sun is older than the big sands. *(omits god)*

    C. The temple of the sun god is newer than the desert. *(message has increase old, not opposite of old)*

    D. The temple of the sun god is older than the desert. *(CORRECT)*

    E. The desert is older than the sun temple. *(omits god)*

1. What is the best interpretation of the coded message: 2(12, 7), K(B11)
    A. The temple guard is a woman who kills big snakes.
    B. The temple guard is a woman and a snake killer.
    C. The woman guarding the temple killed snakes.
    D. The woman guarding the temple kills snakes.
    E. The temple guardian killed the big female snake.

2. What is the best interpretation of the coded message: 1, BC, 10(D, 3H)
    A. In Egypt, the pharaohs sleep under a pyramid.
    B. Egyptian pharaohs are buried under pyramids.
    C. Egyptians buried pharaohs under a pyramid.
    D. The big Egyptian pharaoh sleeps under the Great Pyramid.
    E. Many Egyptians put the pharaoh to rest under the pyramid.

3. What is the best interpretation of the coded message: 8, L16(MD), L(LH)
    A. The river is flooding the building.
    B. The river is flooding the pyramid.
    C. The river is flooding the city.
    D. The river is washing over the city.
    E. The river is washing over the pyramid.

4. What would be the best way to encode the following message?
Message: Don't sleep while guarding the pharaoh's camel.
    A. G10, 12(C17)
    B. G10, 12, L17
    C. E(G10), 12(L17)
    D. E12, G10, C17
    E. E(G10), 12(C17)

5. What is the best interpretation of the coded message: L(LA), B2, F(M9, K), J8
    A. In olden times, the women sacrificed to the god of the river.
    B. Ancient people sacrificed to the river god.
    C. In very ancient times, women sacrificed to the river god.
    D. In olden times, women took and killed for the god of the river.
    E. Ancient people sacrificed the river god.

6. What is the best interpretation of the coded message: B1(2, M2), F4, L(3H)
    A. The ancient Egyptians built the Great Pyramid.
    B. The Egyptians built the Great Pyramid.
    C. The Egyptians built a three-sided building.
    D. The ancient Egyptians built a big triangle.
    E. The Egyptian couple built a big pyramid.

Table of Codes

Operators & General Rules	Specific Information Basic Codes
A = old	1 = Egypt
B = increase	2 = woman
C = pharaoh	3 = triangle
D = under	4 = build
E = command	5 = sand
F = past	6 = sun
G = negative	7 = temple
H = place	8 = river
J = god	9 = leave
K = kill	10 = sleep
L = big	11 = snake
M = opposite	12 = guard
	13 = perfume
	14 = jar
	15 = find
	16 = wash
	17 = camel
	18 = brain
	19 = wheat

7. What would be the best way to encode the following message?

Message: Wash the pharaoh and leave his brain in the jar.

      A. E16, C, E9(19C, 14)

      B. E16, C, 9(19C, 14)

      C. 16, C, 9(19C, 14)

      D. E16, C, 9(19, 14)

      E. 16, C, H(19C, 14)

8. What is the best interpretation of the coded message: 18, BL, 8(3)

      A. The triangle of rivers floods the wheat.

      B. The triangle of rivers washes the wheat.

      C. More wheat grows in the river delta.

      D. Wheat grows big in the river delta.

      E. Wheat was bigger in the three rivers.

9. What would be the best way to encode the following message?

Message: The new man lost the camels by the river.

      A. MA(M2), F(M15), B17, D8

      B. MA(M2), F(M15), B17, 8

      C. MA(M2), (M15), B17, 8

      D. BA(M2), (M15), 17, 8

      E. BA(M2), 15, 17, 8

10. What is the best interpretation of the coded message: L(11, 11), 12, 7, J2(B18)

      A. The temple guard left two big snakes for the goddess of farming.

      B. Big snakes guard the god's temple, and a woman grows wheat.

      C. The temple of the goddess of growing wheat is guarded by snakes.

      D. The temple of the goddess of farming is guarded by snakes.

      E. Two big snakes guard the temple of the goddess of farming.

11. What is the best interpretation of the coded message: C, L10, 12, M(L10)

    A. The pharaoh has a long sleep, while the guard is fully awake.

    B. The pharaoh sleeps well, but the guard does not.

    C. The guard stays awake so the pharaoh can sleep.

    D. The guard does not sleep, while the pharaoh has a good night.

    E. The pharaoh slept longer than the guard.

12. What is the best interpretation of the coded message: ML2, F15, 14(13), 16H

    A. While washing, the girl found a jar of perfume.

    B. The small woman finds an old jar of perfume in the shower.

    C. The girl found a jar of perfume in the bathroom.

    D. While washing, the woman found a jar of perfume.

    E. The small woman found perfume near the washing basin.

After doing your preliminary research, you discover the code is in fact much more complex than you originally thought. The additional codes and information complete the table as follows:

Table of Codes—Complete Code

Operators & General Rules	Specific Information Basic Codes	Complex Information Additional Information	Reactions/Outcomes Emotions
A = old	1 = Egypt	101 = crocodile	201 = lucky
B = increase	2 = woman	102 = hippopotamus	202 = fertile
C = pharaoh	3 = triangle	103 = lead	203 = fearful
D = under	4 = build	104 = eye	204 = cruel
E = command	5 = sand	105 = wrap	205 = joyous
F = past	6 = sun	106 = ride	206 = rare
G = negative	7 = temple	107 = robe	207 = daring
H = place	8 = river	108 = tear	208 = false
J = god	9 = leave	109 = marry	
K = kill	10 = sleep	110 = fire	
L = big	11 = snake	111 = chair	
M= opposite	12 = guard	112 = gold	
N = study	13 = perfume	113 = book	
P = make	14 = jar	114 = boat	
Q = blue	15 = find	115 = reed	
	16 = wash		
	17 = camel		
	18 = brain		
	19 = wheat		

13. What is the best interpretation of the coded message: 12(MK), F103, C2, B108
    A. The queen cried when the guard died.
    B. The guard's death led the queen to cry.
    C. The guard's death made the pharaoh's wife cry.
    D. The pharaoh's wife cried when the guard died.
    E. The queen cried when the leading guard died.

14. What would be the best way to encode the following message?
Message: Wrap the eyes with a torn robe.
    A. E105, L104, 107(F108)
    B. E105, B104, 107(108)
    C. 105, (104, 104), 107(F108)
    D. E105, (104, 104), 107(F108)
    E. 105, B104, 107(108)

15. What is the best interpretation of the coded message: 102, K114, 106(MD), 8
    A. The hippopotamus destroyed a boat crossing the river.
    B. A hippopotamus killed the people on a boat on the river.
    C. The hippopotamus is destroying a boat crossing the river.
    D. A hippopotamus is killing sailors crossing the river.
    E. Sailors killed a hippopotamus crossing the river.

16. What is the best interpretation of the coded message: 101(203), 11(B204, LBK)
    A. A crocodile is afraid of a snake that kills very cruelly.
    B. A crocodile is afraid of a very dangerous snake.
    C. A crocodile is afraid of a nasty, very venomous snake.
    D. A crocodile fears a very highly cruel and deadly snake.
    E. A crocodile fears a very cruel and very highly murderous snake.

17. What is the best interpretation of the coded message: C, MF(106), 112(114), MD, H(6, 9D)

    A. The pharaoh will ride a golden boat over the horizon.
    B. The pharaoh rode his golden boat over the horizon.
    C. The pharaoh rode his golden boat beyond the sun.
    D. The pharaoh will ride his golden boat over the moon.
    E. The pharaoh rode his golden boat during an eclipse.

18. What would be the best way to encode the following message?

Message: A young girl found in the reeds is lucky.

    A. 201, F15, 2(ML, BA), (115, 115)
    B. 201, F15, 2(ML, MA), B115
    C. 201, F15, 2(BL, MA), B115
    D. 201, 15, 2(ML, MA), (115, 115)
    E. 201, 15, M2(L, A), (115, 115)

19. What is the best interpretation of the coded message: Q102, 2(202)

    A. A blue hippo makes a woman fertile.
    B. Blue hippos bring pregnancy.
    C. A woman who sees a blue hippo is fertile.
    D. The fertile hippo is blue and female.
    E. Blue hippo, fertile woman.

20. What is the best interpretation of the coded message: J6, P110(103), P112(111)

    A. The god of the sun burns lead to make a golden chair.
    B. The sun god makes fire sit in a chair.
    C. The sun god leads fire into a golden seat.
    D. The god leads the sun's fire to make a golden chair.
    E. The god leads the sun's fire to make a seat of gold.

Table of Codes—Complete Code

Operators & General Rules	Specific Information Basic Codes	Complex Information Additional Information	Reactions/Outcomes Emotions
A = old	1 = Egypt	101 = crocodile	201 = lucky
B = increase	2 = woman	102 = hippopotamus	202 = fertile
C = pharaoh	3 = triangle	103 = lead	203 = fearful
D = under	4 = build	104 = eye	204 = cruel
E = command	5 = sand	105 = wrap	205 = joyous
F = past	6 = sun	106 = ride	206 = rare
G = negative	7 = temple	107 = robe	207 = daring
H = place	8 = river	108 = tear	208 = false
J = god	9 = leave	109 = marry	
K = kill	10 = sleep	110 = fire	
L = big	11 = snake	111 = chair	
M = opposite	12 = guard	112 = gold	
N = study	13 = perfume	113 = book	
P = make	14 = jar	114 = boat	
Q = blue	15 = find	115 = reed	
	16 = wash		
	17 = camel		
	18 = brain		
	19 = wheat		

21. What is the best interpretation of the coded message: M16(107), M208(104), G201(2, 103, 7)

    A. An unfortunate priest truly sees an unwashed robe.

    B. An unwashed robe indicates an unlucky priestess.

    C. An unfortunate priestess sees too late that her robe is dirty.

    D. A dirty robe is a true sight of an unfortunate priestess.

    E. An unlucky temple has a leader with an unwashed robe.

22. What is the best interpretation of the coded message: BL(M203), MF, B114(106), M, B12(204, BK)

    A. The very brave navy will ride against the cruel guards.

    B. Extreme courage will carry the navy against the viciously murderous army.

    C. The boats will ride their bravery against the murderous guards.

    D. The navy's courage will carry them to oppose the deadly army.

    E. The very courageous boats will ride over the cruelly murderous army.

23. What would be the best way to encode the following message?

Message: Egyptology finds the truths of lost history.

    A. N1, 15, M206, FH(FM15)

    B. N1, 15, M208, FH(FM15)

    C. N1, 15, B(M208), FH(FM15)

    D. N1, 15, B(M206), FH(M15)

    E. N1, 15, B206, FH(M15)

24. What is the best interpretation of the coded message: B101, FK102, B(M2), FK(B101)

    A. The crocodiles killed the hippopotamus before the men could kill the crocodiles.

    B. Crocodiles killed hippopotamuses; men killed crocodiles.

    C. Crocodiles and men are killers of hippopotamuses and crocodiles, respectively.

    D. While crocodiles killed hippopotamuses, men killed crocodiles.

    E. The crocodiles killed the hippopotamus, and the men killed the crocodiles.

25. What is the best interpretation of the coded message: 12, 109(2), 7(MD8)
    A. The woman guard is marrying at the temple across the river.
    B. The guard and woman are marrying at the underwater temple.
    C. The guard and woman are marrying at the temple across the river.
    D. The guard is marrying the woman at the temple above the river.
    E. The guard's wife is at the underwater temple.

26. Which of the following would be the most useful and second most useful additions to the codes in order to convey the message accurately?

Message: The slaughterhouse is scary, dirty, dark and smelly.
    A. slaughter
    B. fright
    C. filth
    D. dark
    E. smell

27. Which of the following would be the most useful and second most useful additions to the codes in order to convey the message accurately?

Message: The pharaoh's tutor found books about fashion and culture at the library.
    A. tutor
    B. book
    C. fashion
    D. culture
    E. library

28. Which of the following would be the most useful and second most useful additions to the codes in order to convey the message accurately?

Message: True love is not common in life or in legend.
    A. true
    B. love
    C. common
    D. life
    E. legend

STOP. IF YOU FINISH BEFORE TIME IS UP, CHECK ANY QUESTIONS YOU HAVE MARKED FOR REVIEW. YOU MAY GO BACK TO QUESTIONS IN THIS SECTION ONLY.

This section contains 17 theoretical scenarios, each involving a medical or dental professional, or a student preparing for a career in medicine or dentistry. Your task is to read the scenario carefully, and then make a series of judgements about possible options for responding to the situation in the scenario. There are two types of scenarios in this section:

Appropriateness: These scenarios will ask you to rate whether possible responses to the scenario are appropriate or inappropriate.

Importance: These scenarios will ask you to rate whether certain factors are important or not important to consider when responding to the scenario.

The first part of the section will contain Appropriateness scenarios; the final part of the section will contain Importance scenarios. Be sure to answer based on the appropriateness or importance of the response/factor to the person who is named in the question under the scenario. Evaluate the responses/factors independently of each other; do not assume that there will be a response/factor corresponding to each answer choice for each scenario.

Answer all 71 items in Section 5, selecting one of the possible answers and circling the letter corresponding to the appropriate answer in your test book.

When you are finished with this section, you may use any remaining time to review your work in this section only. Once you complete this section, you are finished with the Diagnostic Test. You may then assess your results using the scoring tables that follow.

You will have 26 minutes to answer the questions. It is in your best interest to select an answer for every item as there is no penalty for wrong answers.

Set your timer for 26 minutes, turn the page and begin the section.

Samia and Hayley are final-year medical students. Their schedule includes a planned session of helping the junior doctors with work on the wards, followed by a tutorial. That morning, Samia receives a phone call from Hayley asking her to pass on the message that Hayley is unwell with diarrhoea and therefore cannot come in to the hospital today. On her way home, Samia is surprised to see Hayley working behind the counter at the local bakery.

How **appropriate** are each of the following responses by <u>Samia</u> in this situation?

1. Report Hayley to the medical school for lying about her illness
    - A. A very appropriate thing to do
    - B. Appropriate, but not ideal
    - C. Inappropriate, but not awful
    - D. A very inappropriate thing to do

2. Report Hayley to the bakery shop owner, as she shouldn't be working there when she is unwell
    - A. A very appropriate thing to do
    - B. Appropriate, but not ideal
    - C. Inappropriate, but not awful
    - D. A very inappropriate thing to do

3. Ignore the situation and hope that it does not happen again
    - A. A very appropriate thing to do
    - B. Appropriate, but not ideal
    - C. Inappropriate, but not awful
    - D. A very inappropriate thing to do

4. Ask Hayley why she said she could not come to hospital if she was well enough to work in the bakery
    - A. A very appropriate thing to do
    - B. Appropriate, but not ideal
    - C. Inappropriate, but not awful
    - D. A very inappropriate thing to do

5. Ask Hayley the next day how she is feeling and whether she managed to get out and about at all the previous day
    - A. A very appropriate thing to do
    - B. Appropriate, but not ideal
    - C. Inappropriate, but not awful
    - D. A very inappropriate thing to do

Tameka is a junior doctor at a university hospital. One of the medical students whose work she supervises, Shaun, has joined her as Tameka asks a patient, Mrs Oswald, to sign the consent form for surgery to correct a bowel obstruction. Mrs Oswald is booked into theatre later in the day, and the need for the surgery is critical. Mrs Oswald says she is not sure about the surgery as she is terrified of needles, and does not think she can handle being anaesthetised. She asks if she can be hypnotised instead. Shaun sneers, and says that if Mrs Oswald is so superstitious, maybe they can hypnotise her bowel and avoid surgery altogether.

How **appropriate** are each of the following responses by **Tameka** in this situation?

6. Apologise to Mrs Oswald for the rude remark from her student

    A. A very appropriate thing to do

    B. Appropriate, but not ideal

    C. Inappropriate, but not awful

    D. A very inappropriate thing to do

7. Tell Shaun his comment is unhelpful, and ask him to apologise

    A. A very appropriate thing to do

    B. Appropriate, but not ideal

    C. Inappropriate, but not awful

    D. A very inappropriate thing to do

8. Explain to Mrs Oswald that they could hypnotise her before she is anaesthetised

    A. A very appropriate thing to do

    B. Appropriate, but not ideal

    C. Inappropriate, but not awful

    D. A very inappropriate thing to do

9. Instruct Shaun to keep his personal views to himself

    A. A very appropriate thing to do

    B. Appropriate, but not ideal

    C. Inappropriate, but not awful

    D. A very inappropriate thing to do

Lisa is a final-year medical student and has been busy revising for her exams. She overhears several of her peers from her year group discussing a piece of coursework that is due in soon. When she questions them, it transpires the coursework was set a few weeks ago, with all the details included in an email that she did not receive.

How **appropriate** are each of the following responses by <u>Lisa</u> in this situation?

10. Ask a peer to forward the original email to her and complete the coursework before the deadline
    - A. A very appropriate thing to do
    - B. Appropriate, but not ideal
    - C. Inappropriate, but not awful
    - D. A very inappropriate thing to do

11. Contact the course administrator and ask for an extension to complete the coursework
    - A. A very appropriate thing to do
    - B. Appropriate, but not ideal
    - C. Inappropriate, but not awful
    - D. A very inappropriate thing to do

12. Concentrate on revising for exams, as she did not receive the email with the coursework assignment
    - A. A very appropriate thing to do
    - B. Appropriate, but not ideal
    - C. Inappropriate, but not awful
    - D. A very inappropriate thing to do

13. Contact the course administrator and find out if the email should have been sent to her, and if there may have been other important emails she did not receive
    - A. A very appropriate thing to do
    - B. Appropriate, but not ideal
    - C. Inappropriate, but not awful
    - D. A very inappropriate thing to do

14. Email the head of the medical school to complain that the course administrator is incompetent
    - A. A very appropriate thing to do
    - B. Appropriate, but not ideal
    - C. Inappropriate, but not awful
    - D. A very inappropriate thing to do

A consultant enters the lobby of the hospital where he works, and is approached by a patient he does not recognise. The patient starts shouting at the consultant that the hospital is worse than a zoo, and the doctors are not fit to operate on animals.

How **appropriate** are each of the following responses by **<u>the consultant</u>** in this situation?

15. Tell the patient he is mistaken
    A. A very appropriate thing to do
    B. Appropriate, but not ideal
    C. Inappropriate, but not awful
    D. A very inappropriate thing to do

16. Ask a porter to assist the patient
    A. A very appropriate thing to do
    B. Appropriate, but not ideal
    C. Inappropriate, but not awful
    D. A very inappropriate thing to do

17. Invite the patient to sit down and have a chat
    A. A very appropriate thing to do
    B. Appropriate, but not ideal
    C. Inappropriate, but not awful
    D. A very inappropriate thing to do

18. Ask the patient not to shout, and to explain his exact concerns
    A. A very appropriate thing to do
    B. Appropriate, but not ideal
    C. Inappropriate, but not awful
    D. A very inappropriate thing to do

A medical student, Matthew, has signed up to do a Saturday night shift in the A&E department as part of his compulsory duties whilst he is on placement there. On Friday, he is reminded by his family that it is his great aunt's 90th birthday party that Saturday evening in his hometown and they are expecting him to attend. Matthew had forgotten about the party when he signed up to his Saturday night shift.

How **appropriate** are each of the following responses by __Matthew__ in this situation?

19. Ask a fellow student to swap shifts so Matthew can attend the party and do his shift the following weekend
    A. A very appropriate thing to do
    B. Appropriate, but not ideal
    C. Inappropriate, but not awful
    D. A very inappropriate thing to do

20. Pretend to be ill on Saturday night and not attend the shift
    A. A very appropriate thing to do
    B. Appropriate, but not ideal
    C. Inappropriate, but not awful
    D. A very inappropriate thing to do

21. Email the consultant to explain why he cannot attend the Saturday night shift and volunteer to work on Sunday night or the following Saturday night
    A. A very appropriate thing to do
    B. Appropriate, but not ideal
    C. Inappropriate, but not awful
    D. A very inappropriate thing to do

22. Ask a fellow medical student who is also due to work on Saturday night to make up an excuse for Matthew's absence
    A. A very appropriate thing to do
    B. Appropriate, but not ideal
    C. Inappropriate, but not awful
    D. A very inappropriate thing to do

23. Do not go to the party and attend the Saturday night shift
    A. A very appropriate thing to do
    B. Appropriate, but not ideal
    C. Inappropriate, but not awful
    D. A very inappropriate thing to do

Haroon is a junior dentist at a large dental practice. A patient, Mrs Rahman, complains that she has had to wait 2 weeks for an appointment for a toothache. Haroon steps out to check with the receptionist, and finds the receptionist playing solitaire on her computer and typing in a chat window on a social networking site; at the same time, the phone is ringing and a queue of patients are waiting to speak to the receptionist.

How **appropriate** are each of the following responses by **Haroon** in this situation?

24. Instruct the receptionist to answer the phone, and apologise to the patients for their wait

    A. A very appropriate thing to do
    B. Appropriate, but not ideal
    C. Inappropriate, but not awful
    D. A very inappropriate thing to do

25. Demand an immediate explanation from the receptionist for her unacceptable behaviour

    A. A very appropriate thing to do
    B. Appropriate, but not ideal
    C. Inappropriate, but not awful
    D. A very inappropriate thing to do

26. Answer the phone, asking the receptionist to speak with the patients in the queue before doing so

    A. A very appropriate thing to do
    B. Appropriate, but not ideal
    C. Inappropriate, but not awful
    D. A very inappropriate thing to do

27. Take the receptionist to a private space nearby and explain Mrs Rahman's concern about having to wait for an appointment

    A. A very appropriate thing to do
    B. Appropriate, but not ideal
    C. Inappropriate, but not awful
    D. A very inappropriate thing to do

Three medical students, James, Kyle and Avni, regularly visit a patient at home as part of their first-year course. The patient lives 30 minutes away so the students all meet outside the patient's house, having travelled there independently. Kyle is always at least 10 minutes late, and it is starting to annoy James. The third time it happens, Kyle calls and says he will be at least 20 minutes late. James decides he wants to go ahead and meet the patient without waiting for Kyle.

How **appropriate** are each of the following responses by <u>Avni</u> in this situation?

28. Tell James to wait for Kyle so that they can all go together
   A. A very appropriate thing to do
   B. Appropriate, but not ideal
   C. Inappropriate, but not awful
   D. A very inappropriate thing to do

29. Call Kyle and tell him that he should have tried harder to be on time
   A. A very appropriate thing to do
   B. Appropriate, but not ideal
   C. Inappropriate, but not awful
   D. A very inappropriate thing to do

30. Call the patient to apologise and explain that they will be 20 minutes late
   A. A very appropriate thing to do
   B. Appropriate, but not ideal
   C. Inappropriate, but not awful
   D. A very inappropriate thing to do

31. Explain to Kyle that they must start the visit without him, and schedule a time to meet as a group to discuss Kyle's tardiness
   A. A very appropriate thing to do
   B. Appropriate, but not ideal
   C. Inappropriate, but not awful
   D. A very inappropriate thing to do

32. Start the visit without Kyle and tell James to talk to him about the problem
   A. A very appropriate thing to do
   B. Appropriate, but not ideal
   C. Inappropriate, but not awful
   D. A very inappropriate thing to do

Katie is a junior doctor on a cardiology ward at a major hospital. On her day off, she plans to meet a friend for lunch; her friend works on the cardiology ward at another major hospital. On arriving in the ward, Katie sees her consultant sitting in the waiting area with the other patients, reading a newspaper. The consultant does not see her, and he is not wearing scrubs.

How **appropriate** are each of the following responses by **Katie** in this situation?

33. Say hello to the consultant and ask why he is here

    A. A very appropriate thing to do
    B. Appropriate, but not ideal
    C. Inappropriate, but not awful
    D. A very inappropriate thing to do

34. Pretend she didn't see the consultant, unless he brings it up later

    A. A very appropriate thing to do
    B. Appropriate, but not ideal
    C. Inappropriate, but not awful
    D. A very inappropriate thing to do

35. Ask her friend if he knows her consultant

    A. A very appropriate thing to do
    B. Appropriate, but not ideal
    C. Inappropriate, but not awful
    D. A very inappropriate thing to do

36. Find out more about the work her friend is doing at the hospital

    A. A very appropriate thing to do
    B. Appropriate, but not ideal
    C. Inappropriate, but not awful
    D. A very inappropriate thing to do

The infection control nurse asks Tom, a junior doctor, to remove his wristwatch because it is an infection risk. The next day, Neha, a medical student on the ward, notices that Tom is wearing his watch on his wrist again.

How **appropriate** are each of the following responses by <u>Neha</u> in this situation?

37. Report Tom to the infection control nurse
    A. A very appropriate thing to do
    B. Appropriate, but not ideal
    C. Inappropriate, but not awful
    D. A very inappropriate thing to do

38. Ignore the problem, as Neha is just a medical student
    A. A very appropriate thing to do
    B. Appropriate, but not ideal
    C. Inappropriate, but not awful
    D. A very inappropriate thing to do

39. Talk to Tom at the end of the week if he continues to wear the watch
    A. A very appropriate thing to do
    B. Appropriate, but not ideal
    C. Inappropriate, but not awful
    D. A very inappropriate thing to do

40. Quietly say to Tom that he should remove his watch, as it is an infection risk
    A. A very appropriate thing to do
    B. Appropriate, but not ideal
    C. Inappropriate, but not awful
    D. A very inappropriate thing to do

Two junior doctors, Emmanuel and Simone, are working in a busy A&E department. Emmanuel comes out of an examination room and tells Simone that the patient inside is a leader of an extreme right-wing political group known for its anti-immigrant policies. Emmanuel's parents are from Nigeria, and he does not feel comfortable treating this patient. Emmanuel asks Simone if she will take the patient instead.

How **appropriate** are each of the following responses by <u>**Simone**</u> in this situation?

41. Ask Emmanuel if the patient has said anything to make him uncomfortable

    A. A very appropriate thing to do
    B. Appropriate, but not ideal
    C. Inappropriate, but not awful
    D. A very inappropriate thing to do

42. Ask the patient if Emmanuel said anything to make him uncomfortable

    A. A very appropriate thing to do
    B. Appropriate, but not ideal
    C. Inappropriate, but not awful
    D. A very inappropriate thing to do

43. Remind Emmanuel of his duty to treat all patients, regardless of their beliefs

    A. A very appropriate thing to do
    B. Appropriate, but not ideal
    C. Inappropriate, but not awful
    D. A very inappropriate thing to do

Esme is a consultant surgeon. She is on call from home but has been feeling increasingly dizzy and sick throughout the day, to the extent where she has to hold onto walls to walk along the corridor. In the middle of the night, a junior colleague calls to ask her to come in to assist with an unwell patient. Esme usually drives herself to the hospital—a journey of around 30 minutes on difficult country roads. Given how unbalanced she feels, Esme is not sure she could drive for even 5 minutes.

How **appropriate** are each of the following responses by <u>Esme</u> in this situation?

44. Tell the junior colleague that she cannot come in, as she is unwell
   A. A very appropriate thing to do
   B. Appropriate, but not ideal
   C. Inappropriate, but not awful
   D. A very inappropriate thing to do

45. Call a taxi to take her in to the hospital to assist
   A. A very appropriate thing to do
   B. Appropriate, but not ideal
   C. Inappropriate, but not awful
   D. A very inappropriate thing to do

46. Tell the junior colleague to try a different consultant who is not on call
   A. A very appropriate thing to do
   B. Appropriate, but not ideal
   C. Inappropriate, but not awful
   D. A very inappropriate thing to do

47. Call a different consultant who is not on call and ask them to go into hospital in her place
   A. A very appropriate thing to do
   B. Appropriate, but not ideal
   C. Inappropriate, but not awful
   D. A very inappropriate thing to do

48. Drive herself to the hospital to assist
   A. A very appropriate thing to do
   B. Appropriate, but not ideal
   C. Inappropriate, but not awful
   D. A very inappropriate thing to do

A patient asks Luke, a junior doctor, to explain why a new medication has been prescribed. Luke is covering on the ward for another doctor who is away on annual leave, and he has not met this patient before. Luke checks the patient's chart and sees that the doctor has prescribed a medication that Luke is entirely unfamiliar with.

How **appropriate** are each of the following responses by <u>**Luke**</u> in this situation?

49. Explain that the treatment is new, and that he does not know much about it
    - A. A very appropriate thing to do
    - B. Appropriate, but not ideal
    - C. Inappropriate, but not awful
    - D. A very inappropriate thing to do

50. Reassure the patient there is a good reason, and that he will follow up with more information soon
    - A. A very appropriate thing to do
    - B. Appropriate, but not ideal
    - C. Inappropriate, but not awful
    - D. A very inappropriate thing to do

51. Tell the patient he is unfamiliar with this treatment, and the doctor that prescribed it is away
    - A. A very appropriate thing to do
    - B. Appropriate, but not ideal
    - C. Inappropriate, but not awful
    - D. A very inappropriate thing to do

Jitesh is a final-year medical student on geriatric wards. Every afternoon at 3:30pm the junior doctor, Rob, goes home and asks Jitesh to do his paperwork, such as copying out blood results and delivering X-ray requests.

How **important** to take into account are the following considerations for **Jitesh** when deciding how to respond to the situation?

52. Rob is the sole carer for his sick father
    A. Very important
    B. Important
    C. Of minor importance
    D. Not important at all

53. The learning objectives of Jitesh's course state that he should be helping the junior doctors with their jobs to experience the real life of a junior doctor
    A. Very important
    B. Important
    C. Of minor importance
    D. Not important at all

54. The rules of the contract that the doctors sign at the beginning of their jobs within the hospitals state that the junior doctors should be on the wards from at least 9am until 5pm during the week
    A. Very important
    B. Important
    C. Of minor importance
    D. Not important at all

55. 4–5pm is often the busiest time of the day on the wards
    A. Very important
    B. Important
    C. Of minor importance
    D. Not important at all

Nima, a junior doctor, enters the supply cupboard and is surprised to discover Lauren, a medical student, in the process of removing her clothes. Nima asks Lauren what she is doing, and Lauren comments that she does not like changing clothes in the presence of others.

How **important** to take into account are the following considerations for **Nima** when deciding how to respond to the situation?

56. The hospital provides a suitably private location for all staff members to change clothes
    A. Very important
    B. Important
    C. Of minor importance
    D. Not important at all

57. Nima's religious beliefs require her to wear a headscarf
    A. Very important
    B. Important
    C. Of minor importance
    D. Not important at all

58. Lauren does not have any clothes to change into—only the clothes she is removing
    A. Very important
    B. Important
    C. Of minor importance
    D. Not important at all

59. Whether someone besides Lauren was also in the supply cupboard when Nima entered
    A. Very important
    B. Important
    C. Of minor importance
    D. Not important at all

60. Whether Lauren's behaviour is heightened in other ways (slurring speech, breathing rapidly)
    A. Very important
    B. Important
    C. Of minor importance
    D. Not important at all

Abiola is a medical student. She is in the hospital lift one day when she hears two of the junior doctors loudly discussing the sensitive details of a case that they have been involved in.

How **important** to take into account are the following considerations for **Abiola** when deciding how to respond to the situation?

61. The only other occupant of the lift is an elderly man with hearing aids
    A. Very important
    B. Important
    C. Of minor importance
    D. Not important at all

62. The junior doctors do not use the patient's name
    A. Very important
    B. Important
    C. Of minor importance
    D. Not important at all

63. The junior doctors are responsible for Abiola's report at the end of her placement
    A. Very important
    B. Important
    C. Of minor importance
    D. Not important at all

64. Abiola does not know the patient to whom they are referring
    A. Very important
    B. Important
    C. Of minor importance
    D. Not important at all

Two medical students, Violet and Uma, are in the same tutor group, as well as being housemates. One morning, before they have left the house for their tutor group, Violet gets a call that her grandmother is critically ill and has been rushed to hospital. Violet's grandmother is asking for her, and she must leave immediately if she is to catch the next train to her grandmother's town.

How **important** to take into account are the following considerations for **<u>Violet</u>** when deciding how to respond to the situation?

65. Whether she has a phone number where she can reach the tutor
- A. Very important
- B. Important
- C. Of minor importance
- D. Not important at all

66. Whether the tutor would mind if Uma explained her absence
- A. Very important
- B. Important
- C. Of minor importance
- D. Not important at all

67. Whether she will be able to email the tutor from the train before the tutor group starts
- A. Very important
- B. Important
- C. Of minor importance
- D. Not important at all

Meera is starting her first medical school placement in hospital and is paired with Adam, another student. Throughout the first week on the wards, Meera notices that Adam always looks scruffy, with his hair unbrushed, and is not dressed as smartly as she is.

How **important** to take into account are the following considerations for **Meera** when deciding how to respond to the situation?

68. The medical school has firm guidelines about how a student should dress for the wards
    A. Very important
    B. Important
    C. Of minor importance
    D. Not important at all

69. Adam has just split up with his girlfriend of 5 years
    A. Very important
    B. Important
    C. Of minor importance
    D. Not important at all

70. Meera knows that Adam has just reached his overdraft limit on his student bank account and is really short of money
    A. Very important
    B. Important
    C. Of minor importance
    D. Not important at all

71. The students have all signed an agreement declaring that they will follow the guidelines set by the medical school
    A. Very important
    B. Important
    C. Of minor importance
    D. Not important at all

STOP. IF YOU FINISH BEFORE TIME IS UP, CHECK ANY QUESTIONS YOU HAVE MARKED FOR REVIEW. YOU MAY GO BACK TO QUESTIONS IN THIS SECTION ONLY.

Verbal Reasoning

1. B
2. B
3. D
4. A
5. A
6. C
7. C
8. D
9. B
10. C
11. A
12. B
13. B
14. A
15. B
16. C
17. B
18. C
19. D
20. D
21. C
22. D
23. B
24. C
25. C
26. B
27. C
28. A
29. D
30. A
31. A
32. B
33. C
34. B
35. B
36. A
37. A
38. B
39. C
40. C
41. B
42. D
43. A
44. B

Quantitative Reasoning

1. A
2. E
3. C
4. B
5. C
6. B
7. A
8. B
9. D
10. B
11. C
12. C
13. C
14. D
15. B
16. C
17. B
18. E
19. C
20. D
21. C
22. E
23. A
24. D
25. C
26. B
27. D
28. A
29. D
30. E
31. C
32. B
33. A
34. C
35. E
36. D

Abstract Reasoning

1. C
2. C
3. B
4. A
5. C
6. C
7. A
8. B
9. C
10. B
11. B
12. C
13. C
14. A
15. B
16. C
17. A
18. B
19. B
20. C
21. C
22. B
23. C
24. A
25. A
26. B
27. B
28. C
29. C
30. A
31. A
32. C
33. C
34. A
35. B
36. A
37. B
38. C
39. B
40. C
41. C
42. A
43. C
44. B
45. A
46. A
47. C
48. B
49. C
50. B

Abstract Reasoning (continued)

51. C
52. D
53. B
54. A
55. C

Decision Analysis

1. D
2. A
3. C
4. E
5. C
6. B
7. A
8. D
9. B
10. E
11. A
12. C
13. B
14. D
15. C
16. E
17. A
18. B
19. E
20. A
21. D
22. B
23. C
24. E
25. D
26. C and E
27. A and D
28. B and D

Kaplan UKCAT Diagnostic Test Scoring Table: Sections 1–4

1. Count up your number of correct answers in each scored section.

2. Find your approximate score for each section in the table below.

	Number correct	Approximate UKCAT score
Verbal Reasoning	_____	_____
Quantitative Reasoning	_____	_____
Abstract Reasoning	_____	_____
Decision Analysis	_____	_____

3. Add your section scores to find your total score: _____

Approximate UKCAT Score	Number of Questions Answered Correctly			
	Verbal Reasoning	Quantitative Reasoning	Abstract Reasoning	Decision Analysis
300	0–5	0–3	0–6	0–2
330	6	4–5	7–8	3
350	7	6	9–10	4
370	8	7	11–12	5
400	9–10	8	13–14	6
430	11–12	9	15–16	7
450	13–14	10	17–18	8
470	15	11	19–20	9
500	16	12	21–22	10
530	17–18	13	23–24	11
550	19–20	14–15	25–26	12
570	21–22	16–17	27–29	13
600	23–24	18–19	30–32	14–15
630	25–26	20–21	33–34	16
650	27–28	22–23	35–36	17
670	29–30	24	37	18
700	31	25	38-39	19
730	32	26	40–41	20
750	33	27	42–43	21
770	34	28	44–45	22
800	35–36	29	46–47	23
830	37–38	30	48-49	24
850	39–40	31–32	50–51	25
890	41–42	33–34	52–53	26
900	43–44	35–36	54–55	27–28

NB These scores are for approximation purposes only. Scores on the UKCAT are given in 10-point intervals, so actual scores will vary slightly from this scheme. This table is designed to err on the side of caution, so in most cases a similar performance on the UKCAT would result in a slightly higher score.

Situational Judgement

1. D
2. D
3. D
4. B
5. A
6. A
7. A
8. A
9. B
10. A
11. B
12. D
13. A
14. D
15. C
16. C

17. A
18. A
19. A
20. D
21. A
22. D
23. B
24. A
25. D
26. C
27. A
28. D
29. C
30. D
31. A
32. C
33. D
34. A
35. D

36. A
37. D
38. D
39. D
40. A
41. A
42. D
43. B
44. B
45. D
46. D
47. A
48. D
49. D
50. A
51. C
52. D
53. D
54. A

55. B
56. B
57. D
58. A
59. A
60. B
61. D
62. C
63. D
64. D
65. A
66. C
67. A
68. A
69. D
70. D
71. A

Kaplan UKCAT Diagnostic Test Scoring Table: Section 5

1. Count up your number of correct answers in this section.

2. Find your approximate scoring band for this section in the table below.

	Number correct	Approximate UKCAT score
Situational Judgement	_____	_____

Approximate UKCAT Scoring Band	Number of Questions Answered Correctly
Band 4	0–17
Band 3	18–35
Band 2	36–53
Band 1	54–71

3

Verbal Reasoning

The Task

Verbal Reasoning is the first scored subtest on the UKCAT. The Verbal section includes a total of 11 passages, each with 4 items to answer. You have 1 minute to read the instructions, and then 21 minutes to answer the items. If you divide your time equally among the 11 sets, then you will have just under 2 minutes to complete each set in the Verbal Reasoning section. As you'll see, it will be very difficult to read a full passage and answer the 4 accompanying items in 2 minutes—so you must attack the Verbal section with a strategy that will allow you to attempt all the statements within the allotted time.

The Format

Verbal passages vary in length; most passages are two to four paragraphs, and 200 to 400 words long. The passages are mostly written in a neutral and slightly engaging style, much like articles in a magazine, and can involve virtually any subject matter. Some passages will discuss topics from science or medicine, though these are likely to be a distinct minority on Test Day; most passages will focus on topics from history, the arts or everyday life.

Some Verbal Reasoning items are statements, which you must assess as True, False or Can't tell, based on the passage. Statements are fairly short—most are 10 words or fewer—and as such are relatively straightforward to compare to the passage. The answer choices for Verbal statements are always the same: True, False or Can't tell. It is essential to 'internalise' the meaning of these answers, in the context of Verbal Reasoning:

True: The passage supports the statement.

False: The statement contradicts the passage.

Can't tell: The statement is neither True nor False, or there is not enough information in the passage to evaluate the statement as True or False.

All other Verbal Reasoning items are questions. Each question will have four answer choices, and these will be particular to each question. This makes it very straightforward to distinguish questions from statements (as statements have only three answer choices, and these are always the same). Most questions will require you to select the answer that is true—the answer that is supported by the passage. A few, more difficult questions will ask you to find an answer that contradicts the passage, or is not supported by the passage. Thus, your understanding of True, False and Can't tell Verbal statements will be invaluable in selecting the correct answers to Verbal questions. Each answer choice to a Verbal question is effectively a Verbal statement.

The most obvious challenge in Verbal Reasoning is timing: it is virtually impossible to read the passages fully and answer the questions properly in just 2 minutes per set. If you could manage to read a passage in a minute, you would have only 15 seconds to answer each of the accompanying items. That might be enough time for a simple, straightforward item—but most items will be of medium to advanced difficulty; that is, they will be very tough to assess in 15 seconds.

The other major challenge in the Verbal section is the nature of the task involved—or, to be more precise, the three different tasks. Test-takers who struggle with Verbal tend to confuse the tasks: the most common mistake is to assume that False means the statement is not True. On the UKCAT, a statement is False if it contradicts the passage. This meaning of False is very particular, and differs from the usual meaning of false ('not true'). If a Verbal statement is not True, that does not mean that it is False. A statement must contradict the passage to be False. If a statement is not True and does not contradict the passage, the answer is Can't tell. If a statement does not exactly contradict the passage, then the answer is likely to be Can't tell. Failing to distinguish between False and Can't tell is the second most common mistake in Verbal Reasoning. Thus, a confident understanding of the answer choices is key to Verbal success.

Kaplan Top Tips for Verbal Reasoning

1. Don't read the passage

This may seem counterintuitive, but there are several good reasons not to read the passage:

- *You don't have time*: With 2 minutes per set, you could allow 1 minute to read the passage and then 15 seconds per statement. However, this is not enough time to evaluate most statements. Moreover, it's not enough time to read passages that are 3 paragraphs or longer.

- *Marks come from statements*: Remember, the Verbal section does not assess your ability to read a passage, but your ability to evaluate statements based on a passage. You get a mark for each statement you correctly label as True, False or Can't tell. Reading the passage could help you earn those marks. But it's not the only way, nor is it the best way, given the time constraints of Verbal Reasoning.

- *Each question comes with four statements—the answer choices:* Verbal questions may feel like a fundamentally different format, but in fact they simply require you to apply your skill at assessing statements against the passage. The only difference is that you are given a set of four statements, and (on most questions) must select the one that is True. (A minority of 'negative' questions require you to select the answer that is False or Can't tell, and thus are more difficult.) For this reason, you must learn to assess statements with confidence, as this skill is equally essential for attacking Verbal questions.

- *Speed + accuracy = more marks*: the key to improving your Verbal score is increasing how quickly and how accurately you assess the statements. That is where you'll focus as you practise. You could try reading the passages more quickly, but that would mean reading them less accurately, and would cost you marks on the statements. So a different approach is required.

2. Scan for keywords

This approach has proven the most effective for the thousands of students we at Kaplan have prepared for the UKCAT. Instead of reading the passage:

- Read the statement/question.

- Choose a keyword (or two), and scan the passage for the keyword.

- Pick an answer (or eliminate answers) based on what you find.

A *keyword* is any word or phrase that will help you determine whether the statement is True or False. If the keywords aren't in the passage, then the answer is almost always Can't tell.

Scanning means looking very quickly through the passage for all appearances of the keyword, or related words. Scanning is not the same as reading, but it is a shortcut to save time and make the most of minimal reading: once you find the keyword, read the sentence in which it appears—and just before and after it, if necessary; in most instances, this research will be sufficient to determine that a statement is (or is not) True or False.

It is essential to scan for all appearances of the keyword. If a keyword appears twice in the passage, you may have to combine information from both of its appearances to determine the correct answer. Scanning will help you zero in on the answer to these 'pick 'n' mix' statements.

Some questions will not contain a keyword. For these questions, you must scan for a keyword from each answer choice. We will cover this approach in more detail later in the chapter.

3. If unsure, eliminate

Don't delay once you have scanned the passage and found the relevant information, even when a difficult statement makes it tough to choose an answer. Most commonly, you will be stuck choosing between Can't tell and one other answer. No matter how difficult a statement, you can always eliminate one answer choice:

- If the statement is not supported by the passage, eliminate True.
- If the statement does not contradict the passage, eliminate False.

With two remaining answers, you have a 50% chance of answering correctly. At this point, make a quick judgement call. Most of the time, you'll find yourself uncertain whether there is enough information to justify a statement as True/False. Keep it simple: if there's not enough info, then click Can't tell, flag for review and move on. There are more marks, and easier marks, ahead.

4. Skip the most difficult questions

We will spend some time considering the more challenging types of Verbal questions later in this chapter. You should practise recognising them and deciding how (or whether) to attack them. The most difficult questions can be very time-consuming, and will take more than a minute to answer. Since you have only 30 seconds per question, if you spend, say, 90 seconds on a single question, you will miss out 2 other questions later in the section—and it's likely that those 2 missed questions would be much easier than one that took 90 seconds. If a question looks very difficult or time-consuming, or you find yourself spending a minute or longer, mark an answer, flag for review and move on. Each question is worth one mark, so you will not get any extra marks for spending so much extra time on a single question. But you will run a real risk of missing out easier marks later in the section. Be quick, and be ruthless about skipping the most difficult questions.

5. Check the balance of Verbal questions and statements in the year you sit the UKCAT

The proportion of Verbal items that are questions (rather than statements) has shifted significantly in each of the three years prior to 2013, which is the first year in which a majority of Verbal items were questions. You can confirm the approximate proportion of Verbal questions and statements in the Online Resource Centre (which should be updated each July for the current year's exam), and also in the official practice tests on the UKCAT website, which usually reflect the same proportion of question types that students will expect to see in the current year (again, check this in July). See page ix.

Set your timer for 2 minutes. Write down answers for the 4 statements before time is up!

Born in 1643 in Lincolnshire, Isaac Newton pioneered the study of optics, the properties of light detectable by the human eye, with his insight that white light is made up of the same spectrum of colour as a rainbow. Newton was also the first to demonstrate that gravity was a universal physical force, applied to everything in the universe, in his groundbreaking 1687 study, *Mathematical Principles of Natural Philosophy*. Newton furthered the study of physics in this same work by explaining the three fundamental laws of classical mechanics for the first time.

Following from insights developed by mathematicians over several centuries, Isaac Newton was the first to elucidate the fundamental theorem of calculus and the first to explore differential calculus, as well as its relation to integral calculus. Newton originally developed these concepts of calculus in a 1666 treatise that was not published in full until 1704. There are two reasons that Newton's discovery of calculus remained unknown for so long. First, publishers in the 17th century were wary of texts in the field of theoretical maths, which were so unprofitable that they drove one specialist publisher to bankruptcy. Second, Newton was very tight-lipped about his highly original work in 'the method of fluxions and fluents' (as he called calculus), not mentioning it in print until a brief reference in *Mathematical Principles of Natural Philosophy*.

After commencing study of differential calculus in the 1670s, Gottfried Leibniz, a German mathematician, developed many of the principles of calculus independently of Newton, and was initially given credit for its discovery, with a 1684 publication. However, it is not clear that Newton and Leibniz worked entirely independently, as they had many of the same friends (fellow mathematicians), and occasionally wrote to each other. Calculus as studied and applied today is more similar to the method developed by Leibniz, but this does not diminish Newton's record as an extraordinary innovator of maths as well as physics.

1. White light consists of a spectrum of colour.
    A. True
    B. False
    C. Can't tell

2. Newton was born in Lincoln.
    A. True
    B. False
    C. Can't tell

3. No one studied differential calculus before Leibniz.
    A. True
    B. False
    C. Can't tell

4. Newton was a leading scholar of physics.
    A. True
    B. False
    C. Can't tell

Self-assessment

How did you get on? Hopefully, you finished the statements in the 2 minutes, and answered them all correctly. As you practise with this book, you should **always** read through the explanations for every question, to ensure that you got the right answer for the right reasons. The explanations may also give tips that will help you on later questions with similar twists. If you didn't get them all right, don't despair—in fact, it's good to make mistakes as you practise. Each mistake you make as you practise is one you can avoid on Test Day.

Kaplan Timed Practice Set—*Try the Kaplan Top Tips*: Answers and Explanations

1. (A)

Scan for the keywords 'white light', and you'll find them in the first sentence of the passage. This sentence states that white light is made up of the same spectrum of colour as a rainbow. The statement says the same, so it is true.

2. (C)

Scan for the keywords 'Newton' and 'Lincoln'. Newton is mentioned throughout the passage, but Lincoln is never mentioned. The first sentence states that Newton was born in Lincolnshire, but it does not specify where in Lincolnshire he was born. Thus, based on the passage, we don't know whether or not Newton was born in Lincoln. The answer is therefore (C).

3. (B)

The keywords here are 'Leibniz' and 'differential calculus'. Leibniz appears in the final paragraph, which states that he developed calculus independently of Newton, and that Leibniz started to study differential calculus in the 1670s. However, differential calculus appears earlier, in the second paragraph, where it is mentioned as something that Newton was 'first to explore', and that Newton developed in 1666. Thus, we know from the passage that Newton studied differential calculus before Leibniz; this statement contradicts the passage, so it is false.

4. (A)

Scan for the keyword 'physics' in reference to Newton. The first paragraph specifies that Newton was the first to explain gravity as a universal physical force and that he was also first to explain the fundamental laws of classical mechanics, furthering the study of physics. The passage's final sentence goes even further, stating that Newton was an 'extraordinary innovator' of physics. Innovator is a synonym for leader, so the passage supports this statement. The answer is therefore (A).

Now, let's move on and consider some of the challenges posed by difficult statements.

Inferences

Many challenging Verbal Reasoning statements require you to make inferences from the passage. An inference is something that is not directly stated in the passage, but nearly so. For an inference to be True, it must stay very close to what the passage says. Here is a good rule of thumb about Verbal Reasoning inferences: if you have to work through elaborate reasoning to justify an inference, then your inference is not supported by the passage.

The following three statements involve inferences, based on the passage about Inverness. As you practise, try to evaluate each statement in 30 seconds before reading the answer.

> In 2001, Inverness was granted city status, making it the northernmost city in the UK and also one of the smallest, with a current population of 70,000. Inverness is known as the 'capital of the Highlands', and sits amid hills at the edge of the Great Glen, where the River Ness empties into the Moray Firth. The river is nearly the shortest in Scotland, running a mere six miles from Loch Ness (*Loch Nis*, in Gaelic) to the firth. In fact, the city's Gaelic name, *Inbhir Nis*, literally means 'mouth of the river Ness'. Inverness is a popular base for tourists visiting the many historical sites in the Highlands, along with the perhaps more 'mythical' site of Loch Ness; nearly everyone takes the obligatory boat cruise.
>
> Gaelic has always been widely spoken in the Highlands of Scotland, and Inverness is currently home to a Gaelic renaissance. The city opened a Gaelic primary school in 2007, and expanded capacity to 200 students a few years later. Many street signs in the city are bilingual, though very few adults or children in Inverness (approximately 5% of the population) speak Gaelic. So English speakers needn't worry about communicating with locals when visiting this gorgeous, historic gem of the Highlands.

5. In Gaelic, *Inbhir* means 'mouth of the river'.

   A. True
   B. False
   C. Can't tell

Answer: The keyword '*Inbhir*' is easy to scan for, since it is given in italics. The next-to-last sentence of the first paragraph says that *Inbhir Nis* is Gaelic for 'mouth of the river Ness'. The previous sentence specifies that *Loch Nis* is Gaelic for Loch Ness, so it is safe to infer that *Nis* is Gaelic for Ness. *Inbhir* must therefore mean 'mouth of the river' in Gaelic. This inference from the passage supports the statement, so the statement is true.

6. The River Ness is Scotland's shortest river.

   A. True
   B. False
   C. Can't tell

Answer: Scan for the keywords 'shortest river', and you will find the relevant detail midway through the first paragraph. The passage explains that the River Ness is nearly the shortest river in Scotland. The statement is more extreme than the passage: the River Ness is not the shortest river in Scotland, so the statement is false.

7. Tourists cruise Loch Ness hoping to see the Loch Ness Monster.

   A. True
   B. False
   C. Can't tell

Answer: Scan for 'Loch Ness Monster'—you won't find it in the passage. The final sentence of the first paragraph refers to tourists taking an obligatory boat cruise of the 'mythical' site of Loch Ness, but there is nothing to suggest why exactly the Loch is a mythical site. You cannot infer the Loch Ness Monster without drawing on outside knowledge. Since this statement cannot be assessed based on information in the passage, the answer is (C).

Extreme language can also make Verbal Reasoning statements difficult to evaluate. Extreme language can include absolute words (such as all, never and only) and relative words (such as most, less or nearly). For a statement to be True, its language must be exactly as extreme as the passage. If the statement is more extreme than the passage, the answer is likely to be False or Can't tell. **NB** Exact numbers and categorical verbs (is/are) are used as absolute terms in UKCAT Verbal Reasoning, and therefore count as a form of extreme language.

Here are three statements involving extreme language, based on the passage about Inverness. Once again, try to evaluate each statement in 30 seconds before reading the answer.

8. Most children in Inverness speak Gaelic.

    A. True
    B. False
    C. Can't tell

Answer: Scan for the keywords 'children' and 'speak Gaelic'; they appear in the next-to-last sentence, which states that very few children in Inverness speak Gaelic. 'Very few' means a very small number, and 'most' means a majority. Thus, this statement contradicts the passage, and is false.

9. Virtually all people in Inverness speak English.

    A. True
    B. False
    C. Can't tell

Answer: 'Virtually all' is extreme language—the passage must support the extreme for the statement to be true, or provide sufficient grounds to contradict the extreme for the statement to be false. In this case, the keywords 'speak English' will take you to the last sentences of the second paragraph, which state that Inverness street signs are bilingual, that approximately 5% of people in Inverness speak Gaelic and that English speakers will be able to communicate with locals. Thus, it is safe to infer that the second language on Inverness street signs is English, and that the 95% of locals who do not speak Gaelic speak English. 95% is virtually all of the population; as such, the passage supports the statement, and the statement is true.

10. No city is further north than Inverness.

    A. True
    B. False
    C. Can't tell

Answer: 'No city is further north' is very extreme language. The keyword 'north' leads to the passage's first sentence, which says that Inverness is the northernmost city in the UK. At first glance, it may appear that the passage supports the statement. However, notice the subtle shift in terms—the statement does not say that no city in the UK is further north than Inverness. Since the passage does not mention other cities, it is impossible to say whether there are any cities outside the UK that are further north than Inverness (in which case the statement would be true) or whether there is at least one such city (in which case the statement would be false). Since the statement cannot be assessed based on the passage, the answer is (C).

Set your timer for 2 minutes. Try to mark answers for all 4 statements before time runs out.

The story of Romeo and Juliet, the 'star-cross'd lovers', is one of the most popular of all time, and has been told in several different versions. Best known is the play *Romeo and Juliet,* which nearly everyone reads in school and which introduced such famous lines as 'What's in a name? That which we call a rose by any other name would smell as sweet.' Written and first performed in the 1590s, this highly poetical work of English theatre is set in Italy, where the legend of Romeo and Juliet and their warring families originates.

In the 18th century, the actor and producer David Garrick adapted the original play to remove material considered indecent. Among other changes, he changed references to Rosaline, Romeo's girlfriend at the start of the play, to references to Juliet, so that Romeo already knows and loves Juliet at the start of the play, and the theme is faithfulness rather than love at first sight. The original text was restored in the 19th century, with a sensational production at Sadler's Wells Theatre, London, starring the American sisters Charlotte and Susan Cushman as Romeo and Juliet. 'Gender-bending' is part of the play's tradition: in its early days, men played all the roles. By all accounts Charlotte Cushman was entirely convincing as Romeo. After seeing the Cushmans at Sadler's Wells, Queen Victoria noted in her journal that 'no-one would ever have imagined she was a woman.'

In the 20th century, *Romeo and Juliet* took to the screen in a series of films, including Franco Zeffirelli's 1968 Technicolor epic, which was the first to cast unknown teenagers as the leads and to feature a controversial nude wedding scene, and Baz Luhrmann's 1996 version for the MTV generation, with a soundtrack of pop hits and gun battles instead of swordfights. The most popular film version of *Romeo and Juliet* is *West Side Story*, in which the Jets and the Sharks, rival gangs in New York City, replace the feuding Montagues and Capulets, and Romeo and Juliet become Tony and Maria. *West Side Story* also changes the ending so that one of the central couple survives; this version won 10 Academy Awards in 1961, making it the most acclaimed film adaptation of *Romeo and Juliet* to date. Who knows what twist on *Romeo and Juliet* we'll see next?

11. Queen Victoria never went to the theatre.

    A. True

    B. False

    C. Can't tell

12. Shakespeare wrote *Romeo and Juliet*.

    A. True

    B. False

    C. Can't tell

13. Susan Cushman played Juliet.

    A. True

    B. False

    C. Can't tell

14. Zeffirelli made the only film that cast unknown teenagers as Romeo and Juliet.

    A. True

    B. False

    C. Can't tell

Statements involving inferences and extreme language can be difficult to evaluate quickly. Thus, be sure to review the worked answers in their entirety to ensure that you chose the correct answers for the correct reasons. Doing so will help to build your Verbal Reasoning skills, and help you pick up more marks within the allotted time on Test Day.

Kaplan Timed Practice Set—*Inferences and Extreme Language*: Answers and Explanations

11. (B)

The keywords in this statement are 'Queen Victoria' and 'theatre'. Scan the passage for both, and you will find them in the second paragraph. Sadler's Wells Theatre, London, is mentioned as the home of a sensational production of *Romeo and Juliet* that featured 'gender-bending' casting, with a woman playing Romeo. Queen Victoria saw this production at Sadler's Wells, and found Charlotte Cushman entirely convincing as Romeo. Since the passage states that Queen Victoria saw this performance at the theatre, we know that Queen Victoria went to the theatre at least once in her life. This statement contradicts the passage on this point, and is therefore false.

12. (C)

Here, the keyword is 'Shakespeare'. Scan the passage for his name—it does not appear. Although the passage discusses *Romeo and Juliet* at great length, and discusses Shakespeare's play *Romeo and Juliet* throughout the first two paragraphs, the passage never names him as the author of the play. He can only be identified as the person who wrote *Romeo and Juliet* based on outside knowledge of the details of the play mentioned in the passage. Since this statement cannot be assessed based on information in the passage, the answer is Can't tell.

13. (A)

Scan for the keywords 'Susan Cushman' and 'Juliet'. Susan Cushman appears midway through the second paragraph, which states that the sisters Charlotte and Susan Cushman played Romeo and Juliet in London sometime in the 19th century. The penultimate sentence of that paragraph specifies that Charlotte Cushman played Romeo, so it is safe to infer that Susan Cushman played Juliet. This statement is supported by the passage, so it is true.

14. (C)

Scan for the keywords 'Zeffirelli' and 'unknown teenagers'—both appear in the first sentence of the final paragraph, which states that Zeffirelli was the first to cast unknown teenagers as the leads in a film of *Romeo and Juliet*. Scanning the rest of the passage yields no further reference to casting unknown teenagers as Romeo and Juliet. Thus, on the basis of the passage, it's impossible to say whether Zeffirelli's film is the only one to cast unknown teens as the star-crossed lovers. The answer is therefore (C).

What if the first statement said 'Queen Victoria went to the theatre infrequently'? The answer would be Can't tell, as the passage only mentions a single visit to the theatre by the Queen, with no context for the frequency of her theatre-going. You cannot infer frequency based on other information, such as the fact that the Queen enjoyed the performance, or that she made a note of it in her diary. Such a statement involves a shift from the terms of the passage to the terms of the statement; such a shift makes the statement more difficult to answer, and a good example of some of the most difficult Verbal statements the UKCAT can present.

Verbal Reasoning Questions

The UKCAT will also contain some Verbal Reasoning sets that include a passage and 4 questions. Prior to 2013, only one or two Verbal sets contained questions; in 2013, a majority of Verbal sets contained questions, and it is likely that the Verbal section will be similarly balanced in future. A Verbal question has four answer choices, and only one answer will be correct based on the passage. These questions will stand out from the statements we have practised with so far for a few reasons:

1. They are questions, rather than statements.

2. There are four answer choices, rather than three.

3. The answer choices are not fixed-format; that is, each question will have its own four answers from which you must choose.

By far, the biggest challenge of Verbal Reasoning questions is that they require you to read a lot in order to come up with an answer. The questions and answers are usually full sentences, and will often run to more than one line of text. That is quite a lot of reading, before you have even gone to the passage! As such, Verbal questions are very challenging to answer in 30 seconds each—however, you have a good chance of answering most Verbal questions correctly, in the time allowed, if you follow the usual tips for Verbal statements, with these adjustments:

- Skip the passage—as you have even less time to read it.

- Read the question, and identify keywords that will lead to the correct answer.

- Scan the passage for the keywords. In most cases, the correct answer will paraphrase something that occurs in the passage just before or after the keywords.

- You are looking for the one answer that is supported by the passage. Even though questions may use wording such as 'best supported' or 'most likely to be true', only one answer will be supported by the passage, or true based on the passage. The other answers will either contradict the passage (just like a False statement) or will fall partially or entirely outside it (like a Can't tell statement). Thus, the skills you've practised so far are equally useful for Verbal questions.

- The exceptions to this rule are negative questions—those containing a 'negative' word, such as 'cannot', 'except' or 'least'. On a negative question, answer choices supported by the passage are incorrect. Thus, these questions are like a photographic 'negative' of most Verbal questions, in which the answer supported by the passage is correct. We'll look at these questions in more detail a bit later in the chapter.

Let's practise with the following passage and questions. As always, try to answer each question in 30 seconds before reading the answer.

Pluto was considered the Solar System's ninth planet, and the furthest from the sun, from the time of its discovery in 1930 until 2006, when the International Astronomical Union (IAU) voted to define *planet* for the first time. According to this definition, a planet has three characteristics: it must orbit the sun, be of approximately round shape, and have 'cleared its neighbourhood'—that is, it must be the only body of its size, other than its own satellites, in its region of outer space.

Because its orbit, which is eccentrically elliptical compared to those of the other planets, overlaps significantly with the orbit of Neptune—its nearest neighbouring planet in the Solar System—Pluto fails to meet the third criterion of the definition, and so it is no longer considered a planet, but instead a 'dwarf planet'. This decision by the IAU caused considerable controversy in the popular press at the time it was taken, due to the fact that generations of children had learnt in school that the Solar System includes nine planets; people often have difficulty facing reality when further scientific discovery complicates what they had previously thought to be settled, definite fact.

The IAU's decision to 'demote' Pluto from planet to dwarf planet was not taken lightly, and became necessary due to the discovery of a number of objects in the Kuiper Belt—the region of outer space that extends some 55 astronomical units beyond the orbit of Neptune. (An astronomical unit equals the distance from the Earth to the sun—so the Kuiper Belt extends very far out indeed!) A space object discovered in 2003 and since named Eris (after the ancient Greek goddess of discord) has a greater diameter than Pluto, with 25% more mass; both Pluto and Eris are thought to consist of the same mixture of ice and rock. Scientists could not justify calling Pluto a planet and Eris a Kuiper Belt object; since Eris was larger than Pluto, why shouldn't it also be a planet? The matter was further complicated by the fact that a second Kuiper Belt object, Makemake, discovered in

2005, is only slightly smaller than Pluto. Due to their significantly smaller mass and their resulting weaker gravitational pull, dwarf planets such as Pluto, Eris and Makemake are unable to clear other nearby space objects—either by repelling them, or by colliding and absorbing much of their mass, and thus growing larger and increasing their gravitational pull—and so are unlikely ever to become planets.

For these reasons, the IAU considered three options for defining planets at its meeting in 2006: the first would have increased the number of known planets to twelve, keeping Pluto and adding Eris, Makemake and Ceres, long known as the Solar System's largest asteroid; the second would have defined a planet as being one of the nine planets discovered as of 1930; the third was the definition ultimately approved. Despite popular sentiment, scientists could not justify defining planets according to what was already known, as ongoing improvements in technology continue to allow us to observe the deepest reaches of the Solar System with increasing accuracy. The major problem with the first definition is that its broad nature could allow for an astonishing number of planets, once the expanse of the Kuiper Belt is further explored: since the Kuiper Belt is thought to contain 70,000 or more icy objects, it's very possible that some of these will be as large as—or much larger than—Pluto. Given the extreme distance of some of these Kuiper Belt objects from the sun, they are very likely to further challenge our understanding of what is (and is not) a planet.

15. According to information in the passage, what is the primary reason that Pluto is no longer considered a planet?
    A. Pluto is not as round in shape as Eris.
    B. Astronomers voted to limit the number of planets to eight.
    C. Pluto is too far from the sun to be considered a planet.
    D. Pluto's orbit is unusual in shape, and intersects Neptune's.

Answer: The keywords in this question are 'Pluto' and 'no longer considered a planet'—these appear near the end of the first sentence of the second paragraph. The early part of the sentence explains that Pluto is no longer considered a planet because its orbit is eccentrically elliptical, compared to the other planets' orbits, and that its orbit overlaps significantly with that of its neighbour, Neptune; for this reason, Pluto fails the third criterion of the IAU's definition of planet. Answer (D) is a very close paraphrase of the reason that Pluto fails to qualify as a planet under the new definition, so it must be correct. On Test Day, you'd simply click (D) and move on to the next question. To improve your understanding of how Verbal questions work, take a moment and try to find support for the remaining answer choices. You could take much longer than a moment, but you won't find support. Only the correct answer on a Verbal question is true, based on the passage.

16. The passage best supports which of the following statements about Eris?
    A. Eris is smaller than Neptune.
    B. Eris is nearer to the sun than Pluto.
    C. Eris is currently classified as a dwarf planet.
    D. Eris is approximately round in shape.

Answer: The keyword in this question is 'Eris', which is mentioned several times in the third paragraph and once in the final paragraph. Since there are so many references to Eris, check a keyword from each answer choice to see if the answer is supported by the passage. The keyword in the first answer is 'Neptune', but Neptune is never mentioned in connection with Eris, so the comparison in (A) is not supported; eliminate (A). The sun is never mentioned in connection with Eris, so eliminate (B) for the same reason. The keyword 'dwarf planet' appears in the final sentence of the third paragraph, which states that Pluto, Eris and Makemake are dwarf planets; (C) is therefore correct, and there's no need to check (D). (If you did check (D), you'd see that Eris's shape never comes up in the passage.)

17. The writer of the passage would most likely agree that which of the following was the ultimate cause of the public controversy that met Pluto's demotion from planet to dwarf planet?

    A. People have trouble aligning new scientific discoveries with what they 'know'.

    B. Children are taught that there are nine planets.

    C. Astronomers did not explain their decision in terms that the public could understand.

    D. Most people think a 'Kuiper Belt' is something worn with trousers.

Answer: The keywords here are 'ultimate cause', 'public controversy' and 'Pluto's demotion'. Scanning for these leads to the final sentence of the second paragraph. Here, the writer of the passage attributes the controversy caused by the IAU's decision to define Pluto as a 'dwarf planet' rather than a 'planet' to the fact that people have trouble dealing with scientific discoveries that complicate what they had previously thought to be settled fact. Answer (A) paraphrases this point very concisely, and is therefore correct. (B) might be a tempting wrong answer, in that the author mentions that generations of children had learnt in school that there are nine planets; however, notice the subtle shift in (B) that makes it wrong: (B) instead talks about what children are taught, in the present tense, and therefore does not match the passage. The remaining answers involve the terms used by astronomers, which are mentioned in the passage but not indicated as leading to public controversy due to their incomprehensibility, and trousers, which are not mentioned in the passage.

Difficult Questions

Difficult questions will appear throughout the Verbal section. Most passages with questions will have at least one difficult question. Most difficult questions will include one or more of the following characteristics:

- There is no keyword in the question. In such cases, you must scan for a keyword from each answer, checking these against the passage one at a time and eliminating until you find the answer that is supported by the passage.

- The question contains a keyword, but you can't find the keyword anywhere in the passage. When scanning, you should always keep an eye out for related words and phrases, but even the best scanner may miss out a particular synonym. This can be a problem when the word in the passage is especially short, or when the correspondence to the keyword in the question is not especially obvious. The fail-safe in these instances is to check for a keyword from the answer choice, and scan for support in the passage—though be careful, as it is more time-consuming to scan for each answer. Try not to spend much more than 30 seconds on each question, even when scanning for all four answers.

- The correct answer is an inference from the entire passage. Such questions will often not contain a keyword, but you may have trouble finding support in the passage for any of the answers, as the correct inference may only be apparent if the passage is read in-depth. These questions are fairly rare, so don't fret about them. If you have checked all the answers and can't find support in the passage, make your best guess quickly and move on. It's best not to waste any extra time with such questions, as more time is not likely to yield a correct mark.

- The question contains a 'negative' word, such as not, cannot, least or except. These negative questions will be covered in the next section. They can be the most difficult to conceptualise, as the answer to a negative question will usually be something that is not true. On a negative question, the true answer choices—those supported by the passage—will normally be incorrect.

Here are three difficult questions, based on the passage about Pluto and the Kuiper Belt. Once again, try to answer each question in 30 seconds before reading the answer.

18. Which of the following conclusions is justified by the passage?

    A. The Kuiper Belt is not part of our Solar System.

    B. We have not fully explored the depths of the Solar System.

    C. It will be many years before the actual number of planets is known.

    D. We know very little about other planets.

Answer: This question does not contain any keywords, so scan for a keyword from each answer choice and eliminate until you find the answer that is supported by the passage. The keywords 'Kuiper Belt' appear several times in the final two paragraphs, but the passage never clearly states whether the Kuiper Belt is in fact part of our Solar System. There's no clear support for (A), so eliminate it. (If you were to read the final two paragraphs in-depth, you would find enough information to infer that the Kuiper Belt is part of our Solar System, but this would not be clear from a quick scan.) The keywords in (B) are 'depths' and 'Solar System'; these occur together in the second sentence of the final paragraph, which states that new technological developments keep allowing us to explore the deepest reaches of the Solar System with increasing accuracy. Since the passage says that we are continuing to explore the depths of the Solar System, then (B) must also be true; (B) is a valid inference from the passage, and is therefore correct. There is no need to check (C) and (D) against the passage—though if you did, you would find they are not supported.

19. Which of these statements must be true?
    A. Eris is the smallest dwarf planet in the Solar System.
    B. Neptune is further from the sun than Pluto is.
    C. Makemake was discovered after Eris.
    D. Neptune and Pluto are the only planets whose orbits intersect.

Answer: Again, there is no keyword in the question, so check each answer against the passage until you find the one that is supported. The keywords 'Eris' and 'smallest dwarf planet' lead to the third paragraph, which mentions that Pluto, Eris and Makemake are dwarf planets in our Solar System, and that Eris is larger than Pluto. Thus, Eris cannot be the smallest dwarf planet in the Solar System, since at least one dwarf planet is smaller. Eliminate (A). The keywords in (B) are 'Neptune', 'Pluto' and 'the sun'. The passage's first sentence explains that Pluto was the ninth planet and furthest from the sun from 1930 to 2006; the first sentence of second paragraph states that Pluto's orbit overlaps with Neptune's, which means that, at times, it's possible that Neptune could be further from the sun than Pluto. However, this inference is as uncertain as it is elaborate, since there is no way of knowing from the passage whether Neptune is currently further from the sun than Pluto is. Thus, while (B) could be true, we cannot say based on the passage that (B) must be true; eliminate (B). The keywords in (C) are 'Makemake' and 'Eris'. These both appear in the third paragraph, which says that Eris was discovered in 2003 and Makemake in 2005. (C) is supported by the passage, and is therefore correct. There is no need to check (D) against the passage.

20. According to the passage, a common measurement used by space scientists involves:
    A. the radius of the sun.
    B. the length between a planet and a star.
    C. the weight of ice.
    D. the distance between the sun and another star.

Answer: The keywords in this question are 'common measurement' and 'space scientists'. The word 'measurement' never appears in the passage, so look for other words related to measuring or common measurement words. The answer choices give good examples to scan for: radius; length; weight; distance. The keyword 'distance' appears in the third paragraph, in the bracketed remark that defines an astronomical unit as equal to the distance from the Earth to the sun. Answer (B) is a close paraphrase for this detail from the passage, so (B) is correct.

Note that once again, when there was difficulty in scanning for keywords from the question, the only approach is to go to the answer choices and find keywords there. It's essential to do so whenever you are stuck with a difficult Verbal question. The one thing you must avoid at all times is getting drawn into reading the passage in-depth—this is an easy trap to fall into with difficult questions, and one that could cause you to run out of time before you've got through all the passages. Practise pacing yourself with Verbal questions, so you can try to keep to 2 minutes per passage set. This will mean guessing based on partial work, or even skipping the most difficult questions—but this is the only approach that will ensure you have a chance to attempt all 11 passage sets on Test Day.

Negative Questions

Most students find negative questions to be the hardest questions in Verbal Reasoning. This is because the correct answer to a negative question will not be supported by the passage; on a negative question, answers that are supported by the passage will be incorrect. The nature of the correct/incorrect answers will vary, depending on the exact negative word in the question:

- If the question asks for an answer that 'cannot be true', then the correct answer must be false. That is, the correct answer will contradict the passage. Incorrect answers will be supported by the passage, or not included in the passage.

- If the question contains the word 'except', then the incorrect answers will normally be things that are supported by the passage. The correct answer could contradict the passage, or could be something not included in the passage. Answers supported by the passage will normally be incorrect. (We say 'normally' in this instance, as all the published examples of 'except' questions are framed this way, i.e. so that the correct answer is something that is not true based on the passage. But there is always the possibility, however unlikely, that the UKCAT could throw up a twist involving 'except' on Test Day—so double-check any 'except' question to make sure that it works this way.)

- If the question contains the word 'least', then the correct answer will not be supported by the passage. The incorrect answers will normally be supported by the passage. Even though the question says 'least', it is not a matter of comparing answers to see which is the 'less' appropriate—only one answer will not be supported by the passage, and will often contradict it.

Try applying these tips about negative questions to the following passage and questions. As usual, try to keep yourself to no more than 30 seconds per question.

For over a hundred years, swimmers have been crossing the English Channel, the 350-mile-long stretch of water that separates Great Britain from the northern shores of France. Captain Matthew Webb made the first recorded attempt in 1875 when he swam the 21-mile distance across the Strait of Dover in 21 hours, 45 minutes. Webb's successful crossing was the beginning of a trend: 811 people have successfully swum across the Strait of Dover since Webb, a total of 1,185 times. In 1927 the Channel Swimming Association was founded as the governing authority of this relatively new sport. The association authenticates claims to channel swimming and keeps track of crossing times and provides regulations for approved swims. For example, the CSA's rules prohibit any assistance other than having nourishment handed to the swimmer (though direct contact is not allowed, even in this instance), and the CSA stipulates the acceptable swimming costumes and use of 'grease' (to protect the exposed parts of the body from the cold waters of the Channel). Each swimmer must also have a pilot in a nearby boat who ensures the swimmer's safety and provides assistance in an emergency situation, as well as feeding the swimmer by hand or feeding pole; if the swimmer leaves the water for any reason, the swim must be aborted.

To date, the record for the fastest Channel crossing by a swimmer belongs to Trent Grimsey, an Australian, who swam from Dover to Cap Gris-Nez, France, on 8 September 2012 in exactly 6 hours, 55 minutes, besting the previous record by nearly 3 minutes. Grimsey, who was aged 24 at the time of his historic Channel swim, had previously won a number of international open water swimming competitions in Argentina, Brazil, California, New Zealand, Queensland (his home state in Australia) and Italy, where he set a record of 6 hours, 29 minutes in the Maratona del Golfo Capri-Napoli. Grimsey retired from competitive swimming in August 2013.

The previous record was set by Petar Stoychev, a Bulgarian swimmer who is also the eight-time winner of the Open Water World Championship. Stoychev made his record-breaking crossing on 24 August 2007 in 6 hours, 57 minutes, 50 seconds, beating his previous time by over twenty minutes. Russian swimmer Yuri Kudinov, Stoychev's long-time rival, swam the Channel on the same day, starting just 18 minutes after Stoychev and finishing less than 30 minutes after the Bulgarian broke the world record. Stoychev's time broke a record set only two years before by Christof Wandratsch, who completed the feat in 7 hours, 3 minutes. Neither Stoychev nor Kudinov knew the other would be attempting the crossing that day until hours before they began. The two were neck and neck for most of the race, and Stoychev later confessed that he imagined he would hold the world record for only a few minutes before watching it be awarded to Kudinov. Grimsey and Stoychev are the only people to have swum across the English Channel in under 7 hours, an extraordinary feat of physical endurance.

21. Which of the following cannot be true?
    A. Stoychev thought Kudinov would break his record.
    B. Webb's first swim across the Channel was not regulated by the CSA.
    C. Stoychev and Kudinov are Bulgarian rivals.
    D. Fewer than 1,000 people have swum across the Strait of Dover.

Answer: This is a negative question, asking for something that cannot be true; the correct answer will contradict the passage. There aren't any keywords in the question, so scan for keywords from each answer and compare to the passage, until you find the one that contradicts the passage. The keywords in (A) are 'Stoychev' and 'Kudinov', which appear in the final paragraph; the fifth sentence of this paragraph supports (A), so (A) is incorrect. The keywords in (B) are 'Webb' and 'CSA'; these occur in the first paragraph, which states that Webb swam across the Channel in 1875 and that the CSA was founded in 1927. From this information, it is safe to infer that (B) is true, so (B) is incorrect. (C) contains the same keywords as (A); checking the final paragraph, you will notice that Stoychev is Bulgarian but Kudinov is Russian. (C) contradicts the passage, and is therefore the correct answer. There is no need to check (D) against the passage.

22. All of the following statements about Trent Grimsey must be true EXCEPT:
    A. He swam competitively in many countries.
    B. He broke a record that had been set just over 5 years earlier.
    C. He no longer competes in open water swimming events.
    D. He is one of three swimmers to cross the English Channel in under 7 hours.

Answer: This negative question contains the word except; three of the answers will be true (supported by the passage), and therefore incorrect. The correct answer will be the one that is not supported by the passage—it could contradict the passage, or could include information that is not in the passage. The question also contains a helpful keyword, the name Trent Grimsey. Grimsey's name appears in the second paragraph, and at the very end of the passage. The second paragraph lists several countries where Grimsey swam competitively, so (A) is supported by the passage; thus, (A) is incorrect. The same paragraph mentions that Grimsey broke the record for swimming across the Channel in September 2012; the next paragraph states that the previous record was set in August 2007. Thus, (B) is supported by the passage and is also incorrect. Answer (C) is a close paraphrase of the final sentence of the second paragraph, so it is incorrect. The correct answer must be (D), and the details in the final paragraph allow you to infer that only two swimmers—Grimsey and Stoychev—have swum across the English Channel in under 7 hours. (D) is false, and therefore correct.

23. The author would least likely agree with which of these claims about approved swims across the English Channel?
    A. They may involve direct contact between the swimmer and his pilot.
    B. Swimmers may use 'grease', subject to regulation.
    C. The choice of swimming costume for such swims is restricted.
    D. Swimmers may not participate without a pilot in a nearby boat.

Answer: Most passages, like this one, will not include direct statements of the author's opinion. Thus, you can infer that the author would agree with anything that is supported by the passage. The author would be least likely to agree with something that contradicts the passage, so that is what you are looking for here. The question contains the keywords 'approved swims', which appear in the first paragraph. The rest of that paragraph explains several of the rules of approved swims. Comparing these details from the passage to the answer choices, you will find that (B), (C) and (D) are supported by the passage, but (A) contradicts it—direct contact with the swimmer is never allowed in approved swims. (A) is therefore correct.

24. Which of these conclusions about open water swimmers is not supported by the passage?
    A. They are capable of extreme accomplishments due to their physical prowess.
    B. They compete in many different countries.
    C. They never swim more than two hours without taking a break on a boat.
    D. They compete to break world records set by other swimmers.

Answer: This question contains a negative word, 'not', so any answers supported by the passage will be incorrect. The question also includes the keywords 'open water swimmers'; since these swimmers are discussed throughout the passage, it will be quicker and easier to scan for keywords from each answer choice. The keywords 'extreme accomplishments' and 'physical prowess' lead to the passage's final sentence, which uses similar words to describe the 'extraordinary feat' of Grimsey and Stoychev; (A) is supported by the passage, so it is incorrect. (B) mentions many different countries, and there is a list of countries where Grimsey won open water swimming competitions in the second paragraph; (B) is also supported, and thus also incorrect. The keywords 'two hours' never appear in the passage, and the keywords 'taking a break on a boat' contradict the rules of the CSA in the first paragraph, which does not allow for the swimmer to leave the water for any reason. (C) is not supported by the passage, so it is correct.

Set your timer for 2 minutes. Attempt to answer all 4 questions before time is up. If you have trouble with a question, try to eliminate one or two answers, then make your best guess.

In 2011, a total of eight ancient boats were discovered in a quarry near the Flag Fen archaeological site, located immediately south-east of Peterborough in the Cambridgeshire fens. In 2013, carbon dating revealed that the boats were from 1600 BC, a full two centuries earlier than the original approximation. The boats, made from lime, oak or maple, were buried extremely deep underground, and were so well built that they were virtually intact and, if allowed onto water, would still be buoyant. This unusual, historical treasure trove led the archaeologists to take the exceptional (and costly) decision to transport the boats from the quarry to their facility at Flag Fen without first cutting the boats into chunks, which required a system of pulleys and special transport equipment reinforced with scaffolding poles to ensure that the boats were not damaged.

The boats had been deliberately submerged to the bottom of what was then a creek, in what is believed to be a Bronze Age ritual of some religious significance. The area of the fens where the boats were found had been criss-crossed with creeks and rivers during the Bronze Age, and the custom of the time was to sink offerings to the gods underwater. Many daggers and jewels were found near the boats, leading archaeologists to believe that the site may have been of religious as well as commercial importance over 3,000 years ago. Some of the boats were well used by fishermen and must have been brought some distance inland in order to be sunk in the creek, and others appear to have been built only for that purpose. We know that they deliberately sank the boats because the transoms—the pieces of wood that close off the rear of the boat—had been removed.

The craftsmanship of the boats is extraordinarily practical and versatile, even by today's standards. The shipwrights used tools made of bronze to carve the tree trunks and shape the boats, some of which were hewn until only as thick as a finger but which were so resiliently buoyant that they were able to float when rain filled the archaeologists' trench. The boats are now on display in a chilled container within a barn on the Flag Fen site. The technician responsible for conserving the boats must spend eight hours a day spraying them with water and removing impurities; once this process is complete, the boats will be injected with a special wax with preservative powers and then dried out, a process that will take two years to complete.

Why did they sink the boats? The likeliest explanation is that an extended period of climate change led to a worrying rise in sea levels, so that the terrain of the fens became increasingly waterlogged over a very small number of years. As a consequence, the mostly agrarian society was not able to grow crops, and was at risk of starvation. The ritual sinking of the boats was thus likely intended to be a profoundly desperate offering to appease the gods and stop the seas from rising.

25. The passage suggests that the Bronze Age is most likely called 'the Bronze Age' because at that time people:
    A. used coins primarily made of bronze.
    B. constructed a series of prominent bronze statues.
    C. worked with bronze implements.
    D. first discovered bronze.

26. Which of the following conclusions cannot be true?
    A. Water once played a part in a religious custom.
    B. Climate change is only a contemporary concern.
    C. The Cambridgeshire fens were not always waterlogged.
    D. Some ancient people deliberately sank boats.

27. All of the following statements about the recently discovered boats are true except:

    A. They were carved from oak or other trees.
    B. Some of the boats are capable of floating.
    C. They were first estimated to date to 1600 BC.
    D. Some of the boats were fishing boats.

28. The author of the passage would most likely agree with which of these assertions?

    A. The Flag Fen boats could be used by fishermen today.
    B. Archaeologists were wrong to chop up the Flag Fen boats.
    C. Flag Fen was the most significant religious site in the Bronze Age.
    D. Conserving ancient boats is a slow, painstaking process.

Passages with Verbal Reasoning questions are the most time-consuming and challenging on the UKCAT. Unprepared test-takers fall into the trap of reading everything, which can easily take 3 to 4 times as long as the time you actually have for the set. Despite the reading involved, you still have only 2 minutes per set. Scanning for keywords and selecting the answer choice that must be true based on the passage—a skill that you have practised on Verbal Reasoning statements—should be sufficient to get you to the correct answer for most Verbal Reasoning questions in 30 seconds. The more quickly and accurately you scan, the more marks you will earn in this section—even on the hardest questions!

Kaplan Timed Practice Set—*Verbal Reasoning Questions*: Answers and Explanations

25. (C)

Scan for the keywords 'Bronze Age', which appear twice in the second paragraph. None of the information here corresponds to the answer choices, so scan for a keyword from each answer choice. The keywords in (A) and (B), 'coins' and 'statues', do not appear in the passage; eliminate (A) and (B). The keywords 'bronze implements' in (C) lead to the third paragraph, which states that the Flag Fen shipwrights used tools made of bronze. This detail from the passage supports (C), which is therefore correct. If you were not confident about this, you might also check (D) against the passage, but there is nothing in the passage to clarify whether bronze was first discovered in the Bronze Age.

26. (B)

There isn't a keyword in this question, and it's a negative question. The correct answer will be something that contradicts the passage; any answers that are supported by the passage are incorrect. The keywords in (A), 'water' and 'religious', are found in the second paragraph, which explains that the boats were deliberately submerged underwater in a ritual of religious significance; the custom of the time was to sink offerings to the gods underwater. (A) is supported by the passage, so it is incorrect. The keyword in (B), 'climate change', appears in the final paragraph. The Flag Fen boats date to an extended period of climate change which resulted in the fens becoming increasingly waterlogged in a very short time. Thus, (B) contradicts the passage, as climate change was a concern in the Bronze Age. (B) is correct.

27. (C)

This question contains a negative word, 'except'. Thus, the three incorrect answers will be supported by the passage; the correct answer will contradict the passage, or will involve information that is not in the passage. The keywords 'oak or other trees' lead to the first paragraph, which states that the Flag Fen boats were made of oak, lime or maple; (A) is supported by the passage, so it is incorrect. The keyword 'floating' in (B) is found in the third paragraph; archaeologists found that some boats could float in rainwater. (B) is supported by the passage, and thus incorrect. The keyword '1600 BC' occurs in the first paragraph; carbon dating revealed the boats are from 1600 BC, two centuries earlier than first thought. Thus, the boats were first estimated to date to 1400 BC. (C) contradicts the passage, so it is the correct answer.

28. (D)

This question asks what the author would agree with, so the answer choice that is supported by the passage will be correct. There isn't a keyword in the question, so scan for a keyword from each answer to find support in the passage. The Flag Fen boats are mentioned throughout the passage, so scan for 'fishermen today', the keywords in (A). Fishermen in the Bronze Age are mentioned in the second paragraph, but fishermen today are not mentioned; while the boats could float, this does not mean that they are sturdy enough to be used by fishermen, so (A) is not supported by the passage. The keywords in (B), 'archaeologists' and 'chop up', lead to the end of the first paragraph. Archaeologists decided not to cut up the boats into chunks, so (B) contradicts the passage. The keywords in (C), 'religious site' and 'Bronze Age', guide you to the second paragraph, which explains that the fen was a site of some religious significance. The statement in (C) is much stronger, and is not supported by the passage. This means that (D) must be correct; indeed, the keywords 'conserving ancient boats' lead to the third paragraph, which details the meticulous two-year process of preserving the boats.

On the next four pages, you will complete a timed Kaplan UKCAT quiz, consisting of 4 Verbal Reasoning passage sets. If you pace yourself, and spend no more than 2 minutes per set, you should be able to attempt to answer every item. Even if you find yourself running out of time near the end, do your best to eliminate at least one answer choice and make your best guess. It is essential that you get into the mindset of marking an answer for every question, and that you practise doing so as you complete several sets under UKCAT time pressure.

As you have seen so far, Verbal statements and questions come in a range of difficulties, and all are worth one mark. If a statement or question is especially difficult, it is essential not to waste time on it. Such items are designed to draw in unprepared students, and ensure they get a poor result.

Before you begin the Kaplan UKCAT quiz, let's consider some of the key issues in Verbal Reasoning that unprepared (or underprepared) test-takers misunderstand time and again on the UKCAT:

The more elaborate your reasoning, the more likely it is to be wrong. The test-maker knows you only have 30 seconds (at most) per statement, so you are not expected to come up with an elaborate explanation to justify your answer. If you feel complicated reasoning is required, then scan the passage again for a different (or related) keyword—it is very likely that you've missed something the first time round. Or that the answer is Can't tell.

Statements can only be True or False based on what is in the passage. Support from the passage in the form of a paraphrase or an inference is required to make a statement True; similarly, a statement must contradict a detail or inference from the passage in order to be False. That is why scanning for keywords is so essential, and why you must be prepared to eliminate appropriately whenever you don't find support or contradiction (or both).

Most questions ask you to find the answer that is True (except for negative questions). Each Verbal question presents you with four statements—the answer choices—and you must normally select the one that is supported by the passage. That is, you must find the one answer that is a True statement. Negative questions are the exception to this rule, as any answers that are True will be incorrect.

Scan the entire passage for all references to your keywords, or related words. This point may seem a bit obvious, but you would be surprised how many test-takers stop scanning as soon as they find a single reference to their keyword. Sometimes, you will have to combine information from two separate references to make an inference, or to discover that the passage gives contradictory information.

Proceed carefully when the passage or the statement uses extreme language. Extreme language can be very subtle, and a shift from passage to statement could result in an unexpected answer (e.g. a statement that appears to be very similar at first glance could be False or Can't tell instead of True). Reading before and after the keyword in the passage, and checking for any other references to the keyword, will help ensure that you pick up these marks.

Remember the many reasons why 'Can't tell' can be the correct answer. The most common reason is that the statement includes a keyword that is not mentioned in the passage (e.g. 'Shakespeare wrote *Romeo and Juliet*'). Also popular, and far more challenging, is a statement that includes terms from the passage, but adds a further term that is not mentioned in (or inferable from) the passage. Another way of thinking about these statements is that they do not have adequate support from the passage to be true, but can't be false because they don't contradict the passage. Often, it is fairly straightforward to see that you can eliminate one answer straightaway on such statements (e.g. most test-takers would eliminate False straightaway on the Shakespeare statement, and then decide between True or Can't tell). Elimination is the key to saving time, and earning marks.

Set your timer for 8 minutes. Try to evaluate all 16 statements and questions, and mark an answer for each before time is up. If a statement is difficult, try to eliminate one answer and then make your best guess, so you can keep to 2 minutes per set.

Because the British government has never undertaken a large-scale campaign to 'put a Briton on the moon', few people know much about the British space programme. Unlike many other national space initiatives, the British space programme's official focus was always on unmanned satellite launches, and, in fact, the UK has banned human space flight since 1986. All British astronauts who have travelled in outer space during the ban have done so with funding from non-governmental sources, either as 'space tourists' or by acquiring American citizenship and joining the NASA programme.

Interest in a British space programme, though, began much earlier. The British Interplanetary Society, founded in 1933, instigated early research in the field and developed the UK's military interest in a space programme. Throughout the 1960s and 1970s, the UK launched a number of satellites and rockets: some on the Isle of Wight, some in Woomera, Australia, where a joint Australia–UK weapons- and aerospace-testing facility was located. More than 6,000 rockets were launched from Woomera, including the hypersonic rocket Falstaff and the satellite-launching rocket Black Arrow. The Ariel programme saw the UK develop and launch six satellites from 1962 to 1979, in collaboration with NASA; the final four spacecraft in this series were designed and built in the UK. In this same era, the UK did not play a role in the 'Space Race' between the world's two military superpowers that led to the first men setting foot on the moon, in a series of American-commanded missions that captured the world's imagination from 1969 to 1972. Since the rise of manned space flight, both the USA and the Soviet Union (and, later, Russia) have included astronauts from Europe and other parts of the world on space missions.

The official programme of UK satellite launches was cancelled in the early 1980s, but in 1985 the British National Space Centre was founded to coordinate UK space activities. Today, the UK Space Agency, founded in Wiltshire in 2010, has replaced the British National Space Centre and assumed responsibility for government policy and budgets for space exploration. In the next 20 years, the agency aims to increase the size of the UK space industry from £6 billion to £40 billion, creating over 30,000 jobs. Central to this plan is the new £40 million International Space Innovation Centre in Oxfordshire, which will investigate climate change and space system security.

29. The UK did not compete in the 'Space Race'.

    A. True ✓
    B. False
    C. Can't tell

30. No Briton has set foot on the moon.

    A. True ✓
    B. False
    C. Can't tell

31. Most UK rockets have been launched in Australia.

    A. True
    B. False
    C. Can't tell ✓

32. Manned space flights will now launch from Oxfordshire.

    A. True
    B. False
    C. Can't tell ✓

Scientists believe that the world is long overdue a serious influenza pandemic. These occur every so often when a strain of the virus possesses the correct combination of proteins to be both infectious and dangerous. These proteins are also used to describe the strain—for example, avian influenza, originating in birds, was also known as H5N1. Pandemics can be very deadly—the 'Spanish flu' pandemic in 1919 was responsible for the deaths of 20 to 40 million people, more than died in the First World War.

In 2009, a new strain of influenza, H1N1, became prominent in Mexico before spreading rapidly around the world. Known as swine flu, due to its origin in pigs, this strain of flu was highly transmissible from person to person, and fears grew that, if the virus was also dangerous, hundreds of thousands of people could die. Whilst some people seemed to suffer severely with the infection, most people seemed to have only mild symptoms lasting a few days.

Two different vaccines against this strain of flu were quickly developed and offered to those people at particular risk, such as pregnant women, health-care workers and people with certain health problems. This led to concern amongst the general population that rushing production could mean that the vaccines were not safe, and there was widespread anxiety about side effects, even though these were rare. However, many people decided that, on balance, it was a risk that they were prepared to take. Fortunately, as the winter flu season progressed, there were nowhere nearly as many serious cases of influenza as predicted, leading many people to believe that we have narrowly escaped another catastrophic pandemic.

33. Which of the following best describes the writer's view of the primary reason that the 2009 outbreak of H1N1 influenza was not as deadly as expected?
    A. Most cases were mild, and lasted for less than a week.
    B. People at high risk for H1N1 influenza were all vaccinated.
    C. The general public decided not to take the H1N1 vaccine.
    D. People who suffered most severely died quickly at the start of the outbreak.

34. The passage best supports which of the following statements about flu pandemics?
    A. They have killed more people than the World Wars.
    B. The next one will occur in the next five years.
    C. They can be averted by rushing vaccines into production.
    D. They can kill millions of people.

35. According to the information in the passage, what is it precisely that causes influenza outbreaks to develop into pandemics?
    A. An influenza strain originates in birds or swine, before passing to humans.
    B. An influenza strain develops with both dangerous and infectious proteins.
    C. An influenza strain arises on the borders of a major international conflict.
    D. An influenza strain grows stronger because the public declines an available vaccine.

36. The writer of the passage would most likely agree with which one of the following statements?
    A. The deadliest strains of flu usually emerge in Spanish-speaking countries.
    B. Avoiding contact with birds and pigs will keep you safe from deadly strains of flu.
    C. Concerns about side effects from the H1N1 vaccine were overblown.
    D. People are most vulnerable to the flu in the winter.

Johannes Vermeer (1632–1675) is now considered to be one of the Old Masters of Dutch painting, though only 35 of his paintings exist and very little is known about his life. Other than information in government registers and a handful of comments by other artists, Vermeer's life was so unknown (and thus inscrutably mysterious) that he was called 'the Sphinx of Delft' in the 19th century; as such, it was common to try and infer the truth about Vermeer from his paintings, as if his use of colour and light and his focus on middle-class subjects could reveal anything certain about the man who painted them. Most of what we now know about Vermeer was extensively researched in the city archives of Delft and published in the early 1980s.

Vermeer's early works were influenced by Caravaggio and Carel Fabritius, another Delft painter active in the early 1650s who was interested in the camera obscura. The Delft painters' guild made Vermeer a master in 1653, and he married in the same year. In the following two decades, Vermeer painted almost all of his extant works, which are in the mature style associated with him, such as *Girl with a Pearl Earring*, *The Music Lesson*, *The Milkmaid* and *Girl Reading a Letter at an Open Window*. This last painting was incorrectly attributed to Rembrandt for some time, until it was correctly recognised as a Vermeer in 1880. Vermeer lost everything near the end of his life and died penniless, having had to sell off the last of his paintings in his possession—though the precise reasons for his penury are lost to history.

Most of Vermeer's surviving paintings are from this mature period and feature interior scenes of tranquil domestic activity, such as reading, writing, drinking and playing musical instruments. The rooms in Vermeer's paintings are mostly dark, and he draws in the viewer's eye with his signature effect, a very distinctive 'pearly' light, achieved with miniature globules of white paint, so that the light appears to stream from a window at the left of every painting. The pearly light almost seems to gleam against the drab middle-class realities that Vermeer depicts. Objects within each painting, such as pianos and paintings, further guide the eye and define the constraints of the domestic sphere. Vermeer is also known for his use of cornflower blue and gold as common accent colours, giving his work a timeless elegance.

37. The passage suggests that the best-known feature of Vermeer's mature paintings was:

    A. his predominant use of white, gold and cornflower.

    B. an unusual, almost glowing, pearlescent light.

    C. his inclusion of musical instruments or paintings in every painting.

    D. his focus on servants and housework.

38. Which of the following was not included in any of Vermeer's paintings?

    A. windows

    B. jewellery

    C. letters

    D. seascapes

39. Based on the passage, it is correct to infer that Vermeer was called 'the Sphinx of Delft' because:

    A. he was viewed as an enigmatic artist in the 1800s.

    B. nothing was known about his life.

    C. he was the most prominent painter from Delft.

    D. his facial features resembled those of the Sphinx.

40. The author of the passage would most likely agree with which of these conclusions?

    A. You cannot determine facts about an artist from his techniques.

    B. Vermeer was uncomfortable with the everyday realities of middle-class life.

    C. The facts of an artist's life are irrelevant to an understanding of his work.

    D. Vermeer's wife was a milkmaid.

Cork is used in a variety of products, the most familiar of which is a wine stopper—or cork! The material's natural compressibility and near-impermeability make it ideal for this purpose, and natural cork is used for about 60% of wine stoppers today. Wine can become tainted during the process of bottling, ageing, storage and transport, and although other factors cause tainting, the stopper is usually held responsible. This association in the mind of the consumer is so strong that a bottle found on opening to have undesirable smells and tastes is usually said to have become 'corked'.

The use of alternative wine closures has grown in an attempt to prevent cork taint. For example, the synthetic cork, designed to look and function like a natural cork, avoids the risk as it is made from a resin that does not contain trichloroanisole. However, alternative closures themselves bring their own disadvantages. Wine experts have noted that a synthetic cork can impart its own slight chemical flavour to wine, replacing one type of cork taint with another. Screw-top bottles provide an alternative free of the risk of cork taint, but present an entirely new problem: consumers associate a screw-top bottle with poor quality wine, regardless of its price, vintage or reputation.

41. Wine in screw-top bottles is of poor quality.

    A. True
    B. False
    C. Can't tell

42. Synthetic cork eliminates cork taint completely.

    A. True
    B. False
    C. Can't tell

43. Most wine is bottled with natural cork.

    A. True
    B. False
    C. Can't tell

44. Vintage is most important when choosing a bottle of wine.

    A. True
    B. False
    C. Can't tell

STOP. IF YOU FINISH BEFORE TIME IS UP, CHECK ANY QUESTIONS YOU HAVE MARKED FOR REVIEW. YOU MAY GO BACK TO QUESTIONS IN THIS QUIZ ONLY.

29. (A)

Scan for the keywords 'Space Race', which appear in inverted commas midway through the second paragraph. The passage states here that the UK did not play a role in the 'Space Race'; this statement paraphrases this closely, and is therefore true.

30. (C)

The keywords 'on the moon' lead to the last sentences of the second paragraph, which say that the first men set foot on the moon in a series of US-commanded missions from 1969 to 1972, and that both the USA and the Soviet Union included European astronauts on space missions since the rise of manned space flight. Thus, the passage leaves open the possibility that a European astronaut may have been included on one of the missions to the moon; however, it is not clear whether or not a European was included, and it is also not clear whether or not any such European astronauts would have also been British. Based on the passage, then, the answer is Can't tell.

31. (C)

This statement is unusual, but scan for the keywords 'UK rockets' and 'Australia'. The third sentence of the second paragraph mentions that the UK launched a number of satellites and rockets in Woomera, Australia; the following sentence specifies that more than 6,000 rockets were launched from Woomera. Thus, the UK launched quite a lot of rockets in Australia; however, the passage does not mention any figures for UK rockets launched from other locations, nor does it clarify whether or not the 6,000-plus rockets launched from Woomera are a majority of UK rockets launched. The answer is therefore (C).

32. (B)

Scan for the keywords 'manned space flight' and 'Oxfordshire'. Oxfordshire is mentioned only in the final sentence, as the location of a new space centre. This paragraph does not indicate whether manned space flights will launch from the Oxfordshire facility. Scanning the rest of the passage for 'manned space flight' will reveal a reference to 'human space flight' midway through the first paragraph; the UK has banned such flights since 1986. Thus, we can infer that manned space flights will not launch from Oxfordshire. This statement contradicts the passage, so the statement is false.

33. (A)

The keywords '2009', 'H1N1 influenza' and 'not as deadly as expected' lead to the second paragraph, which states that, although some people suffered severely with H1N1 infection, most people had mild symptoms lasting a few days. (A) paraphrases this very closely, and is therefore correct. The remaining answers are not supported by the passage.

34. (D)

Scanning for the keywords 'flu' and 'pandemic' is not entirely helpful, as these appear several times in the passage. Scanning for keywords from the answer choices is fairly quick in this instance, since the answers are relatively short. Answer (A) has the keywords 'World Wars', which leads to the detail in the first paragraph that the Spanish flu pandemic in 1919 killed more people than the First World War. There are no statistics about the deaths from the Second World War, so (A) cannot be correct. The keywords 'five years' from (B) do not appear in the passage, which does not indicate precisely (or generally) when the next flu pandemic will occur, so (B) is wrong. The keywords 'rushing vaccines into production' do not lead to support in the passage for answer (C). Thus, the only remaining answer is (D), and the keywords 'millions of people' lead to the figure of deaths from the Spanish flu pandemic in the first paragraph. (D) is therefore correct.

35. (B)

The keywords 'develop into pandemics' lead to the first paragraph, which explains that flu pandemics occur when a strain of the virus has proteins that are both infectious and dangerous. Answer (B) matches this word for word, and is therefore correct.

36. (C)

This question is more challenging, as it does not give any keywords to scan. Instead, check for keywords from each answer choice. The keywords 'Spanish-speaking countries' in (A) lead to references to Spanish flu in the first paragraph, and to Mexico, where the H1N1 strain was first prominent in the 2009 outbreak, in the second paragraph. It is not clear from these details that the writer believes that deadly flu strains originate in Spanish-speaking countries, so eliminate (A). The keywords 'birds' and 'pigs' in (B) lead to references to avian flu in the first paragraph and swine flu in the second; neither part of the passage indicates that you could avoid these strains of flu by avoiding birds and pigs, so eliminate (B). The keywords 'side effects' and 'vaccine' in (C) lead to the final paragraph, which states that there was widespread concern about side effects with the H1N1 vaccine, though these were rare. Thus, (C) is a safe inference based on the passage, and is correct. (For the record, (D) has the keyword 'winter', which leads to the final paragraph—which does not support (D).)

37. (B)

The keywords 'Vermeer's mature paintings' lead to the first sentence of the final paragraph, which states that his signature effect was a distinctive pearly light that almost seems to gleam. (B) is a close paraphrase for this detail from the passage, so (B) is correct.

38. (D)

Details about Vermeer's paintings are given in the second and third paragraphs; scan these for any words that match the answer choices. Since this is a negative question, the three answers that are supported by the passage will be incorrect. Vermeer's paintings include *Girl with a Pearl Earring* and *Girl Reading a Letter by an Open Window*, so jewellery and letters were included in his paintings; eliminate (B) and (C). The keyword 'window' appears in the final paragraph, where it is mentioned as a common feature of Vermeer's paintings; eliminate (A). Seascapes are never mentioned in the passage, so (D) must be correct.

39. (A)

The keywords 'the Sphinx of Delft' appear in inverted commas in the first paragraph, so they are rather straightforward to scan for. The sentence that mentions this term also explains that it was used because Vermeer's life was so unknown and thus inscrutably mysterious in the 19th century. (A) is a close paraphrase for the passage, so it is correct. Beware of (B), which is a classic example of a wrong answer trap that is stronger than the language in the passage. The passage says that there was some information about Vermeer's life in government registers, so the claim in (B) that nothing was known about his life contradicts the passage.

40. (A)

This question asks about the author's opinion, but there is no keyword in the question; you must scan for a keyword from each answer. The keywords 'determine facts' and 'techniques' in (A) lead to the first paragraph, which states that it was common to try and infer the truth about Vermeer from his use of colour and his subjects, as if these could reveal anything about the man who painted them. The 'as if' comment is a strong statement of the author's opinion, and (A) is a very accurate description of this same idea. (A) is therefore correct. If you were not sure of this, you could check the other answers; you'd find nothing in the passage to support (B), (C) or (D).

41. (C)

The keywords 'screw-top bottle' appear in the passage's final sentence, which states that consumers associate such bottles with poor quality wine, regardless of the wine's price or other attributes. Thus, based on the passage, we can infer that wine in screw-top bottles may be good quality or poor quality—the quality of the wine is not necessarily connected to the screw-top bottle. Thus, on the basis of the passage, the answer is Can't tell.

42. (B)

Scanning for 'synthetic cork' and 'cork taint' leads to the start of the second paragraph; synthetic cork is being used in an effort to avoid cork taint. However, a few lines later, the passage states that synthetic cork can result in another type of cork taint. Thus, synthetic cork does not eliminate cork taint completely. This statement says it does, so the statement is false.

43. (A)

The keywords here are 'most wine' and 'natural cork'; scan for statistics, and the figure of 60% in the first paragraph will stand out. Natural cork is used for 60% of wine stoppers today. Hence, the passage supports the statement, and the statement is true.

44. (C)

Scan for the keyword 'vintage', and you'll find that it only appears at the very end of the passage, as one of the attributes that consumers might consider in determining the quality of a bottle of wine. The passage does not give a basis for comparing the importance of vintage relative to other criteria for choosing a bottle of wine: the passage doesn't say that vintage is the most important attribute, but the passage also doesn't say that another factor is the most important. Since the statement is not supported by the passage, and does not contradict it, the answer is Can't tell.

4

Quantitative Reasoning

The Quantitative Reasoning section is the second scored subsection on the UKCAT. It comes straight after the Verbal Reasoning section, so it is important to have a strategy that allows you to power through the questions, despite perhaps feeling somewhat fatigued.

Again, you have 1 minute to read the directions, and then you have just 22 minutes to tackle 36 questions in sets of 4; most of these 9 sets will be accompanied by data. This section requires you to formulate and solve numerical problems by selecting relevant information—information that can be presented to you in the data in a variety of ways. On average, you must complete each question in about 30 seconds, or each set in 2 minutes.

The majority of sets in this section have data presented in charts, graphs, tables or diagrams, with varying amounts of accompanying text. There are usually one or two sets that do not have any visual data, and only a couple of lines of written information. The topics covered are extremely varied, but a range of key ideas come up frequently. These will be covered later in the chapter.

Each question in the Quantitative Reasoning section has five multiple choice answers, from (A) to (E). The format of the answer choices depends on the questions asked, but you may be required to calculate a number, or select an option (for example, a place, person or time), based on the subject matter in the question. Occasionally, the fifth choice, (E), will be 'Can't tell'—as in the Verbal section, this should be selected if there is not enough information presented in order to determine the answer. However, be careful not to assume Can't tell is correct whenever it appears as an answer choice—be sure to check whether the data needed to solve is available first. If there is relevant data available, the answer can't be Can't tell.

During the Quantitative section, you will be able to use an on-screen calculator capable of performing simple functions, including addition, subtraction, multiplication and division. You may type on the keyboard to operate the calculation, which will be much faster than using the mouse to do so. This calculator is likely to be far simpler than the one you are used to using in your school work.

At Kaplan we find that many candidates worry about the mathematics in this section, but this anxiety is misplaced. Most of the maths required in the Quantitative reasoning section is fairly straightforward, and relatively basic—you won't see any trigonometry or calculus! The challenge in Quantitative lies in identifying exactly what each question is asking you to do, confidently manipulating formulae, accurately selecting the correct data to get to the answer, and doing it all within the time constraints of the section. Fortunately, there are a number of techniques that you can employ to enable you to answer the maximum number of questions in the time available.

1. Don't get bogged down in the data

It can be tempting to spend time reading all of the text accompanying sets of data, getting to grips with graphs, and trying to absorb diagrams and tables. With a little over 2 minutes to complete each set, you simply do not have time—especially as much of the data may be irrelevant to the questions. Instead, glance over pictorial data to determine key features:

- The general categories of data involved, and how they relate to each other.
- Labels and units—misreading these is a key pitfall!
- The gist of the information in any accompanying text.

2. Set up calculations to solve accurately

Several maths concepts and formulae come up time and again in the Quantitative Reasoning section. Having these at your fingertips so you can apply them quickly, confidently and accurately will help you to perform to the best of your ability on those questions. There are four basic formulae that come up very frequently on the UKCAT:

- $\text{Percentage} = \dfrac{\text{Part}}{\text{Whole}}$
- $\text{Percentage change} = \dfrac{\text{Difference}}{\text{Original}}$
- $\text{Speed} = \dfrac{\text{Distance}}{\text{Time}}$
- $\text{Mean (average)} = \dfrac{\text{Sum of the terms}}{\text{Number of terms}}$

In addition, you should know and be prepared to use any basic geometry formulae—such as those involving area, perimeter, circumference, and volume of common two- and three-dimensional shapes.

Many of the calculations you must complete in Quantitative Reasoning will require you to work quickly and comfortably with fractions and proportions; remember, a proportion is simply a fraction written side to side, so that $\dfrac{3}{4}$ has the same value as 3:4.

3. Eyeball, estimate and eliminate

The most efficient way to answer some of the questions will not be to calculate them. Eyeballing—comparing data and answers with a rough visual approximation to avoid unnecessary steps—and estimating answers based on rounded figures will help you to move quickly through the section. Eliminating answer choices that must be wrong—too big, too small, 'Can't tell' when the necessary information is available, etc.—is a vital skill to help you reduce the number of calculations you need to do, thus saving time.

4. Minimise the maths

Some of the questions in this section will involve no maths whatsoever. Instead, simply reading the information or eyeballing the data may find the answer. Most of the section comprises questions that involve simple calculations with one or two steps, and a few questions will be more complex, requiring several steps to get to the answer. These complex questions are often excellent targets to guess an answer choice, mark the question for review, move on, and return if there is time remaining.

Time to put some of Kaplan's top tips into practice! Give yourself 2 minutes to work through the Quantitative Reasoning set on the next page, and to write down answers for all 4 questions. Remember, you are allowed a calculator in Quantitative Reasoning, so be sure to use one here. Also, be sure to use scrap paper for any notations, rather than marking on the book itself, when answering practice questions: you can't write on the test itself on Test Day, as the questions appear on the computer screen; it is best to start out with good habits from now on.

Set your timer for 2 minutes. Mark answers for all 4 questions before time is up!

This graph shows the local authorities in England with the greatest percentage rise in population from 1999 to 2009.

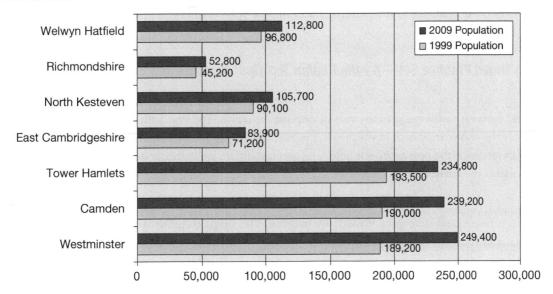

Westminster, Camden and Tower Hamlets are in central London.

Outside England, the largest percentage rise in population in a UK local authority was in Banbridge, Northern Ireland, which grew by 19.3% from 1999 to 2009, though only by 7,700 people.

1. Which local authority saw the greatest rise in population?

    A. Camden

    B. North Kesteven

    C. Tower Hamlets

    D. Welwyn Hatfield

    E. Westminster

2. The population of Tower Hamlets rose by what percentage?

    A. 21.3%

    B. 21.8%

    C. 22.1%

    D. 22.8%

    E. 23.1%

3. What was the average rise in population for the three local authorities in central London?

    A. 46,000

    B. 48,750

    C. 50,233

    D. 53,167

    E. Can't tell

4. What was the population of Banbridge in 1999?

    A. 38,800

    B. 38,900

    C. 39,800

    D. 39,900

    E. 40,000

How did you get on? Hopefully, you finished the statements in the 2 minutes, and answered them all correctly. As you practise with this book, you should **always** read through the explanations for every question, to ensure that you got the right answer for the right reasons. The explanations may also give tips that will help you on later questions with similar twists. If you didn't get them all right, don't despair—in fact, it is good to make mistakes as you practise. Each mistake you make as you practise is one you can avoid on Test Day.

Kaplan Timed Practice Set—*Try the Kaplan Top Tips*: Answers and Explanations

1. (E)

The local authority with the greatest rise in population will be the one with the greatest difference in figures for the two years shown in the graph. Eyeballing the graph, rather than subtracting to find all the exact differences, is the best approach here. The greatest difference is clearly between the two figures for Westminster. The answer is (E).

2. (A)

Percentage rise equals difference divided by original. The original figure is 193,500; the difference is 234,800 – 193,500 = 41,300. The percentage rise is 41,300 ÷ 193,500 = 0.213, or 21.3%, answer (A).

3. (C)

The target here is the average rise in population for the three central London authorities, which are named under the graph as Westminster, Camden and Tower Hamlets. Average equals sum of the terms divided by the number of terms. The number of terms is 3. Subtract the figures for each of the local authorities, writing the differences on your scrap paper:

Tower Hamlets: 234,800 – 193,500 = 41,300

Camden: 239,200 – 190,000 = 49,200

Westminster: 249,400 – 189,200 = 60,200

The sum of the terms is therefore 41,300 + 49,200 + 60,200 = 150,700. The average rise is 150,700 ÷ 3 = 50,233. The correct answer is therefore (C).

4. (D)

The information under the graph states that Banbridge grew by 7,700 from 1999 to 2009, a rise of 19.3%. The target to solve for is the original population of Banbridge in 1999. Since we know the percentage rise and the actual amount of the difference, we can solve for the original using the percentage change formula: Percentage Change = Difference ÷ Original. Plug in the values, and x for the unknown original:

$$0.193 = \frac{7700}{x}$$

Multiply both sides by x, and divide both sides by 0.193 to solve for x: $x = \dfrac{7700}{0.193} = 39,896.4$. This rounds to 39,900, so the answer is (D).

Take a moment to consider the level of maths required for this set, in terms of conceptual difficulty as well as the level of calculation involved. The first question could be answered simply by reading the graph; the second and final questions required a single calculation using one of the common formulae. Only the third question involved a more complex calculation, and this was only more complex as it involved multiple steps. All the questions were conceptually rather straightforward, in that they required setting up and solving a single formula—except for the first, which required no maths at all. It is important to bear this in mind as you prepare yourself mentally for Quantitative Reasoning—most questions will involve a simple calculation, or no maths at all, which means that most questions can be answered in 30 seconds or less.

It is likely that several of the question sets that you will encounter in Quantitative Reasoning will incorporate data in the form of charts, graphs, tables and other visual formats. Some of the techniques that we have discussed already—eyeballing, estimating and working with common formulae—will also be useful in sets that have visual data that is more complicated or confusing than the initial set just considered, and thus questions involving such challenging data will pose further challenges for you when you sit the UKCAT.

When facing a question that requires you to read a chart, graph or table, take a few seconds to quickly familiarise yourself with the visual data:

- What are the labels of the axes?

- What are the units?

- What do the different bars/columns/points represent?

- Is there any supplementary information along with the graph?

This will help you to ensure that you are finding all the data you need to answer the question, and ensure that you do not miss out any relevant information, which can sometimes be tucked into the notes just above or below the visual data. A quick check of the data will also ensure that you do not fall into common pitfalls: misunderstanding the data, misinterpreting categories or labels, or using the wrong scale or unit when working with numbers.

To demonstrate these tips, work through the following four questions, which relate to the graph below. Try to answer each question in 30 seconds before reading the answer.

Beth's boutique sells a leather bag in three colours. She keeps a record of the percentage of each colour sold on each day of a particular week. The shop is closed on Sundays.

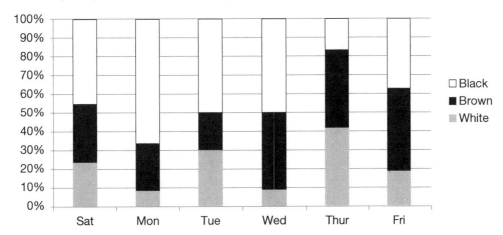

5. What percentage of bags sold on Wednesday were white?

    A. 8%

    B. 12%

    C. 17%

    D. 24%

    E. 50%

Answer: Checking the graph will lead you to a very tricky twist in the legend: the colour of the bars in the graph does not correspond to the colour of the bag represented. Avoiding this pitfall and simply eyeballing the data determines that the grey bar, representing white bags sold, is a little less than 10% of the total for Wednesday. The answer is therefore (A).

6. Fourteen brown bags were sold on Friday. How many white bags were sold?

    A. 3

    B. 6

    C. 18

    D. 24

    E. 36

Answer: The unknown here is the number of white bags sold on Friday. White bags correspond to the grey bar, and the percentage for Friday is about 18%. The legend indicates that the black part of the bar represents the percentage of brown bags sold, which is a few percentage points above 40%, so eyeball this as 42%. The next step is to set up two fractions that equal each other, as the two figures are percentages of the same total, so these part-to-part proportions must be equal (where w is the unknown number of white bags):

$$\frac{42}{14} = \frac{18}{w}$$

You could cross-multiply, or simply reduce the fraction on the left to 3, so that $3 = \frac{18}{w}$ Thus, $w = 6$ the correct answer is (B).

NB This question is more challenging because it requires you to set up two proportions. These are not necessarily difficult proportions, but you must estimate the percentages and set them up quickly to solve in 30 seconds. On Test Day, be sure to set up any such proportions on your noteboard, and take a moment to double-check that you have put everything on the correct sides of the fraction bars before solving. As you practise, make any such notations on scrap paper, so you can get into good noteboard habits ahead of Test Day.

---

7. What percentage of the total number of bags sold on Tuesday and Wednesday were brown?

    A. 19%

    B. 30%

    C. 38%

    D. 60%

    E. Can't tell

Answer: Be careful not to confuse percentages with absolute quantities. Checking the data here, you will notice that the graph does not indicate the actual sales figures for any of the days shown, and the question does not indicate the relative number of bags sold on Tuesday as compared to Wednesday. As such, it is impossible to calculate the individual numbers of bags sold on Tuesday and Wednesday, and the percentages relating to different days cannot be combined in any mathematically meaningful way. Since there is not enough data to solve, the answer is therefore (E). Whenever 'Can't tell' is included in the answer choices, check first to see if there is enough information to solve the question before attempting a calculation. However, do not assume that Can't tell is correct whenever it appears in Quantitative Reasoning: it is a very popular wrong answer trap, designed to catch out students who are certain that they have found a 'sure thing' and an easy shortcut to avoid maths. Always check the data first.

---

8. If the shop sold twice as many bags on Saturday as on Friday, what percentage of bags sold over the two days were white?

    A. 20%

    B. 22%

    C. 41%

    D. 43%

    E. Can't tell

Answer: Although at first glance this question seems similar to the previous one, down to the inclusion of 'Can't tell' in the answer choices, there is a subtle and essential difference: the question includes information about the relative numbers of bags sold on each day, which allows calculations involving the percentages.

On Friday, approximately 18% of the bags sold were white; the percentage for Saturday is about 24%. Since the exact number of bags sold is unknown, it is safe to pick numbers that match the information in the question. Suppose that 100 bags were sold on Friday, and 200 on Saturday; these numbers are acceptable, as total sales for Saturday are twice the total sales for Friday. Thus, 18 white bags were sold on Friday (18 = 18% of 100), and 48 white bags were sold on Saturday (as 48 = 24% of 200). This adds up to a total of 18 + 48 = 66 white bags sold, out of a total of 100 + 200 = 300 bags sold. White bags therefore accounted for 66 ÷ 300 = 0.22, or 22% of bags sold over the two days. The correct answer is (B).

9. Assuming the same number of bags are sold on each day, which chart correctly represents the sale of black bags throughout the week?

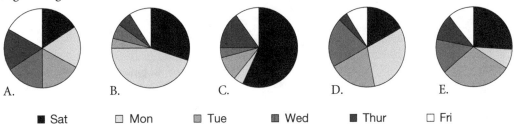

■ Sat   ☐ Mon   ▨ Tue   ▨ Wed   ■ Thur   ☐ Fri

Answer: Questions that feature charts and graphs in the answers are usually highly vulnerable to elimination and eyeballing. Choose a figure from the original data that will be very easy to check against the answers, and use this to eliminate. In this instance, since the question assumes the same number of bags are sold each day, it might be easiest to start with the day that sold the most black bags, which is clearly Monday. Therefore, any answer without Monday as the largest slice of the chart cannot be correct. On this basis, eliminate (A), (C) and (E)—only (B) and (D) remain. Next, eyeball these answers for differences or similarities. In (B), Saturday is by far the next largest slice; in (D), Tuesday, Wednesday and Saturday are all fairly similar in size. In the original graph, Tuesday and Wednesday look to be the same, with Saturday very slightly smaller. The answer must be (D).

As these questions demonstrate, you must be prepared to check the data for each question, and to avoid common traps that are waiting for those who misread the data. You'll also need to improve your speed and accuracy with questions involving percentages (including percentage change), as these are incredibly common on the UKCAT. At Kaplan, we are sometimes surprised to find how many applicants to medical programmes are unable to work quickly and accurately with questions involving percentages—perhaps the skills involved are so basic they have been long forgotten, so they are worth practising in the run-up to Test Day.

Set your timer for 2 minutes. Try to mark answers for all 4 questions before time runs out.

An ongoing school project counts wildlife found in the school pond each summer.

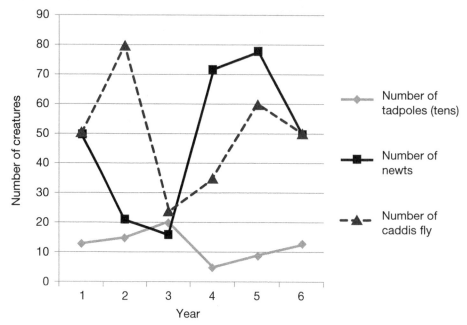

• Tadpoles turn into froglets by the end of the summer, but the children do not count these as they leave the pond immediately.

• 30% of tadpoles will return to the pond as fully grown frogs the next year.

• Frogs that return to the pond are certain to die in the following winter.

10. How many tadpoles were found in Year 4?
   A. 5
   B. 50
   C. 72
   D. 75
   E. 80

11. What is the percentage change in the newt population from Year 3 to Year 6?
   A. 32%
   B. 34%
   C. 68%
   D. 212.5%
   E. 312.5%

12. What was the total number of frogs, newts and tadpoles in the pond in Year 6?
   A. 66
   B. 93
   C. 207
   D. 230
   E. Can't tell

13. In which year was the difference between the newt and tadpole population the smallest?
   A. Year 1
   B. Year 2
   C. Year 3
   D. Year 4
   E. Year 5

If you took a few seconds to familiarise yourself with the graph briefly at the beginning of the question, then hopefully you will have noticed that the black line represents newts, the dashed line represents caddis fly and the grey line represents *tens* of tadpoles—an unusual distinction, and one that is sure to come into play as you attack the questions in this set. You may also have noticed the bullet points underneath the graph, and have noticed that they seem to mention frogs, although you will not have had time to read what these bullet points have to say about frogs in detail. Keep the frogs in the back of your mind until they become relevant to answering a question.

Kaplan Timed Practice Set—*Working with Confusing Data and Percentages*: Answers and Explanations

10. (B)

To answer the first question, simply read the information from the graph—there is no complex calculation required. The grey line lies around 5 at Year 4—but take care to remember that the scale is tens of tadpoles, not individual tadpoles. Thus, the answer is (B).

11. (D)

This question involves a relatively straightforward calculation using the percentage change formula:

$$\text{Percentage change} = \frac{\text{Difference}}{\text{Original}}$$

Reading from the black line on the graph, the newt population in Year 3 is approximately 16, and in Year 6 is about 50. The difference is therefore 50 – 16 = 34. The percentage change is $\frac{34}{16} = 2.125$, or 212.5%. The answer is therefore (D).

If you could not remember the percentage change formula, you could still have a good go at this question. The newt population has more than doubled from Year 3 to Year 6, so the percentage change must be greater than 100%. Realising this allows you to eliminate (A), (B) and (C), leaving you with a 50% chance of guessing the correct answer—far better odds than the 0% chance of getting the mark if you do not click anything at all.

12. (C)

This question may have seemed off-putting because it suddenly mentions frogs, and test-takers who did not notice the frog-related information in the bullet points may be tempted to mark Can't tell as their answer. However, if you had noted the frogs in the bullet points during your quick overview of the data, you will now be able to read about them in a little more detail and discover that 30% of tadpoles from the previous year will return as frogs, but all frogs from years prior to that will have died. In Year 5, there were approximately 9 × 10 = 90 tadpoles, and 30% of these, or 0.3 × 90 = 27, will return in Year 6 as frogs. Adding in the number of newts (50) and tadpoles (13 × 10 = 130), the total number of frogs, newts and tadpoles in Year 6 is 27 + 50 + 130 = 207, so the answer is (C).

13. (E)

This question is a little more tricky, as the lines for newts and tadpoles are difficult to compare through eyeballing. The appealing wrong answer trap is Year 3, as the lines for newts and tadpoles seem to come the closest, unless you remember that the tadpole figure shown in the graph must be multiplied by 10 to give the actual number of tadpoles. Thus, there are 200 tadpoles in Year 3, and fewer than 20 newts—this is actually the greatest difference between the two in the years shown! To find the correct answer, use a modified eyeballing approach, taking care to consider the tadpole figure times 10. The quickest route is to find years where the newt line is high but the tadpole line low, to make up for the factor of 10 in the tadpole line—Years 4 and 5 fit this description. In Year 4, there are about 72 newts and 50 tadpoles, but in Year 5 there are around 78 newts and 90 tadpoles. The answer is therefore (E).

The speed formula is the most commonly tested rate on the UKCAT. Be prepared to rearrange the formula to solve for any one of its constituent parts:

- Speed $= \dfrac{\text{Distance}}{\text{Time}}$
- Time $= \dfrac{\text{Distance}}{\text{Speed}}$
- Distance $=$ Speed $\times$ Time

Many questions involving the speed formula will introduce an extra step—and potential trap—by providing information in inconsistent units, or in units that are inconsistent with the units of the answer choices. To avoid mistakes on such questions, be sure to note the steps required to solve on your noteboard. Include a conversion factor that will divide or multiply out the units that you don't need in the answer, so you are only left with the correct units. For instance, if you are given data in miles per minute $\left(\dfrac{\text{mi}}{\text{min}}\right)$, and you want an answer in miles per hour $\left(\dfrac{\text{mi}}{\text{hr}}\right)$, then multiply the original figure by $\dfrac{60 \text{ min}}{1 \text{ hr}}$, as this will eliminate the minutes and leave the hours in the denominator, where they belong. Conversion factors such as $\dfrac{60 \text{ min}}{1 \text{ hr}}$ can always be included in multiplication, so long as the amounts on the top and bottom of the fraction are equal—this is the same as multiplying by 1.

Be prepared as well for questions that may involve rates other than speed. Any two measurements could be combined into a rate, e.g. books per year, miles per gallon, pence per litre. Solving rate questions will usually involve working with fractions.

Here are five questions involving rates and speed, based on the map shown at the top of the next page. Try to answer each question in 30 seconds before moving on to the answer. Since you may answer some questions quickly, it is okay to spend a bit longer than 30 seconds on one or two that are very challenging—but try to mark an answer even for these in about a minute. Taking much longer as you practise will not help you prepare for UKCAT success.

Marco and Yasmin are going on a driving tour of Wales, with plans to visit the locations shown below:

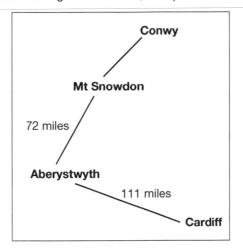

14. If they take 2.5 hours to drive from Cardiff to Aberystwyth without stopping, what is their speed?

    A. 29 mph

    B. 37 mph

    C. 44 mph

    D. 47 mph

    E. 49 mph

Answer: The unknown is speed, which equals distance divided by time. The distance from Cardiff to Aberystwyth is given in the map as 111 miles, and the time is given in the question as 2.5 hours. Thus, the speed = 111 mi ÷ 2.5 hr = 44.4 miles per hour, and the answer is (C).

15. At a speed of 40 mph, what is the driving time from Aberystwyth to Mt Snowdon?

    A. 1 hour, 8 minutes

    B. 1 hour, 32 minutes

    C. 1 hour, 40 minutes

    D. 1 hour, 48 minutes

    E. 1 hour, 54 minutes

Answer: The unknown in this question is time, which equals distance divided by speed. The distance is given in the map as 72 miles, and the speed is given in the question as 40 mph. The time therefore equals 72 mi ÷ 40 mph = 1.8 hours. However, the answers give the time in hours and minutes, so subtract the hour and multiply by a conversion factor to find the remaining minutes: $0.8\,\text{hr} \times \dfrac{60\,\text{min}}{1\,\text{hr}} = 48\,\text{min}$. The total time for the drive from Aberystwyth to Mt Snowdon is therefore 1 hour, 48 minutes, and the answer is (D).

16. If Marco drives from Cardiff to Aberystwyth, and Yasmin drives from Aberystwyth to Mt Snowdon, what percentage of the journey from Cardiff to Mt Snowdon is driven by Yasmin?

    A. 36%

    B. 39%

    C. 42%

    D. 61%

    E. 65%

Answer: Think of percentages as representing a rate, or as a proportion. In this case, the percentage in the answer will represent the portion of the overall journey driven by Yasmin. To solve, set up a fraction with Yasmin's mileage—72 miles—on top, and the total mileage on the bottom: 111 miles + 72 miles = 183 miles total. Thus, Yasmin's percentage is 72 miles ÷ 183 miles = 0.393, or 39.3%. The answer is therefore (B).

NB Wrong answer trap (E) is waiting for those who mistakenly divide 72 by 111, rather than first summing the total mileage before dividing. Expect the UKCAT to present similar traps in Quantitative Reasoning for test-takers who calculate using figures from the data incorrectly.

---

17. How far is Conwy from Mt Snowdon, if the drive takes 52 minutes at a speed of 30 mph?
    - A. 26 miles
    - B. 32 miles
    - C. 37 miles
    - D. 44 miles
    - E. 49 miles

Answer: The unknown in this question is distance, which equals speed multiplied by time. However, there is an added twist, as the units don't match—the time is given in minutes, but the speed is given in miles per hour. The quickest way to solve here is to write the time as a fraction of an hour: since an hour equals 60 minutes, write the time as $\frac{52}{60}$ hr. Then, multiply to find the distance: $30 \text{ mph} \times \frac{52}{60} \text{ hr} = 26$ miles. Answer (A) is correct.

---

18. Yasmin switches on her MP3 player the moment they set off from Cardiff, and counts the songs played during their driving time to Aberystwyth. Their average speed is 37 mph, and exactly 40 songs play on the journey. What is the average length of a song played on the journey?
    - A. 2.75 minutes per song
    - B. 3 minutes per song
    - C. 3.75 minutes per song
    - D. 4 minutes per song
    - E. 4.5 minutes per song

Answer: The answers are given in an unusual rate: minutes per song. Thus, start by finding the time required for the journey from Cardiff to Aberystwyth. Time equals distance divided by speed: 111 miles ÷ 37 mph = 3 hours. Since the answers are given in minutes, convert 3 hours into minutes: $3 \text{ hrs} \times \frac{60 \text{ min}}{1 \text{ hr}} = 180$ minutes. Yasmin played 40 songs on the journey, so the rate of minutes per song is simply 180 minutes ÷ 40 songs = 4.5 minutes per song, answer (E). While this question does involve an unusual rate, keeping an eye on the units involved—and converting at each step as required—is sufficient to get to the correct answer.

Set your timer for 2 minutes. Attempt to answer all 4 questions before time is up. If you have trouble with a question, try to eliminate any answers that seem too large or too small, based on the available data, and then make your best guess before moving on. Come back to any such troubling questions with any remaining time before the 2 minutes is up.

Doris, Mabel and Maud ride their mobility scooters from their sheltered accommodation to the shops, which are 3.5 km away. The mobility scooters normally travel at a constant speed of 10 km/hr.

19. How many minutes will it take the ladies to reach the shops?

    A. 21

    B. 24

    C. 28

    D. 33

    E. 35

20. On the way home, Mabel takes the scenic route. She arrives back at the sheltered accommodation 24 minutes after the others. How far did she travel on her journey home?

    A. 3.1 km

    B. 4.1 km

    C. 4.5 km

    D. 5.7 km

    E. 7.5 km

21. The next day, the battery on Maud's scooter is running low, and it takes her 37 mins to reach the shops. At what speed is her mobility scooter now travelling?

    A. 4.8 km/hr

    B. 5.7 km/hr

    C. 6.3 km/hr

    D. 8.4 km/hr

    E. 9.5 km/hr

22. With a new battery, Maud's scooter can now travel at 14 km/hr. What is the percentage decrease in her journey time from the shops to the sheltered accommodation, compared to her initial journey?

    A. 15%

    B. 21%

    C. 29%

    D. 33%

    E. 35%

Hopefully you were not surprised by the lack of visual data in this set. Whilst most sets in Quantitative Reasoning include at least one chart, graph or table, you are likely to see one or two sets that include no visual data. These may include brief textual information, which may provide essential, if limited, data. Sets with no visual data can generally be answered a bit more quickly than usual sets, and will tend to involve solving for a single rate or percentage. Your work from earlier questions in such sets will often prove useful and save time on later questions, so be sure to note the calculations—including any intermediate figures you came up with in finding the answers—on your noteboard.

Kaplan Timed Practice Set—*Working with Rates and Speed*: Answers and Explanations

19. (A)

This question involves straightforward use of the speed formula. The unknown in this question is time, which equals distance divided by speed: $T = D \div S$. The distance is 3.5 km and the speed is 10 km/hr, so divide: 3.5 km ÷ 10 km/hr = 0.35 hours. To convert to minutes, we multiply by 60: $0.35 \times 60 = 21$ minutes. The answer is therefore (A).

20. (E)

The unknown in this question is distance, which equals speed multiplied by time: $D = S \times T$. Mabel's speed is 10 km/hr, and her time is 24 minutes more than the others, so add: 21 min + 24 min = 45 minutes, or 0.75 hours. Multiply to find Mabel's distance, taking the scenic route: 10 km/hr × 0.75 hours = 7.5 km. The correct answer is (E).

21. (B)

In this question, the unknown is speed: $S = D \div T$. The distance is 3.5 km, and Maud's new time is 37 minutes, which equals $\frac{37}{60}$ hrs, or 0.617 hrs, if you divide out the fraction. To find Maud's new speed, divide: 3.5 km ÷ 0.617 hrs = 5.67 km/hr. The answer is therefore (B).

22. (C)

This question is a little more complex, as it requires multiple steps: to find the percentage change in Maud's journey times, you must first calculate her new journey time with the new battery. Maud's original journey took 21 minutes. With the new battery, the journey time is now 3.5 km ÷ 14 km/hr = 0.25 hours, or 15 minutes. Remember, Percentage Change = Difference ÷ Original, so her percentage decrease in journey time is the difference in the two times divided by the original time. The difference is 21 min − 15 min = 6 min, so the percentage change equals 6 min ÷ 21 min = 0.286, or 28.6%. This rounds up to 29%, so the correct answer is (C).

A few sets in the Quantitative Reasoning section may involve difficult data. Data may be difficult to work with because it is given in unusual or unexpected diagrams, or because the data contains multiple charts, graphs or tables, or lots of bullet points and textual information. Difficult data is anything that is likely to make you spend more time than you should on the questions involved, or anything that looks a bit scary. When faced with difficult data, don't lose your nerve—continue working at the usual pace. If you take more time on questions with difficult data, or if you 'bottle' it, you have fallen for the difficult data trap.

When the data involves geometry, or elaborate figures that can be broken into smaller figures, sketching a quick copy of the diagram on your noteboard can be helpful—you can then add measurements and notations as you calculate. This will help to answer each question in the set, and will save time and frustration, since you are unable to write on the test paper itself.

Try working through the questions that accompany the diagram at the top of the next page, allowing yourself 30 seconds for each question before reviewing the answer. Again, if a question is more time-consuming, you might allow yourself a bit longer, assuming that you have 'banked' time by answering quicker, earlier questions in less than 30 seconds.

Flintborough Town Council is planning a new park. They prepare a scale model (2 m:1 km) to exhibit to the public. The model is 14 m long and 8 m wide, and is horizontally and vertically symmetrical.

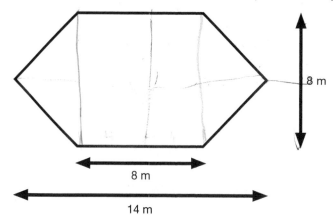

23. What is the area of the model?
    A. 64 m²
    B. 80 m²
    C. 88 m²
    D. 96 m²
    E. Can't tell

Answer: This is a tricky area question, since the model will have to be divided into multiple smaller shapes whose area can be calculated, then added together. Thankfully, the model has horizontal and vertical symmetry, so it can be broken into several possible combinations of conventional shapes, which you can annotate after redrawing the figure on your scrap paper. Eliminate (E); since there is plenty of data here, a numerical answer can be found. Perhaps the simplest approach is to section off the centre portion into a square measuring 8 m on all sides, so this portion would have an area of 8 m × 8 m = 64 m². Since the actual area is larger, eliminate (A). The remaining portions are triangles of equal area; these each have a base of 8 m and a height of 3 m, because 14 m – 8 m = 6 m, and half of this is equal to the height of each triangle. The area of a triangle is 0.5 × base × height, and since there are two equal triangles, their combined area is 2 × 0.5 × 8 m × 3 m = 24 m². The total area is therefore 64 + 24 = 88 m²; the correct answer is therefore (C).

24. The model is to be placed onto a rectangular board. What is the area of the board that will give a minimum border of 50 cm around the entire model?
    A. 72.25 m²
    B. 112.25 m²
    C. 123.25 m²
    D. 128 m²
    E. 135 m²

Answer: In order to ensure a border of 50 cm, or 0.5 m, around the model, a rectangular board would need to include an extra 0.5 m at each end of the model's longest vertical and horizontal measurements. Add in the extra 0.5 m: 14 + 0.5 + 0.5 = 15 m, and 8 + 0.5 + 0.5 = 9 m, so the area of the rectangular board must be 9 m × 15 m = 135 m². The answer is (E).

25. A circular fountain, with an area of 28 m², is planned for the exact centre of the park. How far will it be from the edge of the fountain to the edge of the park, if the shortest possible distance is measured?
    A. 1961 m
    B. 1967 m
    C. 1991 m
    D. 1997 m
    E. 3997 m

Answer: Since the fountain has an area of approximately 28 m², solve for its radius using the formula for area of a circle: $\pi r^2 = 28$ m². Dividing both sides by 3.14 (as an approximation of π): $r^2 = 8.91$ m², or just a bit less than 9 m²; thus, the radius of the fountain is 3 m. The vertical distance from the centre of the model to the edge is 4 m; given the scale of 2 m:1 km, the distance in the actual park will be 2 km, or 2000 m. To solve for the distance from the edge of the fountain to the edge of the park, subtract: 2000 m − 3 m = 1997 m. The answer is therefore (D).

NB Wrong answer trap (E), which was waiting for anyone who miscalculated the distances in the actual park on a scale of 1 m:1 km, instead of using the scale given with the original data.

26. Once the park is built, a man runs around the perimeter at a speed of 15 km/hr. How many minutes does it take him to run around the perimeter of the park exactly once?

   A. 50 minutes
   B. 72 minutes
   C. 84 minutes
   D. 90 minutes
   E. 112 minutes

Answer: Once again, sketching out the figure on the noteboard is invaluable in breaking the model into shapes that are easier to use in calculating the perimeter of the park. If you divide the model into a central square and a triangle on each end in your work for Q. 23, you need only take one further step to find the remaining distances needed for the perimeter: divide each large triangle in half, forming two smaller triangles with a height of 3 m and a base of 4 m. Use Pythagoras's theorem to calculate the hypotenuse of this smaller triangle: $3^2 + 4^2 = h^2 = 9 + 16 = 25$. The hypotenuse is therefore 5 m.

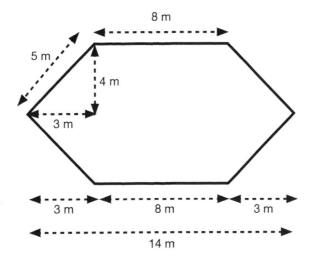

Sum up to find the total perimeter: 8 m + 8 m + 5 m + 5 m + 5 m + 5 m = 36 m. In the park, this distance equals 18 km. To solve for the runner's time, divide distance by speed: 18 km ÷ 15 km/hr = 1.2 hours. As the answers are in minutes, multiply: 1.2 hr × 60 min = 72 min, so the correct answer is (B).

Have a go at a set involving difficult data and geometry under timed conditions. Remember, it's only 2 minutes to attempt this set—try to complete all 4 questions before time is up.

The shark tank at an aquarium has a viewing window with a height of 5 m and a length of 20 m. The tank extends backwards by 3 m. The tank is filed to 50 cm below the brim with water, and there is nothing covering its top.

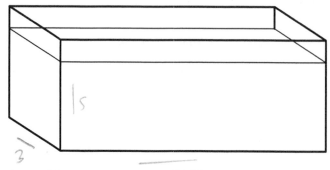

27. What is the volume of water in the tank?
    A. 243 m³
    B. 250 m³
    C. 270 m³
    D. 293 m³
    E. 300 m³

28. On a very hot day, 6 m³ of water evaporates from the tank. What is the percentage change in the depth of the water?
    A. 2%
    B. 4%
    C. 5%
    D. 6%
    E. 9%

29. The shark is 2 m long. It starts with its tail touching one end of the tank and swims at a constant speed of 200 cm per second until its head touches the far side of the tank. How long does it take to traverse the tank?
    A. 5.4 seconds
    B. 7.2 seconds
    C. 8.4 seconds
    D. 9 seconds
    E. 10 seconds

30. The aquarium owners wish to make the glass algae-proof. They must coat the inside and outside of the tank with mould-proofer, which costs £17 per pot. Each pot covers 25 m² of glass. How much will it cost to algae-proof the inside of the tank in its entirety?
    A. £187
    B. £204
    C. £221
    D. £272
    E. £289

These questions were certainly more challenging than those earlier in this chapter. Even on a set with difficult data, you can expect to find at least one or two questions that can be answered fairly quickly. So don't despair if you found it difficult to finish—it's meant to be!

Kaplan Timed Practice Set—*Working with Difficult Data and Geometry*: Answers and Explanations

27. (C)

Volume of water in the tank = length × width × height = 20 m × 3 m × 4.5 m = 270 m³, and the answer is (C). If you mistakenly calculated the volume of the entire tank, rather than the volume of the water, you would have fallen for answer trap (E).

28. (A)

The area of the surface of the tank is 20 m × 3 m = 60 m². If the volume of water has dropped by 6 m³, then the depth of water that evaporated must be 6 m³/60 m² = 0.1 m. Percentage Change = Difference ÷ Original, and the original depth of water in the tank was 4.5 m; divide to find the percentage change: 0.1 m ÷ 4.5 m = 0.0222, or 2%. The answer is therefore (A).

29. (D)

The unknown here is the time required for the shark to swim across its tank, so use the speed formula to solve: Time = Distance ÷ Speed. The shark's speed is given as 200 cm/sec, which equals 2 m/sec. Since the shark is 2 m long and starts with its tail touching one wall of the tank, the shark does not swim the total distance of 20 m, but rather swims 20 m – 2 m = 18 m. To solve, plug these figures into the speed formula: Time = 18 m ÷ 2 m/sec = 9 sec. The correct answer is (D).

30. (B)

Drawing a quick sketch of the plan of the tank would help to ensure that you don't miss out each segment of glass that must be algae-proofed:

The total area to be covered is the bottom, plus two sides, plus the front and back, which are also equal. The total area of these is (20 × 3) + 2(20 × 5) + 2(3 × 5) = 60 + 200 + 30 = 290 m². Divide to find the number of pots required: 290 m² ÷ 25 m² per pot = 11.6. This means that 12 pots of mould-proofer are needed, giving a total cost of 12 × £17 = £204, answer (B).

Well done! You have now looked at the examples of the common types of data, questions and challenges that are found in the Quantitative Reasoning section, and practised the strategies necessary to work through all of these systematically and efficiently. Over the next few pages, you will tackle four Quantitative Reasoning sets under timed conditions. By eyeballing, estimating and minimising the maths wherever possible, you should have enough time to attempt—and to mark an answer for—every question in the Kaplan UKCAT quiz.

Remember to be aware of questions that seem overly complicated or that you are struggling to complete, and get used to guessing an answer, marking for review, and moving on—just as you will do on Test Day—to ensure you submit answers for as many questions as possible.

Students who are less familiar with the test format may find themselves bogged down on an especially difficult or time-consuming question, missing the opportunity to answer questions later in the section that may have earned them more marks and a higher overall score.

Before beginning the Kaplan UKCAT quiz, take a few moments to review some of Kaplan's tips that will help you maximise your performance on the quiz—and also on Test Day:

Not every question requires complex calculation. Several questions in any given Quantitative section can be answered by simply reading data, by eyeballing or estimating, or by making a straightforward calculation involving just one step.

Three-part formulae pop up again and again. Confidence in setting up and solving three-part formulae is essential to success in this section. The most common formulae are speed, mean and percentage change—which may be used alone or in combination.

Use the noteboard. Making notes on the noteboard can help to maintain accuracy when setting up calculations and solving, and will also help on questions involving figures, where a rough sketch onto which you can fill in measurements, etc., as they are calculated will save time and reduce the chance of making simple mistakes. Use scrap paper as you continue to practise to simulate the noteboard, rather than writing directly on the questions themselves—you won't be able to do so on Test Day.

Take care with related concepts. As some of these examples have shown, it is easy to get caught up in questions and to not notice simple shifts in focus such as percentages vs real numbers, generalising specific cases to larger populations, etc. It is important to maintain awareness of this whilst powering through the section.

Eliminate. Elimination of wrong answers—those that are too small/large, those that are in the wrong units, those that are odd when the answer must be even, etc.—will help to minimise maths and find the fastest route to the correct answer.

Check the Online Resource Centre and the UKCAT website for details of any test changes in the year you sit the exam. The Quantitative section has not undergone any significant changes in a number of years, but that does not mean that there won't be test changes in the year you sit the UKCAT. Be sure to check for these ahead of time, to minimise the risk of any rude surprises on Test Day. See page ix.

Set your timer for 10 minutes. Try to answer all 16 questions, and mark an answer for each, before time is up. As you work through the section, try to answer each question in 30 seconds, so you can keep to 2 minutes per set. If you can generally keep to this timing, you will have an extra minute or two, which you can then use on some of the more difficult or time-consuming questions.

Mrs Tiwari runs a clothes shop. She buys the dresses as she needs more stock, paying £130 for batches of ten dresses, and sells each dress for £25.

31. If Mrs Tiwari sells 17 dresses, what profit has she made per dress?

    A. £7.96
    B. £8.75
    C. £9.18
    D. £9.71
    E. £9.98

32. In a summer sale, Mrs Tiwari advertises a 15% discount on all items. What is the percentage change in profit on a sale dress compared to a non-sale dress, assuming all dresses in stock are sold?

    A. 15%
    B. 22%
    C. 24%
    D. 27%
    E. 31%

33. Mrs Tiwari exports 40 dresses to a shop in Belgium at full price. She must pay a customs tax of 12% on the first £500 paid to her, and 8% of any further money she receives on the sale of the dresses. What is the total profit that she makes on these dresses?

    A. £380
    B. £420
    C. £445
    D. £475
    E. £520

34. The Belgian shop sells each dress for 32 euros. The exchange rate is £1:1.12 euro. What is the difference in price for a dress between the Belgian shop and Mrs Tiwari's shop during the sale?

    A. £5.20
    B. £7.32
    C. £8.04
    D. £9.12
    E. Can't tell

Paul's Paints are running a deal on white, blue and red paint. Blue paint costs £6.20 per litre, red paint £5.51 per litre and white paint £2.11 per litre. They will mix the paints in equal parts (1:1 mixture) to create new colours, as shown. Each mixture costs £3 extra for the time taken, plus £1.59 to clean the machine.

	Blue	Red	White
Blue	Blue	Purple	Pale Blue
Red	Purple	Red	Pink
White	Pale Blue	Pink	White

To improve sales, Paul offers to further mix 2 parts of each colour created with 1 part of either blue, red or white paint to make seven new colours. The extra charges for time and cleaning remain the same as for the simple mixtures.

	Pale Blue	Pink	Purple
Blue	Cornflower	Mauve	Indigo
Red	Mauve	Rose	Violet
White	Sky	Blush	Mauve

35. Niamh wishes to buy 5 litres of pink paint. How much will it cost her?

    A. £19.05
    B. £21.05
    C. £23.64
    D. £27.45
    E. £38.10

36. Yosuke purchases 3 litres of cornflower paint. What is the total cost?

    A. £8.31
    B. £7.32
    C. £8.04
    D. £14.51
    E. £19.10

37. A litre of paint will cover 1.5 m². Magali's bedroom is 3 m × 5 m, and the ceiling is 2.5 m high. She wishes to paint the walls in mauve and the ceiling in white. How many litres of paint does she require?

    A. 26 L
    B. 27 L
    C. 36 L
    D. 37 L
    E. 42 L

38. Chris is very bored in the shop one day, and decides to experiment. He mixes 6 litres of indigo paint with twice as much mauve paint, and then adds 3 litres each of rose, blush and sky coloured paint. How much would 1 litre of the resulting colour cost, excluding time and cleaning costs?

    A. £3.64
    B. £4.61
    C. £6.92
    D. £13.64
    E. £14.92

The following graph shows the number of pupils, divided by sex, in each class for AS-level subjects at a sixth-form college.

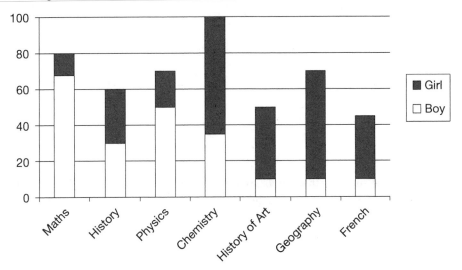

39. How many more boys study Chemistry than girls study Maths?

    A. 23
    B. 25
    C. 30
    D. 35
    E. 37

40. What percentage of History of Art students are girls?

    A. 50%
    B. 60%
    C. 70%
    D. 80%
    E. 90%

41. Half of all Economics students are boys, and there are 10 more girls studying Economics than French. What is the total number of Economics students?

    A. 45
    B. 70
    C. 90
    D. 110
    E. Can't tell

42. Half of the girls studying Chemistry also study Biology, and one-third of the girls studying Geography also study Biology; there are 10 more girls who study Biology, who do not also study Chemistry or Geography. How many boys study Biology, if there are two-thirds as many boys as girls studying Biology?

    A. 29
    B. 35
    C. 42
    D. 63
    E. 95

Salim walks 6 km due west from Axelbury to Castle Point. He stops for an hour to eat lunch in Banchurch, which is equidistant between the two. Upon arriving at Castle Point, Salim realises that he walked twice as fast after lunch as he did before lunch.

43. If Salim's total journey took 3 hours and 15 minutes, inclusive of lunch, what was the average speed at which Salim walked?

    A. 2 km/hr

    B. 2.67 km/hr

    C. 3 km/hr

    D. 3.33 km/hr

    E. Can't tell

44. Castle Point is up a hill, meaning that it is 420 m further above sea level than Axelbury. If Salim walked at a rate of 2 km/hr before lunch, at what rate did Salim gain elevation in metres per minute? (Assume that the hill rises at a constant rate.)

    A. 2.3

    B. 3.5

    C. 4.6

    D. 6.5

    E. 9.2

45. Eagleton is 4 km due south of Banchurch. The area between Axelbury, Castle Point and Eagleton is a designated nature reserve. What area does the nature reserve cover?

    A. 6 km²

    B. 9 km²

    C. 12 km²

    D. 18 km²

    E. 24 km²

46. On the next day, Salim takes a bus 3 km due south to Darroway, and then walks due east 2 km to meet a friend. They decide to race straight back to Axelbury, leaving at 2pm. They both travel at a constant speed. Salim takes 75 minutes, at which point his friend is 1 km from Axelbury. At what time will the friend arrive?

    A. 3.15pm

    B. 3.17pm

    C. 3.19pm

    D. 3.34pm

    E. Can't tell

STOP. IF YOU FINISH BEFORE TIME IS UP, CHECK ANY QUESTIONS YOU HAVE MARKED FOR REVIEW. YOU MAY GO BACK TO QUESTIONS IN THIS QUIZ ONLY.

31. (D)

Mrs Tiwari must have bought two batches of dresses in order to have sold 17, so she has paid 2 × £130 = £260. She earned 17 × £25 = £425 from the sale of the 17 dresses. £425 − £260 = £165 profit. Divide to find the profit per dress sold: £165 ÷ 17 = £9.71. The answer is (D).

32. (E)

The tempting answer trap here is 15%, as that is the discount mentioned in the question. However, only the sale price of the dress has changed; the cost price has not, so Mrs Tiwari's profit will have changed by more than 15%. To solve, use the percentage change formula, which first requires you to find the original profit per dress, and the difference in profit per dress during the summer sale. If all stock is sold, then the cost of a dress is £130 ÷ 10 = £13, and the profit (at the original price) is £25 − £13 = £12. During the summer sale, a customer would pay 0.85 × £25 = £21.25 per dress, leaving a profit of £21.25 − £13 = £8.25. Subtract to find the difference in profit during the summer sale: £12 − £8.25 = £3.75. Divide to find the percentage change: £3.75 ÷ £12 = 0.3125, or 31%. The correct answer is (E).

33. (A)

40 dresses sold at full price means that Mrs Tiwari will be paid 40 × £25 = £1000. She must pay 12% of the first £500: 0.12 × 500 = 60. She must also pay 8% of the second £500: 0.08 × 500 = 40. Sum these figures to find the total due in customs tax: £60 + £40 = £100. She will also have paid 4 × £130 = £520 to buy the dresses in the first place, so her total profit is £1000 − £620 = £380. The answer is therefore (A).

34. (B)

The final question asks for the difference in price between the Belgian shop and Mrs Tiwari's shop during the sale. We already calculated the sale price in the second question: £21.25; if you noted this on your noteboard, then you would not have to work it out again here. Next, calculate the Belgian sale price in pounds: 32 euros ÷ 1.12 euros/pound = £28.57. Finally, subtract for the difference: £28.57 − £21.25 = £7.32, answer (B).

35. (C)

Pink paint is made from equal parts of Red and White paint. Red paint costs £5.51, and White paint £2.11, and 1 litre of each will mix to make 2 litres of Pink paint, with a cost of £5.51 + £2.11 = £7.62. Since Niamh wants 5 L of Pink paint, and 5 L = 2 L × 2.5, multiply the cost of 2 L by 2.5 to find the cost of 5 L: £7.62 × 2.5 = £19.05. Don't forget to factor in the extra £3 for time and £1.59 for cleaning costs, resulting in a total of £23.64. The answer is (C).

36. (E)

According to the data, Cornflower paint is one part Blue and two parts Pale Blue (which itself is one part Blue and one part White). 3 litres of Cornflower paint is therefore made up of 1 litre of White paint and 2 litres of Blue paint. The cost of this would be £2.11 + (2 × £6.20) = £14.51. With the additional costs of time and cleaning, the total price is £19.10, so the answer is (E).

37. (D)

The colours in this question are not important, as we only need to calculate the total amount of paint needed, making this question more straightforward than it might appear at first glance. A noteboard sketch of Magali's room will help find the correct answer quickly:

The total area is therefore $2(3 \times 2.5) + 2(5 \times 2.5) + (3 \times 5) = 15 + 25 + 15 = 55$ m². Divide to find the litres required: 55 m² ÷ 1.5 m²/L = 36.7 L. Magali will need 37 litres, answer (D).

38. (B)

At first glance, this question looks like it will involve a great deal of calculation, and therefore it is probably best to guess an answer, mark it for review, and move on, so you can maximise the time that you have to spend on questions where you can find correct answers more quickly. If you had time to solve this question when you came back to it at the end of the Kaplan UKCAT quiz, the fastest way is to note the number of litres of each colour used in the mixture:

- Indigo: 6 L = 4 L Blue + 2 L Red
- Mauve: 12 L = 4 L Blue + 4 L Red + 4 L White
- Rose: 3 L = 2 L Red + 1 L White
- Blush: 3 L = 1 L Red + 2 L White
- Sky: 3 L = 2 L White + 1 L Blue

Sum to find the total litres of the three basic colours, and then multiply for the cost for each:

- Red = 2 L + 4 L + 2 L + 1 L = 9 L; 9 L × £5.51/L = £49.59
- Blue = 4 L + 4 L + 1 L = 9 L; 9 L × £6.20/L = £55.80
- White = 4 L + 1 L + 2 L + 2 L = 9 L; 9 L × £2.11/L = £18.99

Add these three for the total cost, then divide by 27 for the cost per litre: £49.59 + £55.80 + £18.99 = £124.38; £124.38 ÷ 27 L = £4.61 per litre. The correct answer is (B).

39. (A)

This first question is a great candidate for eyeballing. Scanning the graph shows us that girls are in grey, and boys in white. The scale on the y-axis goes up in increments of 20. Approximately 35 boys study Chemistry, and approximately 12 girls study Maths, so the answer is 35 – 12 = 23. The answer is (A).

40. (D)

Another reasonably straightforward question, allowing you to bank time for the more complex questions in the Kaplan UKCAT quiz. The graph shows that a total of 50 students study History of Art, and that 40 of these are girls: $\frac{40}{50} = 0.8$, or 80%, of History of Art students are girls. The answer is therefore (D).

41. (C)

The tempting answer here is Can't tell, as there is no representation of Economics on the graph. However, the question text provides all the information required to deduce the answer, so Can't tell is incorrect. The graph shows that 35 girls study French, so there must be 35 + 10 = 45 girls studying Economics. If these 45 girls = 50% of the Economics students, then there must be 45 boys studying Economics, and the total number of Economics students is 45 × 2 = 90. The correct answer is (C).

42. (C)

The final question in this set is a bit more complicated, so make a note of the various figures involved on your noteboard as you work. There are approximately 66 girls studying Chemistry, so there are 66 × 0.5 = 33 girls who study both Chemistry and Biology. There are approximately 60 girls studying Geography, so there are 60 × 0.333 = 20 girls who study both Geography and Biology. Adding in the 10 further girls who study Biology, but neither Chemistry nor Geography, there are a total of 33 + 20 + 10 = 63 girls who study Biology. The number of boys studying Biology is two-thirds the number of girls, so there are 63 × 0.667 = 42 boys studying Biology. The answer is (C).

43. (B)

In this question, the unknown is speed, so set up the speed formula appropriately: Speed = Distance ÷ Time. Because the question is asking for Salim's average speed for the whole journey, simply calculate his total distance and total time, and plug these into the speed formula. The distance covered is 6 km, and he takes 2.25 hours to walk this distance: 3.25 hours minus 1 hour for lunch. Thus, Salim's average speed is a simple calculation: 6 km ÷ 2.25 hr = 2.67 km/hr. The answer is therefore (B).

44. (A)

To solve for Salim's rate of elevation in metres per minute, find the time spent in the walk before lunch first. The data state that Salim walked 3 km before lunch, and the question specifies that he walked that distance at a rate of 2 km/hr. Time = Distance ÷ Speed, so the time walked before lunch = 3 km ÷ 2 km/hour, or 1.5 hours. Since Salim travelled half the distance to Castle Point before lunch, he has climbed half of the incline, so he has gained 210 m in elevation during the 90 minutes. Divide to find the rate of metres per minute: 210 m ÷ 90 min = 2.3 m/min. Answer (A) is correct.

45. (C)

Drawing a sketch on your noteboard would help with this question:

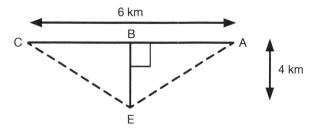

The area of a triangle is 0.5 × base × height, so the area of the nature reserve is 0.5 × 6 × 4 = 12 km². The answer is (C).

46. (D)

Another sketch is helpful here:

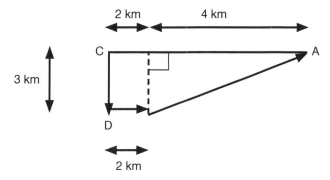

Filling in the distances involved reveals that the distance that Salim and his friend will race over is the hypotenuse of a triangle whose perpendicular sides measure 3 km and 4 km. You may recognise this as a Pythagorean triple—the hypotenuse measures 5 km—or you may need to calculate the length using Pythagoras's theorem.

Since they start out at 2pm, Salim reaches Axelbury at 2pm + 75 minutes = 3.15pm. If Salim's friend is 1 km away from Axelbury when Salim finishes, then he has travelled 5 − 1 = 4 km in 75 minutes, giving him a speed of 4 km ÷ 75 min = 0.053 km/min. The friend will therefore take 1 ÷ 0.053 = 19 min longer to reach Axelbury. Salim's friend will therefore arrive at 3.15pm + 19 min = 3.34pm. The answer is therefore (D).

Abstract Reasoning

The Task

Abstract Reasoning is the third scored subtest on the UKCAT. The Abstract section consists of 55 items, which must be answered in 13 minutes. Prior to 2013, all these items were in the same format, now known as Type 1: they come in sets of 5, with a corresponding Set A and Set B. The test shapes appear one at a time, to the left of Sets A and B. You must evaluate whether the test shapes belong to Set A, Set B or Neither. As with the other subtests, there is 1 minute to read the instructions. This allows 1 minute to complete each set, and it makes the Abstract section the most time-constrained subtest on the UKCAT. Thus, it's essential to approach the Abstract questions with a time-saving strategy in mind.

In 2013, the UKCAT Consortium added three additional Abstract question types (Type 2, Type 3 and Type 4). However, there were minimal examples of the three new Abstract question types in the official practice materials—only 5 out of 55 questions in each official practice test were in one of the new formats—and most students did not see any of the new formats on Test Day in 2013. Thus, at the time of going to press, it is unclear whether the three new question types will appear on the UKCAT in 2014 or subsequent years, or what proportion of the Abstract items may be in the new formats. This chapter will thus focus primarily on Type 1 questions, with some basic tips for the new formats. Be sure to check the Online Resource Centre for an update as to the exact test format (and any additional Kaplan UKCAT test tips and practice questions) in the year you take the test.

The Format

Each Type 1 set is composed of a Set A and a Set B. Set A and Set B both contain six 'boxes'. In Set A, each of the boxes will share one or more attributes. This shared attribute for Set A is termed 'the pattern'. Likewise, Set B's six boxes will also have one or more shared attributes, and Set B will have its own unique pattern. NB Set A and Set B can never have the exact same pattern. The difference may be quite subtle; nevertheless, there will always be a difference between Set A and Set B.

Each Abstract Reasoning 'test shape' is a single box containing various shapes within it. The answer choices for Type 1 questions are always the same: Set A, Set B or Neither. These answers require you to evaluate the test shapes according to the patterns in Sets A and B:

Set A: The test shape fits the pattern for Set A exactly, but not Set B.

Set B: The test shape fits the pattern for Set B exactly, but not Set A.

Neither: Three possibilities may lead to an answer of Neither:

- the test shape does not fit the pattern for either Set A or B;
- the test shape only partially fits the pattern for Set A or B; or
- the test shape fits the patterns for both Set A and Set B.

Type 1 is the only Abstract question type that has answer choices in this format. The format for the other Abstract question types will be explained later in the chapter. The skills you will develop in attacking Type 1 questions will be extremely useful in attacking the other question types—but it is easier to learn these skills by focusing on a single question type. So we'll start with the most common one.

The Challenges

The most obvious challenge in Abstract Reasoning is timing: 55 questions in 13 minutes makes this the fastest paced subsection on the UKCAT. Many test-takers will simply take too long searching for patterns, or will spend a large amount of time on one particular set, and will not finish the section.

The other major challenge in the Abstract section is finding the patterns. No test-takers will have learned any visual pattern finding techniques in school. Some test-takers may feel this is a skill they are either lucky enough to be born with or not. The truth is that visual pattern finding is a skill that can be learned and developed with an understanding of what kind of patterns to look for and with sufficient practice.

Kaplan Top Tips for Abstract Reasoning

1. Don't start with the test shape

There are several good reasons not to start with the test shape:

- *The test shape doesn't help you find the pattern.* The test shape may not have the pattern for either set, so you will waste valuable time if you try to use the test shape to find the pattern.

- *Marks come from finding patterns, not matching.* Occasionally there will be overlap between the patterns for Set A and Set B. A test shape may even look very similar to a box in one of the sets, but actually fit the pattern for the other set. If you try to simply match the test shapes to a similar-looking box in one of the sets, you will lose marks.

2. Start with the simplest box first

This is a fantastic approach that will dramatically improve your pattern finding skills for two reasons:

- *Distracting shapes are minimised.* Not all shapes in the boxes have to be of any relevance to the patterns. Shapes that are not part of the pattern are 'distractors'. The box containing the fewest number of items will have the fewest distractors, and thus will help you focus in on the true pattern.

- *Even the simplest box contains the pattern.* If the simplest box contains only one shape, your task becomes much more straightforward. For example, if a box contains a single shaded triangle in a corner of the box, you now have a clue that the pattern is either about triangles, a shaded shape, or about arrangement in the corner. By checking the other boxes in the set for these same characteristics, you will find the pattern quickly.

3. Learn to search the pattern categories

Once you know what types of patterns are common on the UKCAT, you will spot patterns with ease. Basic patterns involve:

Types—a particular type of shape.

Features—the colour, size and number of a shape.

Arrangement—the position of shapes within the box, as well as relative to each other.

Most UKCAT patterns use one or two of these categories, while some of the most difficult patterns may involve all. Patterns for Set A and Set B will often use the same pattern category. However, the patterns do not necessarily have to be related.

4. If unsure, keep moving on

Spending too much time on one pattern means that you will run out of time and miss easy marks at the end of the section. You should spend no more than 1 minute on each set, which normally includes 30 seconds to find both patterns, then 5 seconds to evaluate each test shape. If you haven't seen the patterns after 45 seconds, it is unlikely that you will see the patterns with more time. At this point, it is crucial to take a guess and mark these questions for review.

The best Abstract test-takers are ruthless in moving forward to finish the section. If you follow the timing guidelines precisely, you will have 2 minutes at the end of the section to return for a second look at the difficult sets you have marked for review. It is quite common for patterns to become obvious with a fresh look.

Don't feel bad if you don't see every pattern. Even Abstract experts will have one or two difficult patterns they can't quite figure out!

5. Make the most of the Abstract practice sets in this book

As you practise with this book, always try to find the pattern and answer the questions within the 1 minute per set guideline. After your timed practice, come back to any sets you found difficult or impossible the first time round, and see if you can get the pattern with a little more time and fresh eyes. Then check the explanations for the pattern. The explanations may also include tips on pattern finding techniques that you will find helpful on later questions.

6. Check the Online Resource Centre for updates

It's essential to ensure you have the most up-to-date information about the Abstract question types, and the approximate balance of question types in the Abstract section in the year you sit the UKCAT. We expect this will be something of a developing situation, with a high likelihood of significant changes on an annual basis. Be sure to check the Online Resource Centre and the test-maker's website, so you are not caught out by unexpected test changes on Test Day. See page ix.

Score Higher on the UKCAT

Set your timer for 1 minute. Write down answers for the 5 test shapes before time is up!

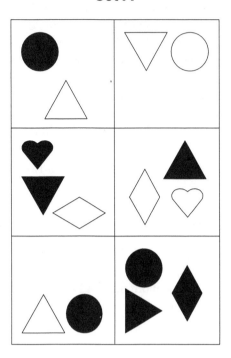

Set A   **Set B**

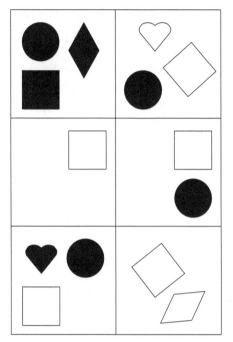

Test Shapes

| 1 | 2 | 3 | 4 | 5 |

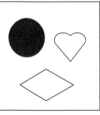

A. Set A	A. Set A	A. Set A	A. Set A	A. Set A
B. Set B	B. Set B	B. Set B	B. Set B	B. Set B
C. Neither	C. Neither	C. Neither	C. Neither	C. Neither

If you found the patterns—well done! If not, don't fret—you're just getting started. In either case, you will want to review the approach to this set using the Kaplan Abstract top tips.

First, ignore the test shape, as it won't help in finding the pattern. Next, focus on the simplest box in either Set A or Set B. The simplest box in either set is the middle left box in Set B, which contains a lone square. Now, check this against the pattern categories. The pattern may involve the type of shape (square) or a feature of the shape (white in colour, or straight sides). Check the other boxes in Set B, and you'll find there is a square in every box, though the colour of the square can be black or white; the arrangement of the square varies as well. Thus, the pattern in Set B appears to be that there is a square in every box; this is a simple type of shape pattern. Now, examine Set A and look for a similar pattern. The only shape that appears in every box in Set A is a triangle. This is the pattern for Set A.

1. (B)

The first test shape contains a square and no triangle, therefore the correct answer is (B).

2. (C)

This test shape doesn't contain either a square or a triangle. As such, it doesn't fit either set, and the answer is (C).

3. (A)

Even though there isn't a box with a lone triangle in Set A, the UKCAT does not include 'at least' patterns. You would not find a pattern where there has to be a triangle and *at least* one other shape. If in doubt, keep the pattern simple. The answer is therefore (A).

4. (C)

This test shape contains a triangle, so you might think it belongs to Set A. However, it also contains a square, which would make it belong to Set B. In this situation, the correct answer is that the test shape belongs exclusively to neither set, so the answer is (C).

5. (A)

The last test shape has a triangle and no square. The answer is (A).

Don't worry if you didn't find this pattern straightaway. With more practice, you will improve with speed as you develop 'trained eyes' of your own.

NB On Test Day, you will see the test shapes one at a time, to the right of Set B. In this book, we have printed all 5 test shapes for each set below Set A and Set B, to facilitate easier and speedier practising. Remember, you will have to click through the test shapes on Test Day, which will take a few seconds more. Whether practising with this book or with a computer-based UKCAT, you might cover the test shapes with your hand until you find the pattern. This will help you to focus on Sets A and B, and ensure that you do not let the test shape distract you from finding the patterns.

Many of the UKCAT Abstract patterns will only involve a pattern from one category. The first practice set was a classic pattern involving type of shape, and just the sort of pattern that you should have at the forefront of your mind when attacking new Abstract sets. Other patterns may involve two or more basic categories. Adding on layers of patterns is one way that an Abstract pattern can become more difficult.

Keep in mind, though, that you are likely to see only one or two really overly complex patterns on Test Day. Don't be drawn into the trap of overinvesting your time to make sure you haven't missed every aspect of the pattern. If the pattern seems simple, it probably is!

Let's have a look at the other pattern categories and how they might be combined on Test Day with another example set. Take 30 seconds to find the patterns.

Set A   **Set B**

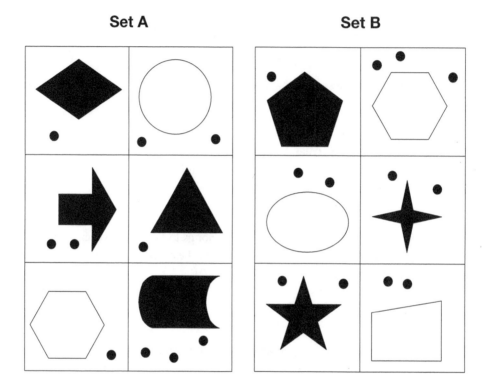

At first glance the pair of sets here seems very similar; the simplest box in each set contains a large shape with one small black circle.

There are actually two ways to use the simplest box in each set. The first is to compare the simplest box in Set A with other boxes in Set A. The second is to compare the simplest box in Set A with the simplest box in Set B. How are they different? For example, looking at the upper left-hand box in each set, you can see that the main difference is in how the shapes are arranged within the box. In Set A, the large shape is above the small black circles; in Set B, the small black circles are arranged above the large shape.

This pattern combines all of our basic categories. We have a type of shape pattern—each box has to contain small circles. Other features are important too. There is a colour element because all the small circles are shaded black. Number and size are also included as there is one large shape in each box. The pattern in how these shapes are arranged is the crucial difference between Set A and Set B.

Consider each of the test shapes in turn. Spend no more than 30 seconds total on the 5 test shapes, and be sure to mark an answer for each.

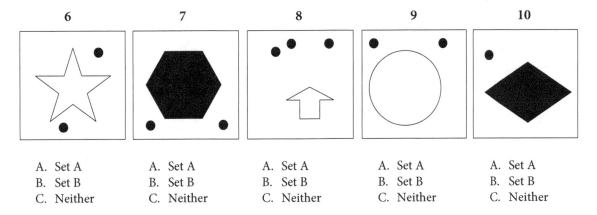

6	7	8	9	10
A. Set A	A. Set A	A. Set A	A. Set A	A. Set A
B. Set B	B. Set B	B. Set B	B. Set B	B. Set B
C. Neither	C. Neither	C. Neither	C. Neither	C. Neither

Answers and Explanations

6. (C)

The first test shape has small black circles above and below the large shape. The answer is therefore (C).

7. (A)

This test shape has a large shape and small black circles below it. The answer is (A).

8. (C)

This test shape has three small black circles; however, there is no big shape. This test shape belongs to neither set; thus, the correct answer is (C). If you hadn't seen the arrangement pattern, you could have still earned this mark by simply noticing that a large shape was required for both Sets A and B. The good news is that there are many marks, like this one, that you can pick up even if you haven't spotted the entire pattern.

9. (B)

This test shape has a large shape with small black circles above it. The answer is (B).

10. (B)

The last test shape looks very similar to a box in Set A. This would potentially trap a student who was trying to match the test shapes to individual boxes in Set A or Set B. Having identified the pattern, this one is quick, straightforward work—the correct answer is (B).

Let's try working through another set on the next page.

Set your timer for 1 minute. Try to find the patterns below in 30 seconds. If you don't spot the patterns after 45 seconds, move on to the test shapes and take a guess.

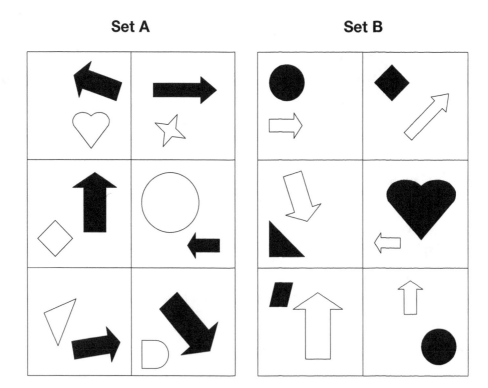

Set A   **Set B**

Test Shapes

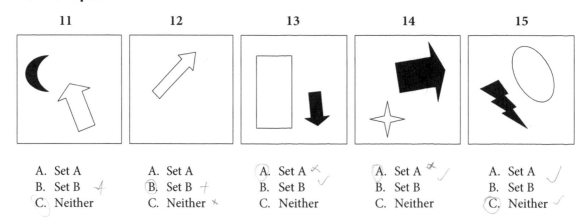

11	12	13	14	15

A. Set A
B. Set B
C. Neither

A. Set A
B. Set B
C. Neither

A. Set A
B. Set B
C. Neither

A. Set A
B. Set B
C. Neither

A. Set A
B. Set B
C. Neither

If you looked for the box with the fewest number of items in Sets A and B, you'll have noticed that all the boxes in both sets have 2 shapes—so there isn't a 'simplest' box in either. And this is indeed part of the pattern: both Set A and Set B have exactly 2 shapes in each box. You might wonder why we would notice a characteristic that both sets have in common as it won't help us differentiate as to whether the test shape belongs to Set A or Set B. In fact, you will be able to determine that some test shapes belong to neither Set A nor Set B based on this number characteristic, so it's definitely worth noticing.

To find the rest of the pattern, check for common categories first. There is one type of shape—an arrow—in every box in both Set A and Set B. Check the other features (colour, size) and arrangement to find the difference between the two sets. The pattern in Set A is that there is a black arrow and a white shape, and in Set B there is a white arrow and a black shape.

11. (B)

The first test shape has a white arrow and a black shape so it belongs to (B).

12. (C)

This test shape has a white arrow, but no second black shape; as such, it cannot belong to either set. The answer is (C).

13. (A)

A black arrow and a white shape mean this test shape belongs to (A).

14. (A)

Again we have a black arrow and a white shape. The answer is (A).

15. (C)

This test shape is lacking an arrow, so it cannot belong to either set. The answer is (C).

Set your timer for 1 minute. Try to mark answers for all 5 test shapes before time runs out.

Set A   **Set B**

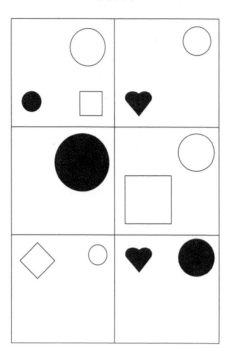 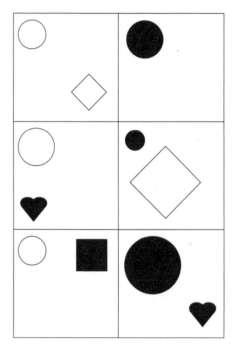

Test Shapes

16	17	18	19	20

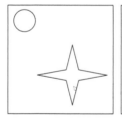 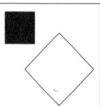 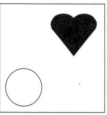 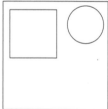 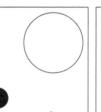

16	17	18	19	20
A. Set A	A. Set A	A. Set A	A. Set A	A. Set A
B. Set B	B. Set B	B. Set B	B. Set B	B. Set B
C. Neither	C. Neither	C. Neither	C. Neither	C. Neither

Starting with the simplest box leads to the marks once again here. The simplest box in both Set A and Set B has a solitary circle. If you check the rest of the boxes in the sets, you will see that there is always a circle in every box. To find the difference between these, consider how the circles are arranged. In Set A, the circle is positioned in the upper right-hand corner of the box, while in Set B the circle is in the upper left-hand corner of the box.

16. (B)

The first test shape contains a circle in the upper left-hand corner of the box, so the correct answer is (B).

17. (C)

This test shape doesn't include a circle. The answer is (C).

18. (C)

The test shape contains a circle, but it is in the lower left-hand corner. The answer is (C).

19. (A)

A circle in the upper right-hand corner corresponds to (A).

20. (A)

Another circle in the upper right-hand corner means that this test shape belongs to Set A.

Basic Patterns Review

Training your eyes to quickly spot the basic Abstract patterns is vital to achieving a good score on Test Day. Let us review some of the most basic patterns:

Type of shape

Features of shapes:

- Number—an absolute number of items or of a particular shape
- Colour—the shading of shapes
- Size—the size of shapes

Arrangement: the position of shapes within the box as well as relative to each other.

Complex Patterns

The patterns seen so far have been relatively simple. The majority of sets on Test Day will have relatively simple patterns, and you can achieve a respectable score by ensuring that you work your way through the entire section picking up all of the easy points. So many UKCAT test-takers are unable to finish the section, due to their inability to find the simple patterns quickly—the more you can do so, the greater advantage you will have over the competition.

Complex patterns are just as vulnerable to strategy, and to a methodical approach by 'trained eyes' that know how to spot them. Be careful, though, as some 'trained eyes' become obsessed with finding complex patterns, and look for complexity in all sets; as a result, they run the risk of not being able to finish the section. So bear in mind that most sets are not complex, and don't fret when you find a pattern that seems too easy, or simple or obvious to be correct. If a pattern seems simple or obvious—that's almost always because it is!

Complex patterns present many different twists. Let us take a look at a few of the most common, and most challenging, examples that you may encounter on Test Day.

Unusual Shapes and Arrangements

Unusual-looking shapes scare test-takers. Be assured that these funny looking squiggles will still conform to the basic categories. Squiggles are a type of shape, and they have features that can be examined.

Unusual arrangement patterns might involve how the shapes are arranged relative to each other. You should always look for an arrangement pattern if the two sets seem to involve identical or nearly identical shapes.

Counting

Number patterns can be very complex. While a basic number pattern includes counting numbers of shapes (e.g. 2 triangles in each box), a more complex number pattern can involve counting other features. Instead of number of shapes, you might have to count the number of sides, intersections, 'spaces', angles or even the number of times you have to take your pencil off the page to draw a shape within a box.

To further complicate matters, a number pattern can also be about whether you have an even or an odd number of something.

Once test-takers know that the sets can contain these sorts of patterns, they suddenly start to see a lot of the tough patterns. However, this comes with a big downside—students start launching into counting everything in a set right away and end up wasting time. You must find a balance. The best approach is to look for basic patterns first, and consider counting if and only if you haven't been able to find a basic pattern.

Take a minute to see if you can find a pattern below, and then assess the test shapes.

Set A   **Set B**

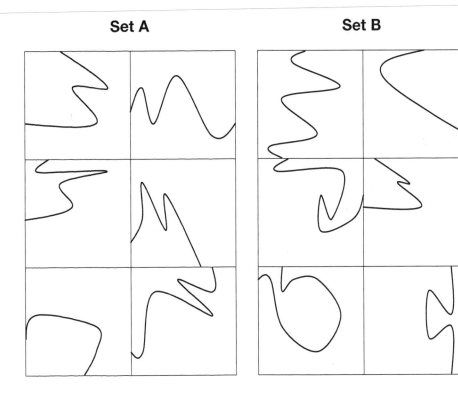

Test Shapes

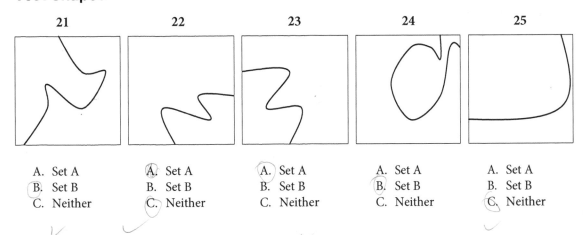

21	22	23	24	25

A. Set A   A. Set A   A. Set A   A. Set A   A. Set A
B. Set B   B. Set B   B. Set B   B. Set B   B. Set B
C. Neither   C. Neither   C. Neither   C. Neither   C. Neither

Answers and Explanations

The first step to find this pattern is to not panic when you see unusual shapes. In some regards, they are a gift because a bizarre shape can't have too many features. Unusual shapes may have a certain number of squiggles or may form a certain number of 'spaces'. They could be concave or convex. They could be symmetrical or asymmetrical. These are the only possible unusual shape features that you should be prepared to consider on Test Day. With one glance, you can see that other features like colour and size can't play any part here.

Not only does this set contain squiggles, but it's even more unusual, as the squiggly lines touch the edges of the box. It is rare to have shapes touching the edges of the box in any set, so this is a big clue to focus in on as a possible part of the pattern.

If you consider where the lines in Set A and Set B start and terminate, you'll see that the only consistency in Set A is that all the lines have one end touching the left-hand border of the box. In Set B, all the lines have one end touching the top border of the box. So this is certainly an unusual arrangement pattern involving highly unusual shapes.

21. (B)

The first test shape has a line that touches the top and the bottom of the box, so it fits into Set B.

22. (C)

The line in this test shape doesn't touch the top or the left of the box, so it doesn't fit into either set.

23. (A)

This test shape has a line that ends on the left and bottom, so it fits into Set A.

24. (B)

This test shape's line ends on the top and right sides of the box. The correct answer is (B).

25. (C)

This test shape's line starts at the top and left of the box, so it fits into both Set A and Set B, which means it belongs exclusively to neither set.

A further way that the UKCAT makes patterns more complex is with conditional characteristics. Conditionals are patterns in which a characteristic of one item in the box dictates a characteristic of another item in the box. For example, you might see a pattern where each box contains a circle and a square, with this conditional: if the circle is shaded, it is positioned above the square; if the circle is not shaded, it is positioned below the square. The pattern in the other set might then be the opposite, or it might be a similar but slightly different conditional—for example, it might involve shading and positioning of shapes that are different from the shapes in Set A. Conditionals can be time-consuming to identify, and even more time-consuming in evaluating answer choices, since you will have to apply the conditionals from Set A and Set B to every test shape.

There are two hints for spotting conditionals. First, if you see arrows, consider if the direction they are pointing is related to the position, shading or type of shape of another shape (or shapes) in the box. Second, if two sets seem almost identical, and you have already checked for an arrangement pattern—check for conditionals!

Remember, conditional patterns are really rather rare on the UKCAT, so only look for them if you can't find anything else.

Take 1 minute to find the conditional pattern in the set at the top of the next page. Make a note of the pattern on your scrap paper, and then spend no more than 30 seconds evaluating the test shapes.

Set A   **Set B**

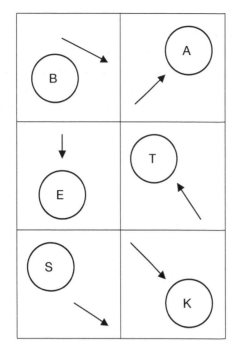
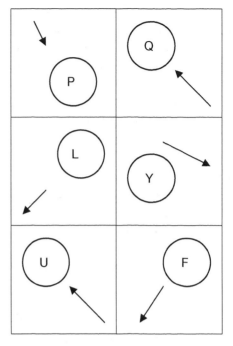

Test Shapes

26	27	28	29	30

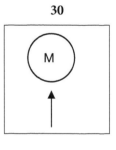

26	27	28	29	30
A. Set A	A. Set A	A. Set A	A. Set A	A. Set A
B. Set B	B. Set B	B. Set B	B. Set B	B. Set B
C. Neither	C. Neither	C. Neither	C. Neither	C. Neither

Answers and Explanations

The most obvious part of the pattern that you will notice straightaway is that all boxes in both sets have an arrow and a circle containing a letter. So the difference between the sets must involve the letters inside the circles, some of which are straight and some of which are curved letters. Since each box also contains an arrow, consider whether the direction of the arrow corresponds to the letter inside the circle. In Set A, if the arrow points at the circle, the letter is straight. If the arrow doesn't point at the circle, the letter inside has curves. The pattern for Set B is the exact opposite: the arrow points at circles with curved letters and not at those containing straight letters.

26. (B)

The first test shape has an arrow pointing at a curved letter. This fits into Set B.

27. (B)

The letter here is straight, and the arrow points away from it. This also belongs to Set B.

28. (A)

The arrow points at a circle containing a straight letter. The correct answer is (A).

29. (B)

The arrow doesn't point at a circle containing a straight letter. The answer must be (B).

30. (A)

The arrow is pointing at a circle containing a straight letter. This corresponds to Set A.

If, after learning about all the common and complex patterns, you find yourself seeing more patterns but running out of time, you are not alone. With newly trained eyes, looking for patterns can be a systematic but very time-consuming process, and the temptation to keep searching until you find every minor nuance in every pattern is irresistible. This may lead you to proceed through Abstract sets at a slower pace, which will result in a lower score. However, as you practice more and more, your speed will improve and you'll find that you can find most, if not all, patterns, rather quickly and accurately.

Once you've become relatively quick, you'll still need to learn when to give up. Almost every UKCAT test is going to contain one or two horrendously difficult patterns that are going to stump even the most brilliant Abstract Reasoning test-takers. The best approach with these sets is to spend up to a minute finding part of the pattern, then use this partial pattern to assess the test shapes. Often, you can eliminate Set A or Set B as a possible answer based on a partial pattern, leaving you with a 50–50 guess. These are good odds, and certainly better than guessing blindly—or panicking and wasting time—on a very hard set.

Take no longer than 1 minute, and see if you can find part of a pattern in the set below.

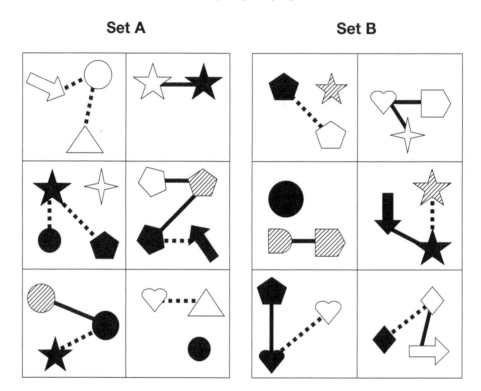

Answer

These sets have lots of different shapes, with unusual shadings, connected by dashed and straight lines. Don't panic, and start with the simplest box first. In Set A, the upper right-hand box has two stars connected by a solid line. Is that pattern repeated elsewhere in the set? Yes—there are two identical shapes connected by a straight line in the middle right and lower left boxes. Compare to the simplest box in Set B; the upper right box has three white shapes—a pentagon, heart and star—all connected by solid lines. Check the other boxes to see if this is a pattern: the lower right box has a white diamond and arrow connected by a solid line; the boxes above and to the left of it each have two black shapes connected by a solid line. Thus, the partial pattern is that the same types of shapes are connected by solid lines in Set A, and the same colour shapes are connected by solid lines in Set B. If that's all you've seen, you can actually make some good eliminations when you move on to the test shapes.

Take 30 seconds to evaluate the test shapes, and make your best guess based on the partial pattern.

Test Shapes

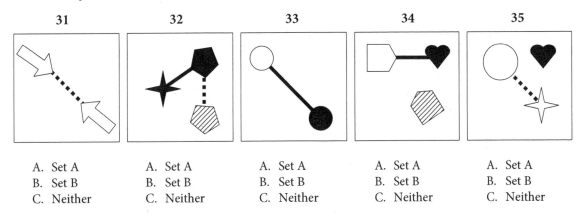

	31	32	33	34	35

A. Set A
B. Set B
C. Neither

A. Set A
B. Set B
C. Neither

A. Set A
B. Set B
C. Neither

A. Set A
B. Set B
C. Neither

A. Set A
B. Set B
C. Neither

Answers and Explanations

Based on the partial pattern, the two white arrows in the first test shape should be connected by a solid line in Set A (because they are the same shape) and also in Set B (because they are the same colour); as such, this test shape cannot fit into either set. The second test shape has two black shapes connected by a solid line, which fits the pattern for Set B; because the two pentagons are not connected by a solid line, it doesn't fit the pattern for Set A, so the answer must be (B). The third test shape has two circles connected by a solid line; the circles are different colours, so the answer must be (A). The fourth test shape does not fit either set, as it has two different shapes of different colour connected by a solid line; the answer must be (C). The final test shape does not have a solid line, but two different shapes of the same colour are connected by a dotted line. This cannot fit the pattern for Set B, so it's a 50–50 guess between (A) and (C).

Even if you only found part of the partial patterns—say, only the detail involving solid lines connecting shapes of the same type in Set A—that would be enough to get the third test shape correct, and to eliminate (A) as an answer choice for the first, second and fourth test shapes (as all of these include identical shapes that are not connected by a solid line). You would have to guess randomly on the final test shape, but would still be able to pick up 2 or 3 marks from the 5 available in this set—far more than you'd get by guessing randomly on all 5 test shapes, or by leaving them unanswered.

For the record: This pattern is incredibly complex, involving many features as well as arrangements. In Set A, if shapes are of the same shading, they are connected with a dotted line. If the shapes are of the same type, they are connected with a solid line. Shapes that aren't the same colour or the same shape as another in the box are not connected. In Set B, if the shapes are of the same type, they are connected with a dotted line. If they are the same colour, they are connected by a solid line. Other shapes are not connected. Thus, the final test shape fits into Set A, as it features two different white shapes connected by a dotted line.

Set your timer for 1 minute. Do your best to find a partial pattern—if not the complete pattern—for each set before the minute is up. It is okay to take the full minute to find the patterns, as this is a very advanced set. If you do so, then give yourself no more than 30 seconds to mark answers for all 5 test shapes. If unsure, eliminate based on a partial pattern and make a guess.

Set A

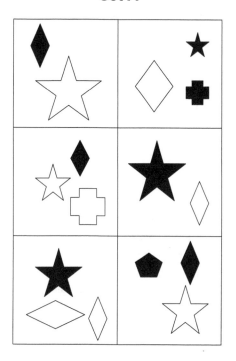

Set B

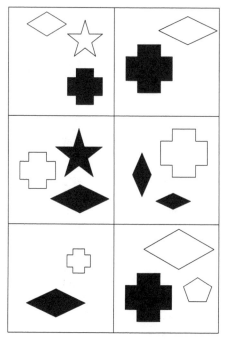

Test Shapes

36	37	38	39	40

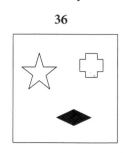 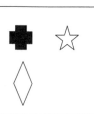 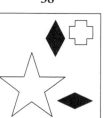 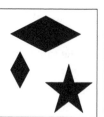 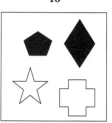

36	37	38	39	40
A. Set A	A. Set A	A. Set A	A. Set A	A. Set A
B. Set B	B. Set B	B. Set B	B. Set B	B. Set B
C. Neither	C. Neither	C. Neither	C. Neither	C. Neither

This set's pattern may be difficult to see because of the distractor shapes, so it helps to start by looking at the box in each set with the fewest number of shapes. In Set A, the upper left and middle right box each have a star and a diamond with longer height than width (a 'tall' diamond). One is white and one is black. In Set B, the upper right and lower left boxes each have a cross and a diamond with longer width than height (a 'wide' diamond). One is white and one is black. Based on this partial pattern, the test shapes would be assessed as follows.

36. (B)

The first test shape has a wide diamond and a cross; one is white and one is black, so this fits into Set B.

37. (C)

The second test shape has a tall diamond and a star; however, both are white, so it does not fit into Set A. There is no wide diamond, so it cannot fit into Set B. The answer must be (C).

38. (C)

The third test shape has a tall diamond and a wide diamond, both of which are black; there's also a star and a cross, both of which are white. As such, the test shape seems to fit into both sets, so it belongs to neither set.

39. (C)

The fourth test shape has a star and a tall diamond, but both are black. Thus, it cannot fit into Set A. Since there is a wide diamond but no cross, it also cannot fit into Set B. The answer must be (C).

40. (A)

The final test shape has a tall diamond that is black and a star that is white, so it belongs to Set A.

In this instance, the partial pattern is enough to determine the correct answers for all the test shapes in the set. The only thing missed out in the partial pattern is the element of arrangement: in Set A, the shape (of the star and tall diamond) that is above the other is black, and the one that is below is white; in Set B, the shape (of the cross and wide diamond) that is above the other is white, and the one that is below is black. None of the test shapes violated this conditional element of the pattern, so you did not need to find it in order to pick up the marks available on this set.

Again, it's essential not to worry about highly complex sets—you are unlikely to see more than one such set on Test Day, and finding a partial pattern based on the basic pattern categories is usually enough to get most, if not all, of the test shapes correct. In the worst case, you may be able to eliminate one answer choice and then make a 50–50 guess between the remaining answers on some test shapes. But doing so is essential to keeping to timing guidelines: normally 1 minute per set, and only slightly longer—no more than 90 seconds—on a very difficult set.

Other Abstract Question Types

The other three Abstract question types each have 4 answer choices, and each answer choice is a test shape. Thus, your skills at assessing test shapes and finding the common features—and to do so quickly—will continue to be essential.

Type 4 Questions

Type 4 questions are virtually identical to Type 1 questions. The key differences:

- You will be asked to select the test shape that fits the pattern for one of the sets.
- The answer choices are 4 test shapes.

Thus, any time you see Set A and Set B, you should start by finding the patterns. We expect that Type 4 questions will come in a set of 5, but be sure to read each question to check whether it is asking about Set A or Set B.

Give yourself 30 seconds to find the patterns in Set A and Set B, then 30 seconds to answer the 5 questions that follow.

Set A   **Set B**

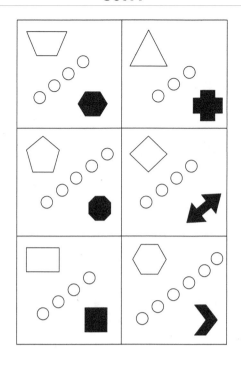
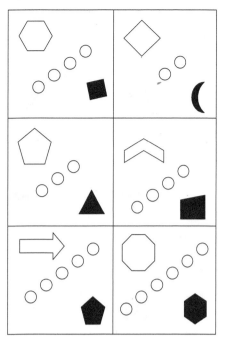

41. Which of the following test shapes belongs in Set A?

A   B   C   D

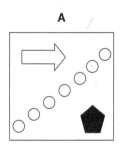 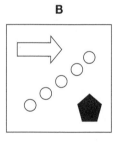 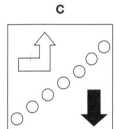 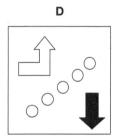

42. Which of the following test shapes belongs in Set A?

A   B   C   D

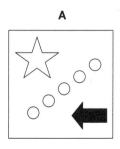 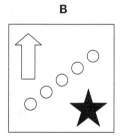 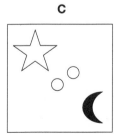 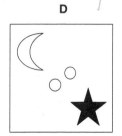

Set A   **Set B**

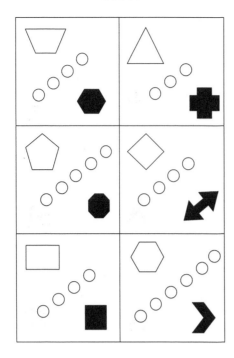 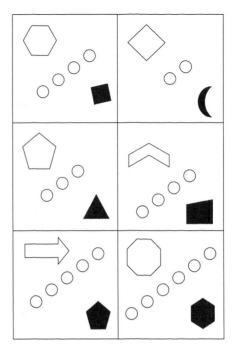

43. Which of the following test shapes belongs in Set B?

A   B   C   D

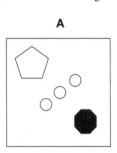 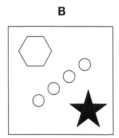 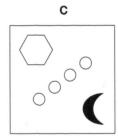 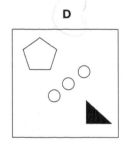

44. Which of the following test shapes belongs in Set B?

A   B   C   D

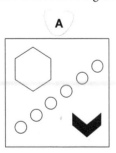 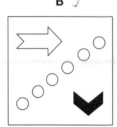 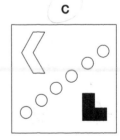 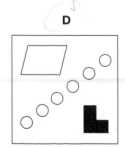

Set A   **Set B**

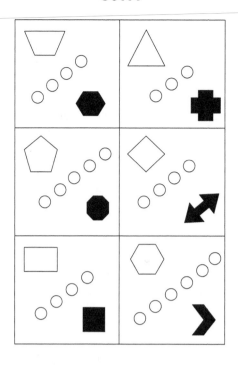

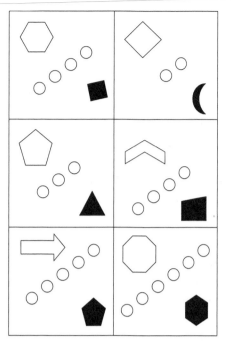

45. Which of the following test shapes belongs in Set A?

A   B   C   D

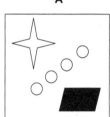

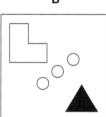

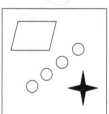

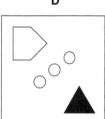

Answers and Explanations

41. (A)

In this set, all the boxes in both sets contain a white shape in the upper left, a black shape in the lower right, and a number of small white circles across the diagonal. In Set A, the number of small white circles is the same as the number of sides on the white shape in the upper left; the number of sides on the black shape is irrelevant to the pattern. In Set B, the number of small white circles is the same as the number of sides on the black shape, and the number of sides on the white shape in the upper left is 2 more than the number of small white circles.

The first question asks about Set A, so compare the number of sides on the shape in the upper left of each box to the number of small white circles. The only answer choice that gives an equal number for both of these is (A), in which there are 7 small white circles and 7 sides on the white arrow in the upper left. Hence, answer (A) is correct.

42. (D)

This question asks for a test shape that belongs to Set A, so the number of sides on the white shape in the upper left must be the same as the number of small white circles on the diagonal. The only answer choices in which these numbers are equal is (D), with 2 small white circles on the diagonal and 2 sides on the white crescent in the upper left, so (D) is correct.

43. (D)

For a test shape to belong to Set B, the number of sides on the black shape must be equal to the number of small white circles on the diagonal. The options here include either 3 or 4 small white circles on the diagonal, but the number of sides on the black shape only corresponds to the number of small white circles in (D), in which there are a black triangle and 3 small white circles. The answer is therefore (D).

44. (B)

This question asks for a test shape that belongs to Set B, so the number of sides on the black shape must be equal to the number of small white circles; unfortunately, this does not eliminate any answers, as both versions of the black shape have 6 sides, and there are 6 small white circles. The other element to the pattern in Set B is that the number of sides of the white shape in the upper left must be 2 more than the number of small white circles, so the correct answer will have 8 sides on the white shape in the upper left. The only choice that has an 8-sided white shape in the upper left is (B), so (B) is correct.

45. (C)

For a test shape to belong to Set A, the number of sides on the white shape in the upper left must be equal to the number of small white circles on the diagonal. The choices here include either 3 or 4 white circles on the diagonal, but the only white shape in the upper left with a corresponding number of sides is the parallelogram in (C); (C) is therefore correct. Note the importance of checking the question to see whether it is asking about Set A or Set B before answering. In this question, if you hadn't checked and had assumed it was Set B, you would have incorrectly selected (D), which fits the pattern for Set B.

Instead of patterns, Type 2 and Type 3 Abstract questions involve progressions—so you must choose the answer that best completes the progression. Progressions involve the same categories as patterns: types of shapes, features of shapes and arrangements. In the official UKCAT practice questions for Type 2 and Type 3, most elements of the progressions involve arrangement and colour, so students generally find that it's a bit easier to 'see' the progressions than it is to see the patterns.

Each Type 2 question will present a series of 4 boxes in a single row. You are asked to select the answer that completes the series. Thus, you must choose the test shape that correctly comes fifth in the progression.

Each Type 3 question will present two pairs of boxes. The first pair of boxes features a progression, in which there are a number of changes from the first box to the second box. The second pair of boxes will have the same progression, only the second box in the second pair is blank; you must choose the test shape that correctly completes it.

Here are some Kaplan UKCAT top tips for Type 2 and Type 3 questions:

- Patterns are about what is the same in the boxes. Progressions are about what is different in the boxes.

- These questions appear individually, rather than in sets of 5. This means you have only 12 seconds per question, so you must work quickly and eliminate ruthlessly. Thus, as soon as you note one element of the progression, eliminate the answer choices that do not present this correctly.

- Do not attempt to identify all elements of the progression before checking the answer choices. Doing so makes each question take a minute or longer.

Attack the next 4 questions, and try to answer all of them in a minute or less. This means no more than 15 seconds per question. **NB** These will include a mix of Type 2 and Type 3 questions, so be sure to look for progressions, rather than patterns!

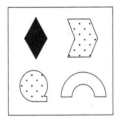 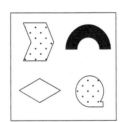 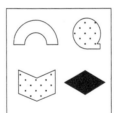 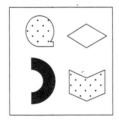

46. Which figure completes the series?

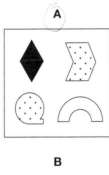
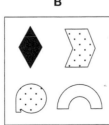
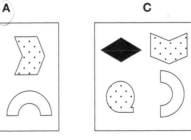
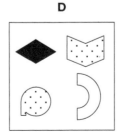

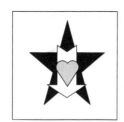

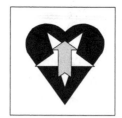
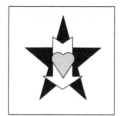

47. Which figure completes the series?

A

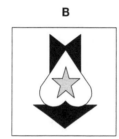

C

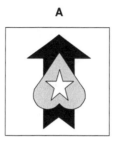

B

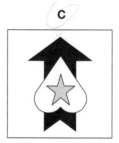

D

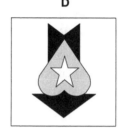

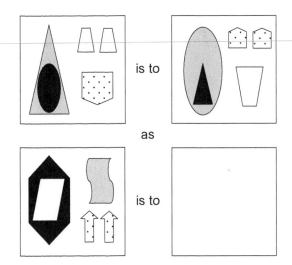

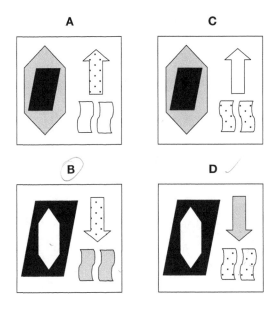

48. Which figure completes the statement?

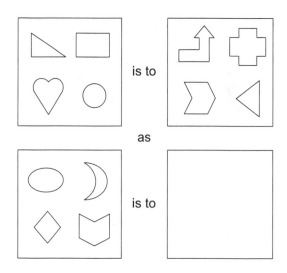

is to

as

is to

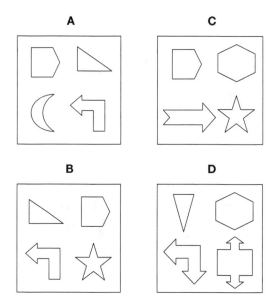

49. Which figure completes the statement?

A

C

B

D

46. (D)

Each box contains the same 4 shapes, which rotate anticlockwise by one position with each subsequent box in the progression. When a shape moves to the lower left position, it rotates 90° to the right. Thus, the correct answer will have the diamond in the upper left, and it will be rotated 90° from its position in the first box; eliminate (A) and (B). The 'Q' shape moves to the lower left after the fourth box, meaning that it will have rotated 90° in the final box. Therefore, the correct answer is (D). There is another element to the progression here, in that the shading moves clockwise by one position with each subsequent box, but it is not necessary to notice this to find the correct answer.

47. (C)

The small shape at the front of each box becomes the medium middle shape in the next box, while the medium middle shape enlarges and moves to the back, and the large back shape becomes the small front shape. The colour is relative to position, so that the front shape is always grey, the middle shape white, and the back shape black. The middle shape is always flipped vertically from its usual orientation. Thus, the correct answer will have a small grey star in front, a white heart pointing upwards in the middle, and a large black arrow pointing upwards in the back. (C) is correct.

48. (B)

The two shapes at the left switch size and position, so that the medium-sized inside shape in the first box becomes the large shape in the second box, and vice versa; these two shapes also switch shading. Thus, the large black hexagon at the left of the third box must become the medium inside shape in the correct answer; since the original medium inside shape is white, the medium-sized hexagon must also be white. Eliminate (A) and (C). The shapes at the right switch position, top and bottom, and retain their original shading; the single medium-sized shape becomes two smaller shapes, and the two smaller shapes become one medium-sized shape. Answer (B) is correct.

49. (D)

Each box contains 4 white shapes, and the shapes in the first and second boxes are entirely different. This means that the type of shape cannot be part of the progression. Compare the shapes in the same relative position in the first and second boxes: the upper left shape changes from a triangle to a bent arrow, the upper right shape changes from a rectangle to a cross, the lower right shape changes from a circle to a triangle, and the lower left shape changes from a heart to a chevron. Each shape in the second box, then, has three times as many sides as the shape in the same position in the first box. The shapes in the third box (going clockwise, starting in the upper left) have 1, 2, 6 and 4 sides, respectively, so the shapes in the correct answer must have 3, 6, 18 and 12 sides. The correct answer is therefore (D). Answer (C) is a trap answer, as each shape in (C) has 4 more sides than the corresponding shape in the same position in the third box; whilst this is a logical progression, it is not the same as the progression from the first box to the second box. You must first find the progression from the first box to the second box, then apply it to the third box to work out the correct answer.

On the next four pages, you will complete a timed Kaplan UKCAT Abstract Reasoning quiz, consisting of 4 sets with 5 test shapes each. Pace yourself, and spend no more than 1 minute per set. Even if you find yourself running out of time near the end, make your best guess based on any partial patterns you can find. It is essential that you get in the mindset of marking an answer for every question, and that you practise doing so as you complete several sets under UKCAT time pressure.

Before you begin the quiz, let's review the Kaplan top tips for Abstract mastery.

Know the common pattern categories. There are only so many building blocks for the patterns that the UKCAT can present on Test Day. Eventually you will develop an 'eye' for all of them. Be sure to consider the types of shapes, features of shapes and arrangement when you first examine each set.

Start with the simplest box in each set. Since the simplest box in each set must contain the pattern, starting with this box will prevent you from becoming lost in distractor shapes and allow you to quickly eliminate pattern categories.

Search for simple patterns first. Don't assume every set is going to be high difficulty. The truth is that you will see many straightforward sets on Test Day. Picking up all (or most) of these marks will ensure you do very well in the Abstract section.

If an aspect of a set seems very unusual, it's probably part of the pattern. If you do see an unusual feature, focus in on it. It is unlikely to have been included to distract you and is almost certainly part of the pattern.

Type 2 and Type 3 questions are about progressions, not patterns. Progressions are about what is different from one box to the next, so these are generally a bit easier to spot than patterns. However, don't fall for the common trap of identifying all elements of a progression before checking the answers. As soon as you see one element of the progression—a change in colour, or a rotation or 'moving' shape—go straight to the answers and eliminate those that do not match that element. The progression in most Type 2 and Type 3 questions will have 4 or more elements, but you can answer virtually any of them by finding only 2 or 3 elements of the progression. Don't do any work beyond the minimum necessary to determine the correct answer.

Be ruthless in moving forward. The wisest test-taker knows when a set has been designed to trap test-takers into wasting time. If you've spent a minute on a set, take a guess and move on. Mark the questions for review and, instead of feeling upset that you couldn't see the pattern, feel happy that you didn't fall into the trap of wasting time, as so many other test-takers will have done.

Set your timer for 5 minutes. Try to evaluate all 20 test shapes and mark an answer for each before time is up. If a pattern is difficult, don't spend much more than a minute; mark an answer, make your best guess and move on to the other sets. Use any time remaining to come back to sets where you had difficulty in spotting the pattern.

Set A   **Set B**

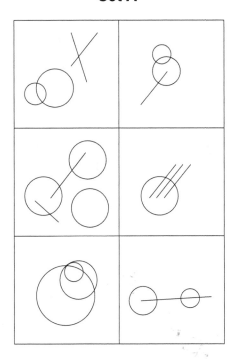 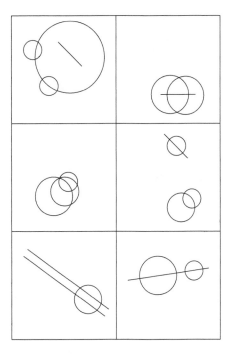

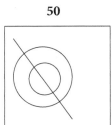 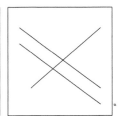

Test Shapes

50	51	52	53	54

A. Set A	A. Set A	A. Set A	A. Set A	A. Set A
B. Set B	B. Set B	B. Set B	B. Set B	B. Set B
C. Neither	C. Neither	C. Neither	C. Neither	C. Neither

Set A   **Set B**

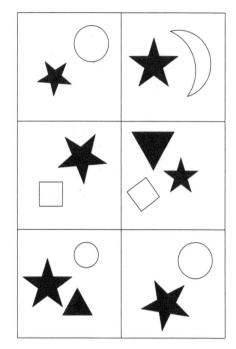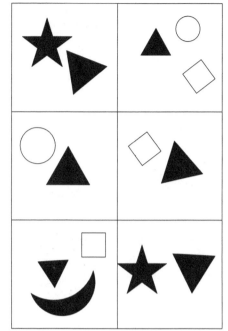

Test Shapes

55	56	57	58	59

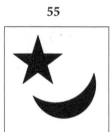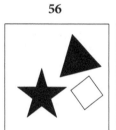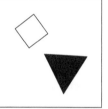

55	56	57	58	59
A. Set A	A. Set A	A. Set A	A. Set A	A. Set A
B. Set B	B. Set B	B. Set B	B. Set B	B. Set B
C. Neither	C. Neither	C. Neither	C. Neither	C. Neither

Set A   **Set B**

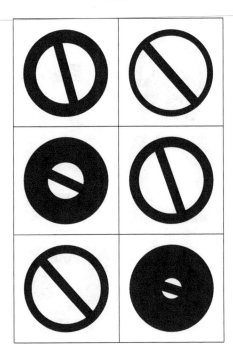 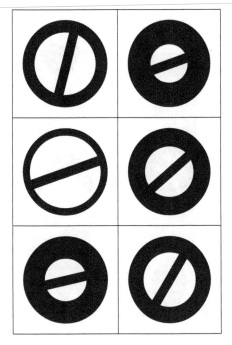

Test Shapes

60	61	62	63	64

 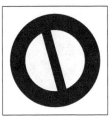 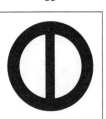 

A. Set A   A. Set A   A. Set A   A. Set A   A. Set A
B. Set B   B. Set B   B. Set B   B. Set B   B. Set B
C. Neither   C. Neither   C. Neither   C. Neither   C. Neither

Set A **Set B**

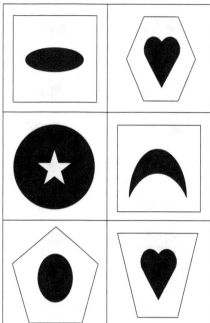 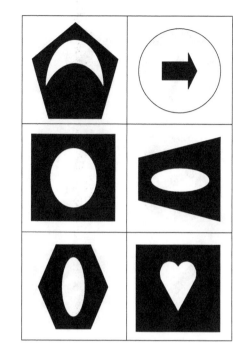

Test Shapes

65	66	67	68	69

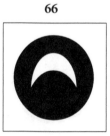  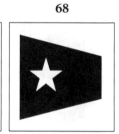 

A. Set A
B. Set B
C. Neither

A. Set A
B. Set B
C. Neither

A. Set A
B. Set B
C. Neither

A. Set A
B. Set B
C. Neither

A. Set A
B. Set B
C. Neither

STOP. IF YOU FINISH BEFORE TIME IS UP, CHECK ANY QUESTIONS YOU HAVE MARKED FOR REVIEW. YOU MAY GO BACK TO QUESTIONS IN THIS QUIZ ONLY.

50. (B)

Both sets contain lots of intersecting circles and lines If you see an unusual characteristic such as intersecting shapes, focus in on that feature as a potential pattern. Both sets contain circles. Each box in Set A includes 3 intersection points, while each box in Set B includes 4 intersection points. The first test shape has 4 intersections, so belongs to Set B.

51. (C)

There are 6 intersections in this test shape, so it belongs to neither set.

52. (A)

This test shape contains 3 intersections, so it belongs to Set A.

53. (B)

This test shape has 4 intersections. Therefore it belongs to Set B.

54. (C)

There isn't a circle in this test shape, and there are only 2 intersections, so this test shape belongs to neither set.

55. (A)

Each box in Set A contains a black star. Each box in Set B contains a black triangle. The first test shape contains a black star and no black triangle, so the correct answer is (A).

56. (C)

This test shape contains both a black star and a black triangle, so it fits the patterns for both sets. The correct answer is therefore (C).

57. (B)

This test shape contains a black triangle and no black star, so it belongs to Set B.

58. (C)

This test shape contains a white triangle, so it doesn't fit the pattern for Set B. The correct answer is (C).

59. (B)

This test shape contains a black triangle and no black star, so it belongs to Set B.

60. (C)

The sets here are very similar looking—remember to consider an arrangement pattern when the sets contain identical shapes. The lines in Set A are downward-sloping, while the lines in Set B are upward-sloping. The first test shape has two crossed lines. This is clearly different from Set A and Set B, so the correct answer is (C).

61. (B)

This test shape has a line that slopes upward. The correct answer is (B).

62. (A)

The downward-sloping line means this test shape belongs to Set A.

63. (C)

The line in this shape is vertical, so it cannot belong to either set. The answer is (C).

64. (B)

This test shape has an upward-sloping line, so the answer is (B).

65. (B)

Both Set A and Set B have a small shape contained within a large shape. Consider conditional patterns in this situation. In Set A, if the shape is curved, it is shaded; if it is straight, it is white. In Set B, if the shape is straight, it is shaded; if it is curved, it is white. The inside/outside feature is irrelevant to the shading. The first test shape has a straight shaded shape with a white curved shape inside. This fits the pattern for Set B.

66. (C)

There is a shaded curved shape and a white curved shape, so this doesn't fit either set.

67. (A)

This test shape contains a straight white shape and a curved shaded shape, so it belongs to Set A.

68. (C)

This test shape contains a shaded straight shape and a white straight shape, so it belongs to neither set.

69. (B)

The white curved shape is contained within a black straight shape. The correct answer is (B).

6

Decision Analysis

The Task

Decision Analysis is the fourth scored subtest on the UKCAT. The Decision Analysis section includes a table of codes with a total of 28 questions. You have 1 minute to read the instructions, and then 33 minutes to review the table of codes and answer the questions, making your best judgement based on your understanding of the code. Part of the way through the section, the table will expand to include additional information in the form of new codes; these will approximately double the number of codes. If you take a minute to review the initial table, and another minute when the additional codes are added, then you will have 1 minute to answer each question in this section. It can be very difficult to evaluate each question and the 5 accompanying answers in a minute, so a strategic approach to this section is essential.

The Format

The Decision Analysis section will present a table of codes with several columns. The table will include a passage explaining the origin of the code, and also a couple of example questions that indicate which answer is correct, and the reasons that the wrong answers are wrong. Reviewing the example questions briefly can be very helpful to see how the code works, especially if there are any difficult operators. There is no need to read the passage, as all of the codes work in the same way, and the specific story is irrelevant to answering the questions.

Approximately two-thirds to three-quarters of the questions in this section will present a message written in code, with parts of the message separated by commas, or grouped together with brackets. You must select the answer that best 'interprets' the coded message into English. The correct answer will not be a literal translation of the message, though noting the literal translation on your noteboard (or in your head, when pressed for time) will help in eliminating answers that omit elements from the coded message, or that include elements that are not in the message. Only one answer will include all the elements from the coded message, with the same groupings, without any extra elements. So you will have to proceed by eliminating the wrong answers. This is what makes the Decision Analysis section so time-consuming.

Most of the remaining questions will be 'reversed'. These will present a message in English and five answers in code. Proceed by elimination, comparing the parts of each answer to the original message and to the table to determine which answer is the best fit for the message.

A few questions will ask you to add two new words to the table of codes. You will have to determine which two of the five answers are the most essential additions for encoding a message. Three answers will not be essential. Again, you will proceed by eliminating these.

In 2013, the UKCAT trialled 'confidence ratings' in Decision Analysis. After answering each question, you are asked to rate your confidence that the answer you gave was correct, on a scale from 1 to 5 (low to high). The ratings are a row of buttons marked 1 to 5 that appear under each question. As this was a trial in 2013, it is not clear if the confidence ratings will be part of Decision Analysis in 2014 or future years, or how your responses to confidence ratings will be used by medical schools. Check the UKCAT website for more information in the year you sit the exam. If confidence ratings are included, then provide them quickly and honestly. It's not worth wasting time worrying about how your ratings will be interpreted. The marks come from answering the questions.

The Challenges

Timing in the Decision Analysis section is much greater than in the other sections, and also somewhat deceptive: because you have an entire minute per question, the timing will likely 'feel' quite a lot slower than in the other sections, and there is the danger that you will slow down your approach a bit too much, in part due to the elaborate nature of some of the messages and codes, and in part due to fatigue. Remember, you will have answered over 100 questions in the hour before Decision Analysis. Take a few seconds to stretch in your seat and rest your eyes during the minute for instructions, so you are fresh for this section.

Decision Analysis is also a bit different from the other sections in that there are three very distinct question types, so three different approaches are required. All questions require you to eliminate, after comparing the messages to the answers and to the table. All also require judgement calls: each question in this section includes a 'best' answer (or answers, in the case of a question that adds new words), but no question will have a 'perfect' answer.

Kaplan Top Tips for Decision Analysis

1. Copy out the codes exactly

This is the initial step for most questions: write out a literal translation on your whiteboard. In doing so, keep the parts of the message separate (with commas) or grouped together (with brackets), as in the original message. When one code modifies another without brackets—for instance, A6—copy it out with brackets, to reflect the modification: A6 = increase(time).

2. Eliminate answers that do not have the same codes (and same groupings) as the message

Once you copy out the codes, compare the answers to the translated message, and eliminate any answers that miss out codes that are in the message. Eliminate as well any answers that include codes that are in the table but not in the message, or that include elements that go beyond what is included in the message. Usually, forms of the verb 'to be' and basic prepositions and directional words (like 'in' or 'on') do not require elements in the code; double-check the table, though, as sometimes directional words are included.

3. Check the operators to see if these create any 'new' terms

Some codes in the 'Operators' column are very powerful, because they can create many new terms. It is worth checking on these when you first see the table, and again when additional info is added. The most powerful operators in this regard are Opposite—which can form the opposite of any code that has an opposite—and Increase; increase (lake) could mean 'a bigger lake', 'more lake', 'lakes' or something larger than a lake (like an ocean), depending on the code and the context of the message. Negative is also a powerful operator, though you should not assume that Negative can form opposites. Negative usually means 'not' or 'bad'.

4. Work with one part of the message at a time

This is the basic approach for 'reversed' questions, which will feature five answer choices with coded messages. Find a part of the coded message that is the same or similar in multiple answers, and determine which version is the best fit, based on the code and original message, for that part of the message. Eliminate the answers that are not a good fit for that part of the message. This approach will also help with questions in the usual format that start with very long messages, and also when you are running out of time. Instead of writing out the entire literal translation, translate one part of the message at a time and eliminate based on that part. Eliminating piece by piece will help save time, and avoid any unnecessary analysis of wrong answers.

5. Check new words against the message and the table

The approach is very similar for questions that ask you to add two new words. First, check that all the answers are needed for the message; eliminate any that are not needed. Next, check the new words against the table to see if any can be represented with the existing codes. This approach is usually sufficient to eliminate all of the wrong answers. If you are left with three or more answers, eliminate those which are less essential to the message.

Now, it is time to put the Kaplan top tips into practice with a timed set over the next few pages.

Set your timer for 5 minutes. Write down answers for the 4 questions before time is up!

Birdwatching Code

You join a local birdwatching society, which meets early every Saturday to observe birds in woodlands near and far. As bird watching requires long hours of waiting in silence, the members of the society communicate with messages written in code. Now that you are a dues-paying member of the society, you are given a table of translations for the code just as you arrive at the local woodland at 7 o'clock on Saturday morning, so you have no option but to determine the code's exact workings without help from the others.

Some of the information will be strange or incomplete but all of the messages contain some logic. You will therefore need to make assessments based on the codes rather than what seems like the most predictable translation. Every code has a best answer that makes the most sense based on all the information presented, but remember that this test requires you to make judgements rather than simply apply logic and rules.

Table of Codes

Operators & General Rules	Specific Information Basic Codes
A = increase	1 = bird
B = opposite	2 = tree
C = three	3 = boy
D = personalise	4 = binoculars
E = far	5 = sun
F = difficult	6 = time
	7 = see
	8 = stay
	9 = noise
	10 = green
	11 = sleep

Example 1

What is the best interpretation of the coded message: D, B7, D4

    A. I did not see any birds with my binoculars. *(bird is in the table, but not in the message)*
    B. I did not see a single bird with my binoculars. *(bird is in the table, but not in the message)*
    C. I could not see with my binoculars. *(CORRECT)*
    D. I was blind without my binoculars. *(without is not represented in the message)*
    E. I was blinded by a person with binoculars. *(person is not a good representation of personalise)*

Example 2

What is the best interpretation of the coded message: A1, A11, BA(5(6))

    A. Birds sleep more in winter. *(CORRECT)*
    B. Birds sleep more in summer. *(no representation of opposite)*
    C. A big bird dreams more in winter. *(dream is not a good representation of sleep)*
    D. A big bird sleeps more with less sun. *(no representation of time)*
    E. Birds sleep more with less sun. *(no representation of time)*

1. What is the best interpretation of the coded message: 3, 7, C1, A2
    A. The boys saw birds in the three trees.
    B. The boys saw three birds in the big tree.
    C. The three boys saw a bird in the big tree. ⸱
    D. The boy saw three birds in the forest.
    E. The boy saw a bird three times in the forest.

2. What would be the best way to encode the following message?
Message: It is very hard to see the green bird in the far tree.
    A. F7, 10(1), E2
    B. F7, 10(1), A(E2)
    C. A(F7), E2, A10(1)
    D. 10(1), A(E2), A(F7)
    E. 10(1), E2, A(F7)

3. What is the best interpretation of the coded message: A3, B4, B(8, B9)
    A. The boys without binoculars would not keep quiet.
    B. The boys with the telescope went quietly.
    C. The man without binoculars will go quietly.
    D. The man with the telescope would not keep quiet.
    E. The boys without binoculars will go with great noise.

4. Which of the following would be the most useful and second most useful additions to the codes in order to convey the message accurately?
Message: At night, the black finch kept the girl awake.
    A. night
    B. black
    C. finch
    D. girl
    E. awake

How did you get on? As you'll see below, elimination is essential to answering Decision Analysis questions. You need to keep an eye on the table of codes as you work, as answer choices may be incorrect simply because they add in elements that are in the table of codes, but not in the message.

Kaplan Timed Practice Set—*Try the Kaplan Top Tips*: Answers and Explanations

1. (D)

The literal translation is *boy, see, three(bird), increase(tree)*. The first element of the message is boy; eliminate (A) and (B), which instead have boys (which would require an additional element, such as increase), and also (C), which has three boys, as the three element in the message modifies bird, not boy. The only difference between the remaining answers is 'three birds' in (D) and 'a bird three times' in (E). Since the table includes time, but it is not in the message here, (E) cannot be correct. The answer is therefore (D).

2. (E)

When the answers contain coded messages, you must work backwards. The quickest way to do this is to compare answers, grouping by grouping. The first grouping in the first three answers is F7, difficult(see), or A(F7), increase(difficult(see)); the final two answers have A(F7) at the end. The message states that it is very hard to see, so increase is required; eliminate (A) and (B). The next element is E2, far(tree), or A(E2), increase(far(tree)). The message includes 'far tree', so eliminate (D). The final element is 10(1), green(bird), or A10(1), increase(green(bird)). The message has a green bird, so the correct answer must be (E).

3. (A)

The literal translation is *increase(boy), opposite(binoculars), opposite(stay, opposite(noise))*. The first element could mean boys or man, so it does not help in eliminating answers. The second element could mean 'without binoculars', but it could not mean 'with a telescope', as a telescope is not the opposite of binoculars. Eliminate (B) and (D). The final element is complicated, so the correct answer will represent the opposite of the concepts within the brackets grouped together. The opposite of noise is quiet, so the final element means the opposite of staying quiet. (C) gives the opposite of stay, go, but keeps quiet as a separate element, rather than including it in the overall opposite. (E) describes the noise as great, but this would require an additional element, such as increase. (A) has a final element that means the opposite of staying quiet, and does not commit any errors, so it is correct.

4. (B) and (C)

To determine the most useful new words, first check to see which answers can be represented by the existing code. Night could be the opposite of sun time, or 6(B5). Girl could be opposite of boy, or B3. Awake could be opposite of sleep, or B11. Eliminate (A), (D) and (E). There is no way to represent black or finch, so the correct answers must be (B) and (C).

Now, let's move on and consider some of the challenges posed by difficult messages.

Many challenging Decision Analysis questions will present messages that are difficult to evaluate in only a minute. Messages can be difficult for any number of reasons:

- They may be very long.
- They may include the same element more than once.
- They may combine elements from the table in complex or unexpected ways.

For many messages, the greatest challenge lies in the long and complicated answers. When evaluating a long or difficult answer, make sure that:

- The answer includes all the elements from the message, with the same groupings (commas and brackets) as the original message.
- The answer does not include any elements that are in the table but not the message.
- The answer does not include any elements that would require elements that are not in the message (or not in the table).

Additionally, for questions that add new words to the code, check whether any of the answers can be used to form other answers, along with existing elements in the code. Sometimes, this is the only way you can reduce the options down to two.

Here are four questions with difficult messages, based on the Birdwatching Code. As you practise, try to eliminate the wrong choices and mark the correct one before reading the answer.

Table of Codes

Operators & General Rules	Specific Information Basic Codes
A = increase B = opposite C = three D = personalise E = far F = difficult	1 = bird 2 = tree 3 = boy 4 = binoculars 5 = sun 6 = time 7 = see 8 = stay 9 = noise 10 = green 11 = sleep

5. What is the best interpretation of the coded message: 7(1), F4, BF(1, A9)

    A. Birdwatching is difficult with binoculars, but easy with bird calls.
    B. Birdwatching is difficult with binoculars, but easy when birds are noisy.
    C. Birds can be easy to hear when they can't be seen.
    D. You can't see birds with binoculars, but you can hear them.
    E. A bird has trouble seeing with binoculars, but has an easy time making more noise.

Answer: The literal translation is *bird(see), difficult(binoculars), opposite(difficult) (bird, increase(noise))*. The first two answers follow the grouping of the first two parts of the message, so hold on to those for now. Of the others, (C) omits binoculars; (D) includes you, but personalise is in the table but not in the message; and (E) mixes the individual elements from the first two parts of the message, so that bird goes with difficult and see with binoculars; eliminate (C), (D) and (E). The only difference between (A) and (B) comes at the very end; since increase modifies noise and not bird, the correct answer must be (A).

6. What is the best interpretation of the coded message: D3, B7, 5, BE

    A. I could not see my son because the sun was near.
    B. My son did not see because the sun was very near.
    C. My son did not see because the sun was near.
    D. The sun was very near, so my son could not see.
    E. The sun was near, so I could not see my son.

Answer: The literal translation is *personalise(boy), opposite(see), sun, opposite(far)*. All the answers give the first part of the message as 'my son', and the second part as 'not see'. Since the message only includes the personalise element once, answers that include it more than once cannot be correct; on this basis, eliminate (A) and (E). The only significant difference among the remaining answers is in how they interpret the final element. The opposite of far is near, but (B) and (D) have 'very near', which would seem to require increase—which is in the table, but not in the message. As such, (B) and (D) must be wrong, and the answer is (C).

7. What would be the best way to encode the following message?

Message: Two birds left in spring.

    A. A10, (BA)C1, B8

    B. A10, 1, 1, B8

    C. 6(5), (BA)C1, B8

    D. 6(5), 1, 1, B8

    E. 6(A10), (BA)C1, B8

Answer: Find the parts of the answers that give different versions of the same part of the message, and compare to see which is the best fit. The first part of each answer appears to represent the concept of spring. The first two answers represent spring as A10, increase(green), the next two as 6(5), time(sun), and the final answer as 6(A10), time (increase(green)). You may recall that one of the examples for this code represented the concept of winter as opposite(increase(sun(time))). Thus, a season would seem to involve the code for time, so eliminate (A) and (B). Time(sun) could be day or summer, not necessarily spring; spring is a time when green things grow, so (E) is the best fit, and therefore correct. Notice that we were able to evaluate without considering the other elements of the answers, which was a major time-saver here.

---

8. Which of the following would be the most useful and second most useful additions to the codes in order to convey the message accurately?

Message: Your dreams are better when birds are good and quiet.

    A. you

    B. dream

    C. better

    D. good

    E. quiet

Answer: All the answers are included in the message, so eliminate any that you can form with the existing code. Quiet appeared in a correct answer for a previous question, so it can be formed with the existing code; eliminate (E). You could be formed by personalise or opposite(personalise), so eliminate (A). Better and good are similar, and in fact you could form better by adding good to the table, and then representing better as increase(good). There is no way to represent dream, so the correct answers are (B) and (D).

Set your timer for 6 minutes. Try to mark answers for all 5 questions before time runs out.

Victorian Detective Code

Your flatmate joins a secret society dedicated to studying the life and habits of a Victorian detective, with a legendary reputation for solving the most mind-boggling and brutal crimes of London's cobble-stoned past. Following the eccentric custom of their nineteenth-century hero, members of the society communicate with messages written in an unusual code. On a lazy Sunday afternoon, you discover that your flatmate has left the table of translations for the code in the lounge. Your flatmate has gone down to the pub for a Sunday roast with many rounds of darts to follow (again, in the detective's custom), so you decide to determine the code's exact workings without any help.

Some of the information will be strange or incomplete but all of the messages contain some logic. You will therefore need to make assessments based on the codes rather than what seems like the most predictable translation. Every code has a best answer that makes the most sense based on all the information presented, but remember that this test requires you to make judgements rather than simply apply logic and rules.

Table of Codes

Operators & General Rules	Specific Information Basic Codes
A = negative	1 = fog
B = increase	2 = fire
C = several	3 = street
D = full	4 = blood
E = royal	5 = house
F = deception	6 = horse
G = murder	7 = man
H = along	8 = girl
	9 = take
	10 = make
	11 = money
	12 = bread
	13 = door
	14 = servant
	15 = diamond

Example 1

What is the best interpretation of the coded message: 7G, 10, 13, D4

A. The murderer made the door bloody. *(no representation of full)*

B. The murderer made the door all bloody. *(CORRECT)*

C. Whoever murdered the man made the door full of blood. *(whoever is not represented in the message)*

D. The murdered man made the door bloody. *(no representation of full)*

E. The murdered man bloodied the door. *(no representation of make or full)*

Example 2

What is the best interpretation of the coded message: A8, A9, 6(AA)

A. The boy took the good horse. *(negative modifies take in the message, but not in the answer)*

B. The horse that the bad boy took wasn't bad. *(negative girl cannot be interpreted as bad boy)*

C. No girl took the good horse. *(negative modifies take in the message, but not in the answer)*

D. The bad girl did not take the very bad horse. *(increase is in the table, but not the message)*

E. The bad girl did not take the good horse. *(CORRECT)*

9. What is the best interpretation of the coded message: C15, A9, E(11(5)), 2

    A. During the fire, diamonds were stolen from the palace.
    B. The fire damaged the palace at a cost of several diamonds.
    C. During the fire, diamonds were stolen from the royal bank.
    D. The royal diamonds were not taken from the bank during the fire.
    E. During the fire, the royal banker stole several diamonds.

10. What is the best interpretation of the coded message: B(C3), D(1, F)

    A. Fog and trickery fill the city's streets.
    B. The streets are fuller of fog than of lies.
    C. The streets are very full of fog and trickery.
    D. All the streets are full of fog and trickery.
    E. All the streets are full of fog and lies.

11. What would be the best way to encode the following message?

Message: The princess took the horse from the stable.

    A. E8, 9(6), 6(5)
    B. E, 9(6), 5
    C. E8, 9, 6, 5
    D. E, 9(6), 6(5)
    E. E(A7), 9, 6, 5

12. What is the best interpretation of the coded message: 14(8), G(7,10(12)), 9(11(7))

    A. The maid took along the banker to murder the baker.
    B. The maid killed the baker and took his money.
    C. The maid took along the banker when she killed the baker.
    D. The baker was killed by his maid because he stole her money.
    E. The maid murdered the baker who stole her money.

13. Which of the following would be the most useful and second most useful additions to the codes in order to convey the message accurately?

Message: A penniless man wants justice, not riches or mansions.

    A. penny
    B. less
    C. want
    D. justice
    E. mansion

Questions involving difficult messages can be challenging to answer in only a minute. Reviewing the worked answers that follow will help to ensure that you chose the correct answers for the correct reasons, and will also show you how to eliminate wrong answers most efficiently. Eliminating quickly and accurately—based on comparisons between the message, the answers and the table of codes—is essential to maximising your marks in this section on Test Day.

Kaplan Timed Practice Set—*Difficult Codes*: Answers and Explanations

9. (C)

The literal translation is *several(diamond), negative(take), royal(money(house)), fire*. Four answers include fire in the first part of the message, which is acceptable—the order of the elements separated by commas does not need to be preserved. However, the groupings within commas and brackets must be preserved, and (D) violates this by regrouping royal and diamond together; eliminate (D). (B) interprets the second part of the message as damage, but damage does not make any logical sense as a representation of negative(take); eliminate (B). The remaining answers interpret the second part of the message as stole or stolen; the decisive difference is in how they interpret the third part of the message: palace, royal bank or royal banker. Royal house could mean palace, but this answer does not include a representation of money; eliminate (A). Bank fits conceptually with money(house), and a banker could be a man who works at a money(house), but the message does not include man. Thus, (E) cannot be correct; the correct answer is (C).

10. (D)

The literal translation is *increase(several(street)), full(fog, deception)*. The first part of the message may seem difficult to work with, so start with the second. Three answers include this as 'full of fog and trickery', or 'fog and trickery fill'; eliminate (B) and (E), which give deception as lies, since lies is plural but deception is not modified by several. (C) says that the streets are very full, but increase modifies several(street), not full; eliminate (C). (A) includes city, but none of the terms in the message or the table represent the concept of city; eliminate (A). The correct answer is therefore (D).

11. (A)

The first term in each answer choice starts with E, so compare these to see which is the best fit for the message. The options are royal(girl), royal, or royal(negative(man)). Royal on its own is not specific enough, so eliminate (B) and (D). Negative(man) could mean woman, but it could also mean boy; as such, it is not specific enough, so eliminate (E). The difference between (A) and (C) is that (C) includes 6, horse, only once; (A) includes it twice, modified by 9, take, and modifying 5, house. (C) would therefore mean something like the princess took the horse from the house; (A) would mean the princess took the horse from the horse-house, and the latter fits logically with the concept of stable, which is in the message. The answer is (A).

12. (B)

The literal translation is *servant(girl), murder(man, make(bread)), take(money(man))*. All the answers interpret the first part of the message as maid and murder(man, make(bread)) as 'murder/kill the baker'. (A) and (C) also include a banker, but there are two problems with this: first, money(man) is not necessarily a banker; second, and more decisively, these answers also include 'along', which is H in the table but is not included in the message. Eliminate (A) and (C). (D) and (E) end with 'stole her money', but this does not fit the message, because money modifies man, and also because take on its own is not sufficient to represent the concept of stealing; the correct answer for question 9 used negative(take) to encode this concept, but negative is not part of this message. Eliminate (D) and (E), and the answer must be (B).

13. (C) and (D)

All the answers are included in the message, so check to see if any can be represented with the existing code. Mansion could be represented as house, 5, so eliminate (E). Penniless could be represented as A11, negative(money), or 'no money'; eliminate (A) and (B). There is no way to represent want or justice with the code, so the answers are (C) and (D).

Good work with these tricky messages! Next, we'll consider some of the factors that make a table of codes difficult, and some of the most challenging codes you might see on Test Day.

Difficult Codes

Decision Analysis messages can be even more challenging when they involve difficult codes. There are a number of things that can make codes difficult:

- Some codes can form many possible new meanings, in combination with various other codes in the table (e.g. Opposite).

- The possible application of some codes can be uncertain or confusing, even once you check the examples (e.g. Can Negative form an opposite, or can it only mean something like 'not' or 'bad'?).

- Some codes can be unusual and form new meanings in unexpected ways.

- Codes can combine in a very idiomatic way; that is, the combined meaning of the codes may go beyond their original meanings, but will have to do so in a way that includes a sense of all the codes included in order for the answer to be correct.

The table of codes will automatically become more complicated when it expands with additional information, which is added sometime in the first half of the section. Normally, the expansion will include two new columns of codes, and may also include new items at the bottom of the existing columns. Whenever the table of codes expands, you should take a minute to look it over, checking for any new codes at the bottom of the original columns, and also taking note of the new codes, particularly if any seem unusual or confusing. Take a minute and look over the expanded Victorian Detective Code:

Table of Codes

Operators & General Rules	Specific Information Basic Codes	Complex Information Additional Information	Reactions/Outcomes Emotions
A = negative	1 = fog	101 = dagger	201 = guilty
B = increase	2 = fire	102 = police	202 = sweet
C = several	3 = street	103 = engine	203 = cross
D = full	4 = blood	104 = Prussian	204 = frightened
E = royal	5 = house	105 = river	205 = hard
F = deception	6 = horse	106 = train	206 = jealous
G = murder	7 = man	107 = love	207 = sad
H = along	8 = girl	108 = push	
J = generalise	9 = take	109 = ink	
K = personalise	10 = make	110 = paper	
	11 = money	111 = mark	
	12 = bread	112 = red	
	13 = door		
	14 = servant		
	15 = diamond		
	16 = finger		
	17 = head		
	18 = foot		

The additional information here includes extra codes in the Operators and Specific Info columns, plus two new columns, Complex Info and Reactions/Outcomes. These are the same types of columns you can expect to see on Test Day. The new operators, Generalise and Personalise, are certainly worth noting; these could take a bit of figuring out, as they were not included in the examples at the beginning.

Here are four questions involving difficult codes from the expanded Victorian Detective Code. Continue to practise by eliminating wrong choices, and try to answer each question in a minute before reading the worked answer.

Table of Codes

Operators & General Rules	Specific Information Basic Codes	Complex Information Additional Information	Reactions/Outcomes Emotions
A = negative	1 = fog	101 = dagger	201 = guilty
B = increase	2 = fire	102 = police	202 = sweet
C = several	3 = street	103 = engine	203 = cross
D = full	4 = blood	104 = Prussian	204 = frightened
E = royal	5 = house	105 = river	205 = hard
F = deception	6 = horse	106 = train	206 = jealous
G = murder	7 = man	107 = love	207 = sad
H = along	8 = girl	108 = push	
J = generalise	9 = take	109 = ink	
K = personalise	10 = make	110 = paper	
	11 = money	111 = mark	
	12 = bread	112 = red	
	13 = door		
	14 = servant		
	15 = diamond		
	16 = finger		
	17 = head		
	18 = foot		

14. What is the best interpretation of the coded message: 102, 9, C16(10, 109(111), 110), 201(7)
   A. Police took the guilty man to sign his confession.
   B. Police made the guilty man take the pen in hand and mark the paper.
   C. Police took the guilty man by the hand to be fingerprinted.
   D. Police fingerprinted the guilty man.
   E. Police took the guilty man's fingerprints.

Answer: The literal translation is *police, take, several(finger)(make, ink(mark), paper), guilty(man)*. All the answers include the first two parts of the message except for (D), which omits a representation of take; eliminate (D). All the answers include the final part of the message as guilty man. Therefore, you must eliminate based on the long third part of the message, which is grouped with brackets into a single element. Several fingers could be a hand, or could combine with the rest of the element to mean fingerprints, as fingerprints are ink marks made on paper by several fingers. The correct answer cannot have both hand and fingerprint, as several(finger) occurs once in the message, so eliminate (C). (A) does not include a representation of several(finger), so eliminate (A). The difference between (B) and (E) is fairly subtle; (E) combines all the codes in the third part of the message into a single concept, which fits with how they are grouped together; (B) keeps them mostly separate, and incorrectly interprets ink as pen. Since ink cannot mean pen—they are not logically the same—(B) cannot be correct. The answer is therefore (E).

---

15. What is the best interpretation of the coded message: 104E, 206, K(6, 112J (C15))
   A. The Prussian king was jealous of my horse and red rubies.
   B. The Prussian duke was jealous of my horse and red jewels.
   C. The Prussian duke wanted to take my horse and red jewels.
   D. The Prussian king envies horses and red jewels.
   E. The Prussian duke was envious of my horse and red rubies.

Answer: The literal translation is *Prussian(royal), jealous, personalise(horse, red(generalise(several(diamond))))*. Royal is not terribly specific, so there is no logical difference between king and duke. The first part of the message does not eliminate any answers. The second, jealous, may also appear at first glance to be used properly in all the answers, but note that 'wanted to take' in (C) includes take, which is 9 in the table, but is not in the message; eliminate (C). The personalise operator applies both to the horse and to the complicated final grouping; eliminate (D), which omits a representation of personalise. The final element, diamonds, would generalise to something like jewels, which fits with the interpretation in (B). Diamonds cannot generalise to rubies, as they are both specific types of jewels, and (A) and (E) both include 'red' as a separate element from rubies. The correct answer is therefore (B).

16. What is the best interpretation of the coded message: 203(7), A107, 8F, A108, 8, 106
    A. The angry man hated the lying girl, so he pulled her from the train.
    B. The man did not love the lying girl, and did not push her from the train.
    C. The angry man did not love the lying girl, but did not push her from the train.
    D. Angry with the unlovable, lying girl, the man pushed her onto a train.
    E. Although angry with the lying girl, the man did not hate her enough to push her from the train.

Answer: When a message is very long, it's usually best to work one term at a time, or otherwise you could risk using most of your minute copying out the literal translation. In this case, the first term, angry(man), is enough to eliminate (B), which does not include angry, and to make us very suspicious of (D), which separates angry and man into different parts of the sentence. The second term, negative(love), might mean hate, if the code allows negative to form an opposite, so keep (A) for now; 'did not love' and 'unlovable' in (C) and (D) are a good fit, but 'did not hate' in (E) requires an extra negative—one to form hate, and another for not—so eliminate (E). 8F, girl(deception), is given as lying girl in all the remaining answers. A108, negative(push), might mean pull (again, if negative equals opposite), and fits well with 'did not push' in (C); (D) is eliminated, as it omits the negative. The final elements, girl and train, are included in both (A) and (C). Of these, (A) seems questionable, as it uses negative to mean opposite twice; however, there is a more solid reason to eliminate (A): it includes 'he' as the subject of pulled, but there is no second representation of man in the message, even though 'girl' is given a second time to represent 'her' in this part of the message. (C) does not include any questionable or missing elements, and is therefore correct. **NB** The two wrong answers that were hardest to eliminate seemed a bit off when their first two terms were evaluated, so you could have eliminated them on that basis if you were tight on time.

17. Which of the following would be the most useful and second most useful additions to the codes in order to convey the message accurately?
Message: The police chief's hardened face is the front door to his heart.
    A. chief
    B. harden
    C. face
    D. front
    E. heart

Answer: All the answers appear in the message, so check to see which can be represented with the existing code. Hard, 205, could be used for harden, so eliminate (B). Police chief could be coded as head(police), 17(102), so eliminate (A). The three remaining answers cannot be represented with the code, so see if one can be used along with the code to form one of the others. You could say that the face is the front of the head; if you add front to the code—as, say, L—you could represent face as front(head), or L17. Eliminate (C), and the correct answers are therefore (D) and (E).

Set your timer for 7 minutes. Try to answer all 6 questions before time is up. If a question is very difficult, try to eliminate as many answers as you can before making your best guess.

Beekeeper Code

You spend the summer working on your uncle's farm as an apprentice beekeeper. On your first day tending the hives, your uncle instructs you to follow the custom of local beekeepers and work in silence. Instead of communicating by speaking, you are to write messages using a table of codes, which your uncle gives you without further explanation before taking up the smoker and setting to work extracting a rather sizable honeycomb. As a result, you decide to let your uncle proceed with his very dedicated work with the bees whilst you determine the code's exact workings without any input.

Some of the information will be strange or incomplete but all of the messages contain some logic. You will therefore need to make assessments based on the codes rather than what seems like the most predictable translation. Every code has a best answer that makes the most sense based on all the information presented, but remember that this test requires you to make judgements rather than simply apply logic and rules.

Table of Codes

Operators & General Rules	Specific Information Basic Codes	Complex Information Additional Information	Reactions/Outcomes Emotions
A = big	1 = bee	101 = queen	201 = busy
B = swarm	2 = honey	102 = drone	202 = hungry
C = female	3 = move	103 = yellow	203 = lazy
D = negative	4 = flower	104 = die	204 = frisky
E = opposite	5 = hive	105 = human	205 = risky
F = keep	6 = give	106 = collect	206 = angry
G = among	7 = make	107 = protect	207 = tired
	8 = eat	108 = wax	
	9 = work	109 = different	
	10 = sting	110 = rush	
	11 = pollen		
	12 = nectar		
	13 = leaf		
	14 = grow		
	15 = fly		

Example 1

What is the best interpretation of the coded message: 1, 3, 4, 4

      A. The bee moved among the flowers. *(among is in the table, but not in the message)*
      B. The bees moved among the flowers. *(among is in the table, but not in the message)*
      C. The bees moved from flower to flower. *(CORRECT)*
      D. The bee moved toward the flowers. *(not a good representation of flower, flower)*
      E. The bee moved pollen from flower to flower. *(pollen is in the table, but not in the message)*

Example 2

What is the best interpretation of the coded message: C1, 9, EC1, D9

      A. Female bees work; male bees don't. *(CORRECT)*
      B. Female bees work more than male bees. *(no representation of negative)*
      C. Female bees work to make male bees not work. *(make is in the table, but not in the message)*
      D. Female bees work; male bees play. *(play is the opposite of work, not negative)*
      E. Female worker bees don't like those who don't work. *(don't like is not represented in the message)*

18. What is the best interpretation of the coded message: F1, F4, 14, 1(F8)
    - A. Beekeepers grow flowers to keep bees eating.
    - B. Keeping bees keeps flowers growing, so bees keep eating.
    - C. Beekeepers keep growing flowers, so the bees they keep can keep eating.
    - D. Keeping bees makes flowers keep growing, so bees keep eating.
    - E. Beekeepers keep flowers growing, so bees can eat.

19. What would be the best way to encode the following message?

Message: A frisky queen is almost the same as a hungry queen.
    - A. 204(101), E(109), 202(101)
    - B. 204(101), 202(101), D(109)
    - C. 204(101), D(109), 202(101)
    - D. 204(101), 202(101), EA(109)
    - E. 204(101), A(109), 202(101)

20. What is the best interpretation of the coded message: 1B, 105, 3(108, D2)
    - A. Bees swarm to move wax, but not honey, when humans attack.
    - B. Bees swarm and attack when humans move wax, but not honey.
    - C. A swarm of bees attacks a human who moves wax, but not honey.
    - D. Bees swarm when a human replaces wax with no honey.
    - E. Bees swarm when humans move wax, but not honey.

21. What is the best interpretation of the coded message: 1, 8(A11), A203, D9
    - A. A bee that eats lots of pollen is given a big break from work.
    - B. A bee that eats a very big pollen gets a big break with no work.
    - C. A bee ate lots of pollen, is extremely lazy and won't work.
    - D. Bees that eat too much pollen are lazy and don't work.
    - E. Bees that eat lots of pollen are very lazy, and do little work.

22. Which of the following would be the most useful and second most useful additions to the codes in order to convey the message accurately?

Message: Humans in cities neglect bees, and risk the ecosystem that gives life.
    - A. city
    - B. neglect
    - C. risk
    - D. ecosystem
    - E. life

23. Which of the following would be the most useful and second most useful additions to the codes in order to convey the message accurately?

Message: The beekeeper's face was left undefended after his mask slipped.
    - A. beekeeper
    - B. face
    - C. defend
    - D. mask
    - E. slip

Hopefully you used the examples to get hints on working with difficult codes. The examples on this set showed that there was no distinction between the singular and plural, and also the correct use of the negative operator as distinct from the opposite operator. A few unusual operators—big, swarm and keep—are not included in the examples, so these required special care. Of these, big has the widest range of possible logical meanings and applications; as with any difficult codes, it is essential to make sure that the range of possible meanings does not include something that would have to be represented by a different code in the table.

Kaplan Timed Practice Set—*Difficult Codes*: Answers and Explanations

18. (B)

The literal translation is *keep(bee), keep(flower), grow, bee(keep(eat))*. The answers here are all very similar, so be careful to eliminate those who include the repeated element 'keep' too many times, or too few. Since keep appears three times in the message, the correct answer must include three representations of keep, and in groupings similar to those in the message. On this basis, eliminate (A) and (E), which each include keep twice, and also (C), which includes keep four times. The only major difference between the remaining answers is that (D) includes make, which is 7 in the code but is not in the message. Thus, (D) cannot be correct, and the answer must be (B).

19. (D)

According to the table, 204(101) is frisky(queen) and 202(101) is hungry(queen); these appear in all five answers, so the other term—meaning 'almost the same'—must be decisive. E(109) is opposite(different), meaning 'same', and D(109) is negative(different), or 'not different'; both would mean 'same', rather than 'almost the same', so eliminate answers (A), (B) and (C). A(109) is big(different), which would mean 'very different'; eliminate (E). EA(109) is opposite(big)(different), or small(different); two things with a small difference would be almost the same, so the answer is (D).

20. (E)

The literal translation is *bee(swarm), human, move(wax, negative(honey))*. All the answers include all the elements from the message, with the same groupings. However, four answers also include elements that are not in the message, and that would be difficult to represent with the code. Answers (A), (B) and (C) include 'attack'; it is not clear how this concept would be represented logically by the code, but it would surely require an extra term beyond what is provided in the message; eliminate these answers. Similarly, (D) includes 'replace', which could be understood as partially representing the concept of move, but would require further elements to have the meaning of replace (as replace does not mean the same as move, but rather something like 'move something for something else'). Since replace is not a good fit for move, eliminate (D). The correct answer is therefore (E).

21. (C)

The literal translation is *bee, eat(big(pollen)), big(lazy), negative(work)*. Since the code does not include an operator that forms the plural of nouns, there is no logical distinction in interpreting the first term as bee or bees. The second part of the message is more helpful; big appears to be an operator that can mean a lot of things, but you can eliminate (B), which interprets big(pollen) as 'very big pollen'; logically, this would require a further code—perhaps something like big(big(pollen)). The third part of the message, big(lazy), fits neither (A)—which interprets lazy as 'break', but these are not logically similar—nor (D), which omits a representation of the 'big' modifying lazy. The final part of the message determines the answer: (E) interprets negative as 'little', rather than a negative, and is therefore wrong. The answer must be (C).

22. (A) and (D)

All of the answers appear in the message, so check to see whether or not any can be represented with the existing codes. Risk is already in the table, as 205, risky; eliminate (C). The presence of the opposite operator allows the formation of two further answers: life could be the opposite of dying, or E104; neglect is the opposite of protect, or E107. Eliminate (B) and (E). There is no clear way to represent city or ecosystem with the code, so the correct answers must be (A) and (D).

23. (B) and (E)

All the answers are included in the message, so check the table to consider if any can be represented with the existing code. A beekeeper is a human who keeps bees, so perhaps this could be represented as something like 105(F1); eliminate (A). Defend means the same as protect, 107; eliminate (C). Of the remaining answers, face and mask are related, as a mask is something that covers or protects the face. Thus, if you add face to the table—as, say, 111—you could encode mask as 107(111). As such, face is more essential than mask, so eliminate (D). There is no way to encode slip using the existing code, so the correct answers are (B) and (E).

Keeping Perspective—Decision Analysis

On the next four pages, you will complete a timed Kaplan UKCAT quiz, consisting of 10 Decision Analysis questions. If you pace yourself, and spend no more than 1 minute per question, you should be able to attempt and answer all of them. Even if you find yourself running out of time near the end, do your best to eliminate one or more answers before making your best guess.

Before you begin the quiz, let's consider some of the challenges in Decision Analysis that lead unprepared (or underprepared) test-takers to waste time and earn a lower score:

When answer choices are very similar, or very unusual, check very carefully against the message and the table. Wrong answers are wrong for only a few reasons: they include one or more elements that are in the table but not in the message; they omit one or more elements that are in the message; they regroup elements from the message; they require elements beyond those included in the message or the table. When answers are very similar, the distinction may come down to a single word that makes an answer wrong for one (or more) of these reasons. When answers are very unusual, they are likely to require extra elements, or to recombine elements from the message—so check very carefully.

Keep track of the possibilities of operators—as well as their limits. When presented with a new (or expanded) table, always check to see whether there is a code required to form plurals, and whether the table includes any powerful operators, such as Opposite, Increase, Negative, Personalise or Generalise. These are among the most common operators, and can result in the greatest possible range of new meanings based on elements in the table. Check the examples to note any limits of these operators, e.g. whether Negative can form an opposite.

Use your noteboard to eliminate answers for every question. This point may seem a bit obvious, but you would be surprised how many test-takers try to eliminate in their head, only to lose track of their work or—in the worst case—waste valuable time accidentally re-reading answers that have already been eliminated. Write out the letters ABCDE and cross out as appropriate, as you eliminate answers. A few seconds of notation will save valuable time—and help you to maximise your marks in this section of the UKCAT. Be sure to practise doing this on scrap paper as you prepare for Test Day.

Check the Online Resource Centre and the UKCAT website for any updates in the year you sit the exam. This will ensure you have the latest information about the confidence ratings, and any minor variations in the section. For example, the number of questions has varied slightly from year to year (switching between 26 and 28), but the question format and the timing (1 minute per question) tends to remain consistent. Even so, you'll want to check online to ascertain the current timing, number of questions and any other variations in the year you sit the UKCAT. See page ix.

Set your timer for 12 minutes. Try to evaluate all 10 questions and mark an answer for each before time is up. If a message is very long, or the answers are very difficult to work with, try to eliminate as many answers as possible before making your best guess. Above all, try to spend no more than 1 minute per question.

Baby Code

Whilst volunteering at the local nursery, you discover that some of the babies appear to be highly intelligent; although unable to speak, these babies have developed a method of communicating in a code, using the numbers and letters found on blocks and other toys to 'write' messages. A few days after your initial observations, a very precocious toddler explains the meaning of each letter and number to you, and you note this in a table of codes (shown below), which represents the range of possible elements the very clever babies use in their messages.

All the messages will contain some logic, though some may seem strange or incomplete. Thus, you must make assessments based on the codes rather than what seems the most obvious translation. Every code has a best answer that makes the most sense based on all the information presented, but remember that this test requires you to make judgements rather than simply apply logic and rules.

Table of Codes

Operators & General Rules	Specific Information Basic Codes
A = multiple	1 = baby
B = generalise	2 = boy
C = strained	3 = sing
D = positive	4 = crawl
E = clean	5 = mouth
F = opposite	6 = apricot
G = Mummy	7 = blanket
H = inside	8 = spoon
J = big	9 = sleep
	10 = warm
	11 = milk
	12 = nappy
	13 = lolly
	14 = silly
	15 = make
	16 = take

Example 1

What is the best interpretation of the coded message: A12, FD (JE)

      A. Nappies were extremely dirty. *(no representation of positive)*

      B. Nappies are very dirty. *(no representation of positive)*

      C. The nappy was not clean. *(no representation of multiple or big)*

      D. Nappies are not very clean. *(CORRECT)*

      E. The nappy was extremely dirty. *(no representation of multiple or positive)*

Example 2

What is the best interpretation of the coded message: B (2, F2), D, A (B13)

      A. Children like chocolates. *(lolly does not necessarily generalise to chocolate)*

      B. Kids like sweets. *(CORRECT)*

      C. Children are sweet. *(no representation of positive or multiple)*

      D. Men like sweets. *(does not include opposite of boy; fails to generalise first term properly)*

      E. Children like lollies. *(fails to generalise final term properly)*

24. What is the best interpretation of the coded message: 1, J4, 16(J11, H5)

    A. A baby who likes to crawl drinks a lot of milk.

    B. A baby takes a lot of milk after a big crawl.

    C. Babies who are big crawlers are also big milk drinkers.

    D. A baby with milk in its mouth took a big crawl.

    E. A baby who crawls a lot drinks a lot of milk.

25. What is the best interpretation of the coded message: F(E12), 15(1), 3(FD), F(J9), 15(1), J3(FD)

    A. A dirty nappy makes a baby cry; a short nap makes a baby cry more.

    B. Short naps make babies cry more than dirty nappies.

    C. A short nap makes a baby like to sing less than a dirty nappy.

    D. A baby that doesn't nap or sing makes for a baby with a dirty nappy.

    E. A dirty nappy makes a baby not sing; a short sleep makes a baby sing more.

26. What would be the best way to encode the following message?

Message: The baby girl likes to sleep with a very warm blanket.

    A. 1(FG), J(D9), 7(J10)

    B. 1(F2), J(D9), 7(J10)

    C. 1(F2), D9, 7(J10)

    D. 1(FG), D9, 7(J10)

    E. 1F(JG), D9, 7(J10)

27. What is the best interpretation of the coded message: G(14(3)), 15(1), 16(8(6))

    A. Mummy sang a silly song to make the baby eat a spoonful of apricot.

    B. Mummy's silly song made the baby take a spoon of apricot.

    C. Mummy made the baby sing a silly song about taking an apricot spoon.

    D. Mummy's silly song made the baby eat a spoonful of apricot.

    E. Mummy made the baby sing silly and take the apricot spoon.

New Information Added

After working for several hours, you discover a second set of symbols and their respective translations. You realise that the new symbols affect the interpretation of the previous symbols, and these are as follows:

Operators & General Rules	Specific Information Basic Codes	Complex Information Additional Information	Reactions/Outcomes Emotions
K = new L = command M = before	17 = pram 18 = book 19 = green	101 = Daddy 102 = finger 103 = cuddle 104 = cot 105 = carrot 106 = count 107 = sheep 108 = bear 109 = dummy 110 = doll 111 = ball 112 = block	201 = yummy 202 = scary 203 = happy 204 = quiet 205 = fun 206 = calm 207 = best

The complete table of codes is therefore as follows:

Table of Codes—Complete Code

Operators & General Rules	Specific Information Basic Codes	Complex Information Additional Information	Reactions/Outcomes Emotions
A = multiple B = generalise C = strained D = positive E = clean F = opposite G = Mummy H = inside J = big K = new L = command M = before	1 = baby 2 = boy 3 = sing 4 = crawl 5 = mouth 6 = apricot 7 = blanket 8 = spoon 9 = sleep 10 = warm 11 = milk 12 = nappy 13 = lolly 14 = silly 15 = make 16 = take 17 = pram 18 = book 19 = green	101 = Daddy 102 = finger 103 = cuddle 104 = cot 105 = carrot 106 = count 107 = sheep 108 = bear 109 = dummy 110 = doll 111 = ball 112 = block	201 = yummy 202 = scary 203 = happy 204 = quiet 205 = fun 206 = calm 207 = best

28. What is the best interpretation of the coded message: G, J(J, 1H), M(K1, 16(FH(G)))

    A. Mummy was pregnant before the new baby was born.

    B. Mummy was very pregnant before the new baby was delivered.

    C. Mummy was big with a baby inside before the baby was born.

    D. Mummy was pregnant before the new baby was delivered.

    E. The new baby was very big inside Mummy before being born.

29. What would be the best way to encode the following message?

Message: Don't eat carrots in bed.

    A. FD, 16(H5), A105, H(J104)
    B. L(FD, 16(H5)), A105, H(104)
    C. FD, 16(H5), A105, H(104)
    D. L(FD, 16(H5)), A105, H(J104)
    E. L(16, A105, (H5)), H(J104)

30. What is the best interpretation of the coded message: M9, 101(103, 1(2)), 1(103, 108(2, 207))

    A. Before bed, Daddy cuddled his baby, who cuddled his best bear.
    B. At bedtime, Daddy cuddled his baby, and baby cuddled his bear.
    C. Before going to bed, Daddy cuddled the baby, who cuddled a bear.
    D. Before a nap, Daddy cuddled the baby boy, who cuddled his bear.
    E. Before sleeping, Daddy cuddled the baby boy, who cuddled his favourite bear.

31. What is the best interpretation of the coded message: K1, FD, C(B(105, 6))

    A. A new baby does not like strained food.
    B. Strained food is not good for new babies.
    C. A new baby doesn't like strained vegetables.
    D. Carrots and apricots are not good for new babies.
    E. A new baby doesn't like anything strained or orange.

32. Which of the following would be the most useful and second most useful additions to the codes in order to convey the message accurately?

Message: The baby girl likes her gentle grandmother and cool sister, but not her rude aunt.

    A. like
    B. grandmother
    C. sister
    D. rude
    E. aunt

33. Which of the following would be the most useful and second most useful additions to the codes in order to convey the message accurately?

Message: Babies planned to free their toys after an older boy took them.

    A. plan
    B. free
    C. toy
    D. after
    E. older

STOP. IF YOU FINISH BEFORE TIME IS UP, CHECK ANY QUESTIONS YOU HAVE MARKED FOR REVIEW. YOU MAY GO BACK TO QUESTIONS IN THIS QUIZ ONLY.

24. (E)

The literal translation is *baby, big(crawl), take(big(milk), inside(mouth))*. The table includes multiple, A, which is required to form a plural noun, as shown in the example questions; eliminate (C), which has babies, since baby is not modified by multiple in the message. The second part of the message is interpreted as 'big crawl' or 'crawls a lot' in three of the remaining answers, which would fit big(crawl); eliminate (A), which misinterprets this as 'likes to crawl', which would require positive while omitting big. The first grouping of codes inside the final brackets, big(milk), is given in (B) and (E) as 'a lot of milk'; eliminate (D), which omits a representation of big with milk. (B) has no representation of the final grouping, inside(mouth), so it cannot be correct. The answer is therefore (E).

25. (A)

The second and fifth terms in this message are identical, and the third and final terms are identical, save for the initial code modifying the final term. Thus, this message appears to involve some sort of parallel structure. 15(1) is make(baby), 3(FD) is sing(opposite(positive)), or sing(negative), and J3(FD) would be something like big(sing(negative)). The first and fourth terms, F(E12) and F(J9), translate literally as opposite(clean(nappy)) and opposite(big(sleep)), respectively. All the answers interpret the first term as 'dirty nappy', except for (B), which incorrectly makes it plural. All of the remaining answers interpret the fourth term as 'short nap' or 'short sleep', except for (D), which mistakenly translates it as negative(sleep). Since the message includes make(baby) twice, an answer that includes this term only once cannot be correct; eliminate (C). Of the final two answers, (A) interprets sing(negative) as 'cry' and big(sing(negative)) as 'cry more', which is consistent and fits with the big that modifies the final term; (E) interprets these as 'not sing' and 'sing more', which is inconsistent and omits the opposite(positive) from the final term. The correct answer is (A).

26. (C)

All the answers start with 1(FG), baby(opposite(Mummy)), 1(F2), baby(opposite(boy)), or 1F(JG), baby(opposite)(big(Mummy)). Of these, only opposite(boy) is necessarily logically equivalent to the concept of girl; eliminate (A), (D) and (E). The only difference between the remaining answers is whether or not the second term, D9, positive(sleep), is modified by J, big. Based on the example questions, positive can mean 'like', so positive(sleep) has the logical meaning 'likes to sleep'. Big is not required to encode the second part of the message, so (B) is wrong. The correct answer is (C).

27. (B)

The literal translation is *Mummy(silly(sing)), make(baby), take(spoon(apricot)*. The message includes sing, 3, only once, but answers (A) and (C) include two representations of 3 (as 'sing' and 'song'); eliminate (A) and (C). In the message, silly(sing) is modified by Mummy, but (E) changes the grouping, so that the baby is the one to sing silly, rather than Mummy; eliminate (E) on this basis. The only difference between (B) and (D) is 'take a spoon' and 'eat a spoonful'; since the message only includes take, 16, and the correct answer for an earlier question encoded 'drink' as 'take inside mouth', it's clear that there are not enough codes to represent the logical concept of eating. The answer is therefore (B).

28. (B)

This message looks very complicated, so start by writing out the literal translation for the first two parts, rather than the entire message: *Mummy, big(big, baby(inside))*. The elements inside the brackets seem to represent the concept of 'pregnant'; eliminate (A) and (D), which include pregnant without modifying the term with the extra 'big' that appears outside the brackets. For the same reason, eliminate (C), which translates the codes inside the brackets literally (as 'big with a baby inside') without modifying them with the extra 'big'. Answer (E) appears at first glance to put the parts of the message in a different order, but note that K is 'new' in the table of codes; K1, in the final part of the message, would therefore mean new(baby). However, (E) includes 'new baby' with the first two parts of the message, rather than in the final combined element, and also omits the earlier representation of baby (the 1 from 1H). As such, (E) cannot be correct; the answer must be (B).

29. (D)

Two of the answers start with FD, opposite(positive), and two include this term modified by L, command. Since the message is a command, the correct answer must include L; eliminate (A) and (C). Since opposite(positive) means negative, and the command is negative, the correct answer must include FD; eliminate (E), which doesn't. The only difference between the remaining answers is in the final term: (B) has H(104), inside(cot), and (D) has H(J104), inside(big(cot)). A bed is not the same as a cot; a bed is bigger than a cot, so the correct answer is (D).

30. (E)

Another very long message, so translate the terms one at a time, eliminating as you go. The first term, M9, is before(sleep). Eliminate (A), (B) and (C), which interpret this term as involving the word 'bed'—the correct answer to the last question demonstrated that this table of codes would encode 'bed' as big(cot), J104, rather than using the code for sleep. The correct answer to a previous question did interpret 9 as nap, so (D) cannot be eliminated based on the first term. The only difference between the remaining answers is in the final part of the message: (D) has 'his bear', and (E) has 'his favourite bear'. The final part of the message, 108(2, 207), translates literally as bear(boy, best). Best could represent the concept of 'favourite', and (D) includes no representation of best. Therefore, (D) cannot be correct, and the answer must be (E).

31. (A)

The literal translation is *new(baby), opposite(positive), strained(generalise(carrot, apricot))*. Eliminate (B) and (D), which mistakenly interpret the first part of the message as a plural; the message does not include the code for multiple, which is required to form plurals. The difference in the remaining answers is found in the final term. Since carrot and apricot are generalised together, the result cannot mean vegetable, as an apricot is not a vegetable; eliminate (C). You could say that carrots and apricots are both orange, but the final term in the message modifies the generalisation with 'strained'; this element would not mean 'strained or orange', so eliminate (E). Carrots and apricots could generalise together as 'food'; the answer is therefore (A).

32. (C) and (D)

All of the answers appear in the message, and like has appeared in previous messages as positive, D; eliminate (A). None of the adjectives in the expanded table match the meaning of 'rude' (or its opposite), so (D) must be one of the answers. Grandmother could be defined as Mummy(Mummy), or big(Mummy); eliminate (B). Sister and aunt cannot be defined with the existing code; however, an aunt is the sister of your parent. Adding sister to the code—as, say, N—would allow you to define aunt as GN or 101N, depending on whether the aunt is the mother's or father's sister. Eliminate (E), and the answers must be (C) and (D).

33. (A) and (B)

All the answer choices appear in the message, so check to see which can be formed by the codes in the existing table. After is the opposite of before, or FM; eliminate (D). Old is the opposite of new, or FK; older might be represented as big(old), or J(FK), so eliminate (E). Toy might seem to be a more challenging concept to represent, unless you notice that the expanded table includes several examples of toys, such as doll and ball; you could thus represent 'toys' as the generalisation of doll and ball, or B(110, 111). Eliminate (C). There is no way to represent the concept of 'plan' or 'free' with the existing codes in the table, so answers (A) and (B) are correct.

7

Situational Judgement

Situational Judgement is the fifth and final section of the UKCAT. Unlike the previous four subtests, you do not receive a scaled score from 300 to 900 in Situational Judgement; rather, you are assessed from Band 1 to Band 4. The band reflects the degree to which the answers you chose match the correct answers as determined by a panel of medical experts: Band 1 means that most of your answers were the same as the panel of medical experts; Band 4 means that very few of your answers were the same. Thus, the task in Situational Judgement is to pick the same answer as the panel of medical experts. You have 26 minutes to answer 71 items, so you must work very quickly.

The Format

The Situational Judgement Test consists of 17 scenarios, each accompanied by 3 to 6 items. The scenarios are drawn from real-life medical and educational situations, and you must consider how a doctor, dentist or student would respond in the circumstances described. Most scenarios will involve a conflict between what a clinician or student is meant to be doing and an interfering issue that arises. The interfering issue could be a problematic behaviour by a patient or a fellow student or clinician, or a 'life issue' that could make it difficult to carry on as normal.

The first part of the section—roughly the first two-thirds of the items—are appropriateness questions, in which you must assess whether possible responses to the situation in the scenario are appropriate or inappropriate. The final part of the section—approximately one-third of the items—are importance questions, in which you must decide whether a series of factors are important or not important in deciding how to respond to the scenario.

Both types of questions include four answer choices, so you must choose a side: appropriate/inappropriate, or important/not important. There is no middle option. Also, you must consider each possible response/factor independently of the others in the scenario. This means that each answer choice can be correct more than once in a given scenario. In fact, when you review the Situational Judgement scenarios in the official UKCAT practice materials, you'll notice that some scenarios have the same correct answer for all possible responses. Thus, it's essential that you consider each response on its own, without any regard for which answers have already been correct in that same scenario.

The Challenges

The most obvious challenge in Situational Judgement is timing: 71 questions and 17 scenarios in 26 minutes means that you have only about 30 seconds to read each scenario, and 10–15 seconds to answer each question. If you work any more slowly, you will run out of time.

The other major challenge in Situational Judgement is the fact that the correct answers are based on principles of medical professionalism that are well known and 'obvious' to the medical experts who have decided the correct answers, but are likely far from obvious to the vast majority of UKCAT test-takers, who are mostly sixth-formers with limited medical experience. Even so, you are likely to have at least a vague awareness of some of these issues, and you can sharpen this relatively easily as you practise ahead of your UKCAT Test Day.

Kaplan Top Tips for Situational Judgement

1. Read the scenario first

This may seem like an obvious point, but we have found that many students initially approach Situational Judgement using their well-honed Verbal Reasoning instincts and go right to the first response option, and then scan the scenario for support. There's a real temptation to do so, as Situational Judgement uses the same visual interface as Verbal Reasoning, with the scenario on the left-hand side of the screen and the response options one at a time on the right-hand side. However, you must always read the scenario before attempting the first response, as you must understand the conflicting issues involved before deciding on appropriateness or importance. If you try to rush and only scan the scenarios, you are highly likely to miss out essential words that could make a huge difference to your understanding of the scenario. It shouldn't take more than 20–30 seconds to read each scenario, so practise for this timing—and for always reading the scenario first—as you revise.

2. Choose a side

As you read each of the response options, get used to making a 'snap judgement' and choosing a side. Decide quickly if the response is appropriate or inappropriate, or if a factor is important or not important. While there will be a few responses or factors that will be very tough to assess quickly, even for the most experienced of medical professionals, the vast majority are relatively straightforward, and you will save valuable time—and maximise your marks—by practising and preparing to choose a side quickly and confidently as often as possible.

3. Know when it's OK to choose (B) or (C)

Unlike in the other sections of the UKCAT, the four answer choices in Situational Judgement do not have an equal probability of being correct. In the official Situational Judgement practice materials from the UKCAT Consortium, answers (A) and (D) are correct about 70% of the time, and answers (B) and (C) are correct about 30% of the time. This means that, most of the time, simply choosing a side will be sufficient to get to the correct answer. The partial marking is likely to help with this as well. It is not entirely clear how the partial marking works—the test-maker has provided no information on this—however, the most logical possibility is that you receive partial marks for giving an answer that is close to the correct answer. For example, if the correct answer is (C) and you choose (D), then you would get partial marks for choosing (D).

It is OK to choose (B) or (C) when the response is less than optimal for some reason, and when the possible negative consequences of that response are not severe. If the negative consequences could be severe, then the correct answer is (D).

4. Learn the key principles of medical professionalism

You will have plenty of time to learn and practise these in real-life settings as you proceed through your medical or dental education, and in your early career as a clinician. However, you are expected to have a basic knowledge of the key principles of medical professionalism in order to obtain a respectable score in Situational Judgement on the UKCAT.

There are two key ways to build your knowledge of these key principles:

1. **Review all the official Situational Judgement practice questions and answers**. This includes all questions in the online UKCAT practice tests available on the UKCAT website, as well as the questions in the official UKCAT practice app. In 2013, the questions and worked answers from the official app are also available in full in the UKCAT Official Guide, a PDF that is available as a free download from the UKCAT website. This PDF provides a great format for obtaining and reading through the official questions and worked answers, so you can start to understand why the correct answers are correct.

2. **Download and review the free booklet *Good Medical Practice*, available from the General Medical Council website.** All the key principles of medical professionalism are drawn from this 36-page booklet. Copies are normally given out to medical students as part of their medical education, so you will get a head start on learning its contents as you prepare for the UKCAT. Whilst this booklet is not explicitly mentioned in the worked answers to the official Situational Judgement questions, you will notice many references to the content of the booklet, and the occasional reference to the General Medical Council. The more time you invest learning these key principles, the more confident and prepared you will be for Situational Judgement questions on Test Day.

Kaplan Timed Practice Set—*Try the Kaplan Top Tips*

Set your timer for 2 minutes. Mark answers for all 5 questions before time is up!

> Lucy is a medical student at the university hospital. Several of the consultants have just returned from a leaving lunch for one of their colleagues. Lucy notices one of the consultants, Dr Perkins, struggling to maintain his balance in the corridor. Dr Perkins stumbles into Lucy, and she can smell whisky on his breath. Lucy asks if everything is all right, and Dr Perkins says he is in a rush, as he has a patient waiting on the operating table.

How **appropriate** are each of the following responses by <u>Lucy</u> in this situation?

1. Take Dr Perkins to one side and suggest he is not in a fit state to interact with patients
    - A. A very appropriate thing to do
    - B. Appropriate, but not ideal
    - C. Inappropriate, but not awful
    - D. A very inappropriate thing to do

2. Inform the patient that the surgery will not take place
    - A. A very appropriate thing to do
    - B. Appropriate, but not ideal
    - C. Inappropriate, but not awful
    - D. A very inappropriate thing to do

3. Email a formal complaint against Dr Perkins to the hospital chairman
    - A. A very appropriate thing to do
    - B. Appropriate, but not ideal
    - C. Inappropriate, but not awful
    - D. A very inappropriate thing to do

4. Seek immediate advice from the consultant who supervises her work at the hospital
    - A. A very appropriate thing to do
    - B. Appropriate, but not ideal
    - C. Inappropriate, but not awful
    - D. A very inappropriate thing to do

5. Check with the surgical nurse to determine whether Dr Perkins is actually about to perform surgery
    - A. A very appropriate thing to do
    - B. Appropriate, but not ideal
    - C. Inappropriate, but not awful
    - D. A very inappropriate thing to do

How did you get on with your first timed set? If you worked efficiently, you should have been able to read the scenario and assess all 5 response options in 2 minutes. If you struggled here, be sure to try to spend no more than 30 seconds reading the scenario in the upcoming sets in this chapter. You'll also want to keep to no more than 10–15 seconds per response option—if you are taking longer to deliberate, then you will miss out quite a lot of items at the end of the section. We'll cover a few more tips to help with pacing in this chapter. For now, here are the worked answers for this first set.

Kaplan Timed Practice Set—*Try the Kaplan Top Tips*: Answers and Explanations

1. (A)

Since it is very clear to Lucy that Dr Perkins is under the influence of alcohol, then it would be just as clear to any patients who he encounters in his current state. Thus, it is highly appropriate for Lucy to take him to one side and suggest that he should avoid interacting with patients. A medical student might feel uncomfortable addressing this issue with a consultant, but Dr Perkins's behaviour here is especially egregious. There is a real risk to public confidence in the profession, not to mention to the patient's life if the doctor were to perform surgery—so Lucy would be entirely correct to intervene in this manner.

2. (D)

It would seriously undermine the patient's confidence in the medical profession to hear from a medical student, rather than a doctor in charge of the patient's care, that surgery will not take place. This response option is therefore highly inappropriate.

3. (D)

Responses that involve formal complaints or written complaints are usually considered very inappropriate. This response is especially so, as there is no guarantee that the hospital chairman would read the email or be able to do anything about it before Dr Perkins heads into the operating theatre. This response does nothing to address the real risk to patient safety and the patient's confidence in the profession, and is not a local solution.

4. (A)

It is always very appropriate for a medical professional to seek advice from a senior colleague, and even more so in the case of a medical student who is encountering an ethically perilous situation for the first time.

5. (B)

This response is not inappropriate, as the surgical nurse is a good person to confirm this detail for Lucy. However, it's less than ideal, as determining whether Dr Perkins actually has a patient scheduled for surgery does nothing to address the fact that the doctor is not in a fit state to see patients.

Appropriateness Scenarios

Most of the items in the Situational Judgement Test ask you to decide the appropriateness of a possible response to the scenario. You must assess each option in an Appropriateness Scenario independently of the others. Thus, you should not assume that each answer choice will be used once, or that there will be one best response among the options given. A scenario could have a series of possible responses that are all very appropriate, or all very inappropriate, or some mix of the two.

You must decide on the appropriateness of the possible responses based on the details in the scenario, and evaluate these according to the principles of medical professionalism. Some of the key principles that come up again and again in the Situational Judgement Test include:

- Doctors and medical students must not do anything to undermine public confidence in the profession, and must act promptly to address a situation in which public confidence in the profession is at risk.

- Doctors and medical students must never act or imply that they have knowledge, expertise or experience beyond their actual level of knowledge, expertise or experience.

- Doctors and medical students should seek advice from a colleague or supervisor if they are unsure of the best course of action.

- Doctors and medical students should seek local solutions to problems that arise wherever possible and practicable.

You can get a full sense of the range of principles of medical professionalism that you may encounter in the Situational Judgement Test on Test Day by reviewing the booklet *Good Medical Practice*.

Try to put the principles of medical professionalism into practice in the following Appropriateness scenario. Spend 30 seconds reading the scenario, then no more than 15 seconds assessing each response before reading the answer.

As he is walking through the ward, a junior doctor, Bao, notices a patient waving him to come to her bedside. Bao approaches the patient, who says that no one will tell her what is wrong with her, and she wants to know if she can get treatment to help her stop feeling tired all the time and getting so many infections. Bao checks the patient's chart, and sees that she is 14 years old and has just been diagnosed with leukaemia.

How **appropriate** are each of the following responses by **Bao** in this situation?

6. Explain immediately to the patient that she has leukaemia, and answer any questions she has about her diagnosis
   - A. A very appropriate thing to do
   - B. Appropriate, but not ideal
   - C. Inappropriate, but not awful
   - D. A very inappropriate thing to do

Answer: From the patient's comments, it is very likely that she has not been informed of her diagnosis. Since Bao is not responsible for her care, it would be very inappropriate for him to share such a diagnosis with a patient who is a child in this way, in the absence of her parents and the doctor responsible for her care. Thus, the correct answer is (D).

7. Ask if there is anything in particular that he can do to help
   - A. A very appropriate thing to do
   - B. Appropriate, but not ideal
   - C. Inappropriate, but not awful
   - D. A very inappropriate thing to do

Answer: This is quite a neutral question, so it is not inappropriate. However, it is less than an ideal response, as the patient has already made a specific request for information about her diagnosis and recommended treatment, so Bao should already have a clear idea of what can be done to help the patient. Answer (B) is correct.

8. Encourage the patient to discuss her concerns together with her parents and the doctor responsible for her care
   - A. A very appropriate thing to do
   - B. Appropriate, but not ideal
   - C. Inappropriate, but not awful
   - D. A very inappropriate thing to do

Answer: This response is highly appropriate, as it guides the patient to initiate this important and necessary conversation with the people who are best positioned to provide the emotional support she will need as she comes to terms with her diagnosis and begins treatment. The answer is (A).

9. Offer to speak to the patient's parents on her behalf
   - A. A very appropriate thing to do
   - B. Appropriate, but not ideal
   - C. Inappropriate, but not awful
   - D. A very inappropriate thing to do

Answer: Bao knows nothing about the patient's family situation; given that the patient is clearly unaware of her diagnosis, Bao should be careful not to do anything that implies that her parents have not told her something, or that there is a reason a discussion might need to be had with the patient's parents that does not involve the patient. It is likely, for example, that the patient's parents have just been told the diagnosis and need a short amount of time to process it themselves so they can be ready to support their daughter. Bao should not do anything that could imply to the patient that her parents are keeping something from her, or that they have done something wrong—so this option is highly inappropriate, answer (D).

10. Offer to speak to the doctor responsible for the patient's care on her behalf
    - A. A very appropriate thing to do
    - B. Appropriate, but not ideal
    - C. Inappropriate, but not awful
    - D. A very inappropriate thing to do

Answer: This is a very appropriate response, as it deflects the patient's concerns to the doctor responsible for her care. This doctor may not be aware of just how anxious the patient is, so speaking to this doctor on the patient's behalf would address her concerns while also ensuring quality of care. Answer (A) is correct.

Importance Scenarios

The final few scenarios in the Situational Judgement Test will ask you to assess the importance of a series of factors in deciding how to respond to the situation in the scenario. Just like with the possible responses to Appropriateness scenarios, you must assess these factors independently of each other. There may not necessarily be a 'best', or single 'very important', factor; there could be multiple very important factors, or multiple 'not at all important' factors.

In assessing the factors, you should only consider the implications to the person deciding how to respond if the factor is true. The principles of medical professionalism will help again here, with a few extra Kaplan top tips:

- Factors that mean the decider would be more aware of the principles of ethics or medical professionalism that have direct bearing on the scenario will generally be important or very important.

- Factors that are external pressures on the decider, with limited (or no) direct relevance to the other people in the scenario, or to the principles of ethics or medical professionalism, will generally be of minor importance or not at all important.

- Factors that relate to the relationship (professional or otherwise) of the people directly involved in the scenario can sometimes be tricky to assess. Don't fret about these—they are tricky for everyone.

- Many of the Importance scenarios will involve doctors or medical students committing (or about to commit) gross misconduct, or other serious ethical or legal breaches. If you're a sixth-former, obviously you are unlikely to be aware of all of the nuances of issues that could be gross misconduct. Several of these (e.g. those that could get you struck off by the GMC) are detailed in *Good Medical Practice*, so it is well worth reviewing this booklet ahead of Test Day.

Put these Kaplan top tips into practice with the following Importance scenario. Be sure to read the scenario before assessing the factors, and be sure to mark an answer for each item before reading the answer. If you are unsure, try at least to choose a side (important or unimportant) and mark an answer on that side.

A medical student, Ruchira, enters the supply cupboard at the university hospital to discover another medical student, Jake, sat there with a credit card in his hand, typing on his laptop. Ruchira can see that Jake is using a website notorious for selling essays to students. Jake closes the laptop quickly, and asks if Ruchira is spying on him.

How **important** to take into account are the following considerations for **<u>Ruchira</u>** when deciding how to respond to the situation?

11. There is no expectation of privacy in the supply cupboard
    A. Very important
    B. Important
    C. Of minor importance
    D. Not important at all

Answer: A supply cupboard is normally open to all staff at the hospital, and students have no expectation of privacy there. This factor undercuts Jake's claim that Ruchira is spying on him, as she has just as much right to be in the supply cupboard as he does. It is therefore a very important consideration. Answer (A) is correct.

12. Jake and Ruchira dated for a few months, until he broke it off with her
    A. Very important
    B. Important
    C. Of minor importance
    D. Not important at all

Answer: Jake appears to be doing something that is highly unethical, and would likely be a breach of university policies about cheating, if he is buying an essay to submit as part of his coursework. Any personal relationship between Jake and Ruchira (current or former) would not mitigate his apparent guilt in any way; however, if Ruchira is Jake's ex-girlfriend, this would be a factor of minor importance in how she might decide how to respond to the situation, as it might explain his suspicion that she is spying on him, for instance. The answer is therefore (C).

13. Jake has a reputation for being honest and doing the right thing
    A. Very important
    B. Important
    C. Of minor importance
    D. Not important at all

Answer: Jake's reputation does not mitigate his current actions, which appear to be highly unethical, in any way. This factor is entirely unimportant. The correct answer is (D).

14. Ruchira thinks the website only sells essays for English and history modules
    A. Very important
    B. Important
    C. Of minor importance
    D. Not important at all

Answer: It would be unethical for a university student to buy an essay to be submitted as part of assessed coursework, whether it was his own coursework or he was buying the essay for someone else. Ruchira could also be wrong in her impression about the website; if she is correct, however, that the essay could not be for Jake's coursework, it could point to a more complicated explanation for what exactly he is up to—so this factor is of minimal importance. Answer (C) is correct.

15. Ruchira led a discussion on ethics at the most recent meeting of her tutor group
    A. Very important
    B. Important
    C. Of minor importance
    D. Not important at all

Answer: If Ruchira recently led a discussion on ethics, then that means that she should be well aware of the ethical responsibilities of doctors and students to behave with integrity at all times. This factor is thus very important. The answer is (A).

On the next three pages, you will complete a timed Situational Judgement quiz, consisting of 3 scenarios and a total of 14 responses/factors. If you pace yourself, and spend no more than 90 seconds per scenario, you should be able to attempt all the scenarios and answer all the items. Even if you find yourself running out of time near the end, do your best to choose a side for each item (appropriate/inappropriate or important/unimportant) and mark an answer on that side.

Before you start the quiz, let's consider some of the challenges in Situational Judgement that cause unprepared test-takers to waste time and earn a lower score:

You must understand the conflict in the scenario before assessing the responses/factors. This may seem a really obvious point, but we find that many students who struggle with Situational Judgement are skimming or glancing over the scenario without 'registering' the key conflict that must be understood in order to assess the possible responses or factors. You should always take 20–30 seconds to read the scenario in full, as you will be able to assess most responses/factors in 10–15 seconds each.

Don't waste time deliberating over any one response/factor. This is perhaps the most vital point. You have only 10–15 seconds for each individual response/factor, so you cannot spend any longer than that in deciding the appropriateness/importance. Always force yourself to choose a side straightaway, and then choose the stronger/weaker answer on that side.

Don't worry about full vs partial marks. The UKCAT Consortium has not released any information (as of this printing in early 2014) regarding how, exactly, the partial marks work. We know that you get full marks if you choose the correct answer; presumably, then, you would get partial marks for choosing an answer that is near (next to) the correct answer. Our best guess (based on years of analysing standardised tests at Kaplan) is that you get partial marks for the other answer on the same side. That is, if B is correct, you get partial marks for A. If we get further information about partial marking from the test-maker, we'll post this in the Online Resource Centre—but you really shouldn't worry about it for now.

Take time to read through *Good Medical Practice*. We have mentioned this several times, as it is really the best guide to the principles of medical professionalism as practised by doctors in the UK. It is a relatively short and easy-to-read booklet, and you will have to read and get to know it very well in any case once you are a medical student—so it's worth putting in a bit of time now, so you can get more comfortable with the range of principles that could be tested in this section of the UKCAT.

Set your timer for 5 minutes. Try to assess all 14 items and mark an answer for each before time is up. If you have trouble with a particular scenario or response/factor, choose a side (appropriate/inappropriate or important/unimportant) and mark an answer on that side. Above all, do your best not to spend more than 15 seconds on any single item.

> Colm and Vicki are junior doctors at a large GP practice. They are the only doctors working in the early evening hours, when Vicki receives a call from A&E at a nearby hospital. Her partner and their young son have been in a car crash and are very seriously injured. Vicki is shaken, and asks Colm if he could see her final two patients of the day, as she must go to the hospital. Vicki hands Colm the patients' records, and he sees that Vicki's handwriting is so impossible to read that he cannot make sense of either patient's notes.

How **appropriate** are each of the following responses by <u>Colm</u> in this situation?

16. Tell Vicki not to worry and that he will take good care of her patients
   A. A very appropriate thing to do
   B. Appropriate, but not ideal
   C. Inappropriate, but not awful
   D. A very inappropriate thing to do

17. Tell Vicki he doesn't feel right about trying to help, as her notes in the patient records are illegible
   A. A very appropriate thing to do
   B. Appropriate, but not ideal
   C. Inappropriate, but not awful
   D. A very inappropriate thing to do

18. Tell Vicki he can't read her handwriting
   A. A very appropriate thing to do
   B. Appropriate, but not ideal
   C. Inappropriate, but not awful
   D. A very inappropriate thing to do

19. See if the receptionist can help decipher Vicki's handwriting
   A. A very appropriate thing to do
   B. Appropriate, but not ideal
   C. Inappropriate, but not awful
   D. A very inappropriate thing to do

20. Ask Vicki to brief him on the reasons for each patient's appointment, along with any underlying conditions or allergies, before she leaves
   A. A very appropriate thing to do
   B. Appropriate, but not ideal
   C. Inappropriate, but not awful
   D. A very inappropriate thing to do

21. Ask Vicki if there's anything else he can do to help
   A. A very appropriate thing to do
   B. Appropriate, but not ideal
   C. Inappropriate, but not awful
   D. A very inappropriate thing to do

Aled is a medical student. His supervisor at the hospital instructs him to perform a certain procedure on a patient while his supervisor observes. Aled has seen the procedure demonstrated several times, and has practised the procedure a few times on an anatomical model, but he has never done the procedure on a living person. As Aled is about to start, the patient asks if he has done this before.

How **appropriate** are each of the following responses by <u>**Aled**</u> in this situation?

22. Ask if the patient would prefer for his supervisor to perform the procedure
    - A. A very appropriate thing to do
    - B. Appropriate, but not ideal
    - C. Inappropriate, but not awful
    - D. A very inappropriate thing to do

23. Explain that he has practised the procedure but has not performed it on a patient, and that his supervisor will observe and can intervene if there is a problem
    - A. A very appropriate thing to do
    - B. Appropriate, but not ideal
    - C. Inappropriate, but not awful
    - D. A very inappropriate thing to do

24. Tell the patient that he has performed the procedure before, and there has never been a problem
    - A. A very appropriate thing to do
    - B. Appropriate, but not ideal
    - C. Inappropriate, but not awful
    - D. A very inappropriate thing to do

Fatima, a consultant at a large hospital, has been asked to help cover on a different ward where there is a staff shortage. Whilst covering on that ward, Fatima opens the door to the supply cupboard and sees a nurse take several bottles of painkillers and put them into her handbag. It looks like the nurse is taking the last bottles of that type of painkiller.

How **important** to take into account are the following considerations for **Fatima** when deciding how to respond to the situation?

25. Fatima's patient requires urgent treatment
    A. Very important
    B. Important
    C. Of minor importance
    D. Not important at all

26. Fatima's brother is a police constable
    A. Very important
    B. Important
    C. Of minor importance
    D. Not important at all

27. Fatima is unlikely to work on this ward again in the near future
    A. Very important
    B. Important
    C. Of minor importance
    D. Not important at all

28. Fatima teaches a module on ethics at the local medical school
    A. Very important
    B. Important
    C. Of minor importance
    D. Not important at all

29. Fatima's patient needs the same painkiller that the nurse is putting in her bag
    A. Very important
    B. Important
    C. Of minor importance
    D. Not important at all

16. (D)

Colm is right to help his colleague, as she is clearly upset by the news about her partner and son and should not be seeing patients in that state. However, there is a real problem in Colm covering for Vicki, as he cannot read her notes in the patient's records, so he has no idea why the patients are coming in for their appointments, or if they have any underlying conditions or allergies. This lack of information could seriously endanger the patients' health if Colm were to see them using Vicki's illegible notes, so this response is very inappropriate.

17. (C)

It is inappropriate for Colm to tell Vicki that he won't help in this situation; however, it is not an awful response, as the reason he gives is the central problem here and puts patient safety at risk. All doctors are required to ensure that the notes they make in patients' records are legible, and it is Vicki's failure to meet this fundamental professional obligation that makes it problematic for Colm to cover for her.

18. (A)

This is a very appropriate response, as it is true and is at the heart of the problem in this scenario.

19. (D)

This response is very inappropriate, as there is no guarantee that the receptionist will be able to help Colm read Vicki's notes. There is also the risk of the receptionist misinterpreting Vicki's handwriting and compromising patient safety as a result.

20. (A)

This response is highly appropriate, as it is a quick and straightforward solution to the problem of Vicki's illegible notes, and will enable Colm to cover for her so she can join her family at the hospital.

21. (A)

This is a very appropriate thing to do, as Vicki may need some other support or help as a result of the emergency.

22. (C)

Aled has been instructed to perform the procedure by his supervisor, so it is inappropriate for him to give the patient the option of having his supervisor take over before explaining his own level of experience with the procedure. Once he answers the patient's question, then this might be an appropriate course of action. However, this response is not awful, as it is clear that the patient doubts that Aled is qualified to undertake the procedure.

23. (A)

This response accurately describes Aled's experience with the procedure, whilst reassuring the patient of his supervisor's support, and it gives the patient the informed choice of whether to allow Aled to proceed. As such, it is a highly appropriate response.

24. (D)

It would be highly inappropriate for Aled to imply that he has performed the procedure on a patient, when in fact he has not practised it on a living person. It is a serious violation of the principles of medical professionalism for a doctor or medical student to state or suggest that they have more experience or expertise than they actually do.

25. (B)

This is an important factor to consider, as Fatima would want to be cautious not to take too long in dealing with the nurse's behaviour at the present moment. However, it does appear that a member of staff is stealing painkillers from the supply cupboard—this must be addressed immediately.

26. (D)

Fatima has a responsibility as a medical professional and a fellow member of staff to address the nurse's actions. The fact that her brother is a policeman is not at all important in deciding how to respond.

27. (D)

The serious nature of the nurse's transgression demands an immediate response. Fatima's responsibility to follow through on this is not diminished at all by the fact that she is unlikely to work on the ward again in the near future.

28. (B)

This factor is important to consider, as it means that Fatima should be aware of the most recent guidance on ethics for medical professionals, and can follow these in responding to the nurse.

29. (A)

This is a very important factor, as Fatima will need to ensure that the painkiller is available for her patient. Thus, it will be all the more essential for her to respond to the nurse urgently and effectively.

Kaplan UKCAT Mock Test

Kaplan UKCAT Mock Test General Instructions

You have 2 hours to complete the Kaplan UKCAT Mock Test. You will need the following items:

- This book.
- A pen or pencil to record your answers.
- Scrap paper for any written calculations and notations.
- A timer (such as one on your watch, mobile or computer).
- A calculator.

Time each section strictly, so you can practise under test-like conditions. Be sure to use the Kaplan top tips wherever possible. You should also try to keep to the timing recommendations for each question or set of questions, but getting comfortable with the Kaplan top tips is the primary goal of the Mock Test. Once you 'internalise' the Kaplan top tips, you will find that your timing improves significantly.

On Test Day, you will have an additional minute to read the directions for each section. That minute cannot be used to answer test questions, so it has not been included here. Time yourself using the timings given once you turn each instructions page and start work on each section.

Answer the questions as quickly and accurately as possible. Now that you have a better understanding of how the UKCAT works, you have every incentive to ensure that you mark an answer for every question in each section.

Record your answers on a sheet of paper, and check them against the explanations in Appendix C once you finish.

NB You cannot write on the test paper on Test Day, because the test is taken on a computer. So be careful not to get into the habit of writing on the practice questions in this book. Make any notations, eliminations, etc., entirely on scrap paper, and not directly on the questions themselves.

Your score on Test Day corresponds to the number of questions you answer correctly. You can find your equivalent score on the scoring table at the end of the test.

This section contains 11 passages, each of which is followed by four items. Some passages in this section will be followed by four statements. Your task is to decide whether each statement logically flows from the information presented in the passage. You have three answer choices for each statement:

True: The information in the statement is stated explicitly in the passage or is a valid inference.

False: The information in the statement contradicts what is stated in the passage.

Can't tell: There is not enough information to determine whether the statement is True or False.

Some passages in this section will be followed by four questions; each question will have four answer choices. Choose the best answer, based on the passage.

Answer all 44 items in Section 1, selecting one of the possible answers and circling the letter corresponding to the appropriate answer in this book.

When you are finished with this section, you may use any remaining time to review your work in this section only. Once you proceed to the next section, you may not return to this section.

You will have 21 minutes to answer the questions. It is in your best interest to select an answer for every item as there is no penalty for wrong answers.

Set your timer for 21 minutes, turn the page and begin the section.

The daughter of a leader of the movement that led to Burmese independence in 1948, Aung San Suu Kyi spent much of her early adulthood studying at UK universities and working for non-governmental organisations, including the United Nations, where fellow Burma native U Thant was Secretary-General. After her mother suffered a severe stroke in 1988, Suu Kyi returned to Rangoon to care for her, and became a leader of the popular resistance to the ruling military junta's brutal suppression of the 8th August protests, which resulted in the killing of thousands of civilians. In the aftermath of this violence, the National League for Democracy (NLD) was founded, with Suu Kyi as its leader. Despite a ban on her involvement, the NLD won 82% of seats in Burma's parliament in the 1990 elections, meaning that Suu Kyi (as head of the party) should have become prime minister.

However, the military junta—whose repressive rule lasted from 1962 until the formal dissolution of the junta in 2011, following the election of a civilian government amidst allegations of military-backed fraud in 2010—ensured that Suu Kyi never became prime minister. Suu Kyi was placed under house arrest for nearly 20 years, starting in 1989 and continuing until the week after the 2010 elections, with only a few short breaks in which her movements were severely restricted and continuously monitored. Aung San Suu Kyi was awarded the Nobel Peace Prize in 1991, but could not travel to Oslo to collect the prize, as she would not have been allowed to return to Burma. For this same reason, Suu Kyi was unable to travel to London when invited to give a series of lectures on democracy and freedom for the BBC in 2011. Instead, producers secretly recorded the lectures in Burma, and Suu Kyi and the BBC did not announce her involvement until the producers and the recordings had safely left the country. Suu Kyi was elected to the parliament of Myanmar (as the junta had re-named Burma) in 2012 and took her seat that year, when she was also finally able to give her Nobel acceptance speech in Oslo. Suu Kyi plans to run for the presidency of Myanmar in 2015.

1. The author would most likely agree that, prior to 2012:
    A. Suu Kyi gave a series of lectures in London for the BBC.
    B. people who visited Suu Kyi in Myanmar were in some danger.
    C. Suu Kyi achieved greater international prominence than any other Burmese person.
    D. people were unable to visit Suu Kyi in Myanmar.

2. Which of these statements cannot be true?
    A. Burma is no longer known as Burma.
    B. Myanmar held elections in 2012.
    C. Suu Kyi never served as prime minister.
    D. Myanmar is ruled by a military junta.

3. Based on the passage, it must be true that the winner of the Nobel Peace Prize:
    A. must be able to travel to Oslo to be eligible for the award.
    B. is not required to collect the award in person.
    C. must be an elected head of state or prime minister.
    D. is not selected by the same committee as the other Nobel prizes.

4. As a consequence of military intervention in Burma in 1990:
    A. the results of elections were not fulfilled.
    B. someone who was not elected became prime minister.
    C. all of the NLD's organisers were placed under house arrest.
    D. there was no real violence against civilians.

Last night's meeting of the county council saw spirited, and, at times, heated debate over the council's decision last month to approve the construction of a supermarket on the site of the village car park in Hiddlesfield. Shopkeepers are particularly concerned about the loss in trade that may result from the opening of a national supermarket in a village of Hiddlesfield's size.

The fishmonger suggested that the council learn the lesson of Aldersham, the neighbouring village, where the council allowed a national supermarket to be built three years ago. Within three months of the supermarket opening, half of the shops in Aldersham's high street had shut, due to the loss in foot traffic. In response, a councillor pointed out that the supermarket had brought dozens of jobs to Aldersham, along with many conveniences and products not previously available in the village.

Hiddlesfield's butcher also spoke very forcefully against the supermarket. She argued that its beef and lamb are sourced from Wales and Ireland, rather than the local farms that her shop favours. The butcher said that the cost to the local economy is far greater than the potential loss of shops on the high street, when the consequences to businesses in the county at large are considered.

5. Most people in Hiddlesfield oppose the new supermarket.

      A. True

      B. False

      C. Can't tell

6. A new supermarket may cause some shops to close.

      A. True

      B. False

      C. Can't tell

7. The butcher supports the new supermarket.

      A. True

      B. False

      C. Can't tell

8. The supermarket recently built in Aldersham was a success.

      A. True

      B. False

      C. Can't tell

Theatres in London's West End—the home of British commercial theatre, and London's equivalent of New York's Broadway—took in revenues of £512 million in 2010, which is £7 million more than their total takings for 2009. However, the rise in revenue is largely due to a rise in ticket prices: West End audiences in 2010 numbered just above 14 million, down slightly from the total for 2009; at the same time, the top ticket price for most West End shows had risen to £60 or more in 2010.

The two new plays that scored a major commercial and critical triumph in the West End in 2011— *Jerusalem* and *Clybourne Park*—were actually transfers, having started their theatrical life in earlier productions at the Royal Court Theatre, among the most innovative of London's subsidised theatres. Such theatres are granted a significant subsidy from Government and Lottery funding, delivered through Arts Council England (ACE). Subsidised theatres receive as much as 35% of their revenue from ACE, which awarded £1.6 billion in subsidy to theatres and other arts organisations in the funding period from 2008 to 2011. After ACE was hit with a 29% cut in its funding for the awards period starting in 2011, subsidised theatres are very concerned about maintaining their high artistic standards while also remaining accessible to the public they serve. These theatres will do all they can to avoid a punishing rise in ticket prices, though some rise is inevitable; ticket sales represent the majority of revenue at UK theatres, even those in the subsidised sector.

These theatres would rightly argue that the practice of theatre involves a collective effort by artists with a wide range of professional skills, and could not succeed without the talents of these actors, writers, directors, designers and technicians—all of whom deserve to be paid for their vital contribution to our culture. Indeed, British plays such as *Jerusalem* and *War Horse*—which started at the subsidised National Theatre, and continue to play in the West End—won the praise of critics and audiences on Broadway. This proves that the best of British subsidised theatre is an essential export, and that subsidised funding has the power to bridge stages across the Atlantic.

9. Which of these statements must be false?
   - A. Some subsidised theatres are in London.
   - B. Most UK theatre funding comes from the audience.
   - C. Some subsidised productions transfer to the West End.
   - D. Most UK theatre funding comes from the Lottery.

10. The passage suggests that British plays are more likely to be a critical and commercial hit on Broadway if they:
   - A. originate at the National Theatre.
   - B. originate at the Royal Court Theatre.
   - C. succeed in the West End.
   - D. feature war, animals or both.

11. It must be true that the figure for total West End audiences in 2010 was:
   - A. less than the comparable figure for 2009.
   - B. more than the comparable figure for 2009.
   - C. less than the comparable figure for 2011.
   - D. more than the comparable figure for 2011.

12. The author would agree with the assertion that:
   - A. theatre is a collaborative art.
   - B. there would be no theatre without public subsidy.
   - C. the best of British theatre originates in the West End.
   - D. the most popular plays in London are imported from New York.

Founded in 1838 as Spring Hill College in Birmingham, Mansfield College was not fully integrated into the University of Oxford until 1995. Today the college, which is home to 210 undergraduates, 130 graduate students and 35 visiting scholars, is Oxford's smallest, except for Harris Manchester, the university's college for mature students. Mansfield has a reputation for friendliness and informality.

Spring Hill College was founded as a Nonconformist college for those who could not attend major national universities such as Oxford or Cambridge, which required allegiance to the Church of England. The college stood in Birmingham for almost 50 years, moving to Oxford after the 1871 Universities Test Act, which abolished religious tests for admission of non-theological students at Oxford, Cambridge and Durham. With the move, the college was also renamed in recognition of its greatest donors, George and Elizabeth Mansfield. Though Mansfield was Oxford's first Nonconformist college, it lost much of its religious character over time, becoming increasingly secular.

Still, signs of the college's religious heritage still stand. A prominent portrait of Oliver Cromwell, the ultimate English dissenter who was killed in 1658, hangs in the Senior Common Room, and in the halls and library of Mansfield hang portraits of the 1662 dissenters who separated from the Church of England after the Act of Uniformity required Anglican ordination for all clergy. Chapel services continue to be performed in the Nonconformist tradition, and the College Chaplain is always from a Nonconformist denomination. The college's religious past has also historically strengthened its ties to universities in the United States, from which the college still carries a long tradition of accepting a number of American junior year abroad students each year.

13. Durham University once required a religious admissions test.

    A. True
    B. False
    C. Can't tell

14. Mansfield is Oxford's smallest college.

    A. True
    B. False
    C. Can't tell

15. The Mansfield College Chapel is not consecrated.

    A. True
    B. False
    C. Can't tell

16. Oliver Cromwell was one of the 1662 dissenters.

    A. True
    B. False
    C. Can't tell

In the last few years, the UK has launched a campaign to conserve water, asking citizens to find small ways to reduce the amount of water they use on a daily basis. The average person in England and Wales currently uses 150 litres of water per day, the equivalent of 264 pints of milk. Most of this water is expended in washing and toilet flushing; in fact, water use has increased by 50% in the last 50 years due to new technological developments. Those numbers are on the rise; the need for fresh water is expected to increase by 30% when the population exceeds 8 billion, which is projected to happen in the next 20 years. The government's goal is to decrease per capita water usage by 20 litres per day. This is easier than most people imagine. For example, turning off the tap while brushing your teeth and cutting down shower time by one minute saves 15 litres of water a day.

Still, the problem is much bigger than these smaller conservation efforts. New studies estimate that UK consumers only see about 3% of the water usage they are responsible for. This is because of what environmental scientists term embedded water, the total amount of water necessary to produce the things we use on a daily basis. For example, a pint of beer contains 74 litres of embedded water, expended in growing the ingredients and running the processes that make the beer. A cup of coffee is worse; its embedded water content is about 140 litres. A cotton T-shirt embeds about 2,000 litres. Many developing countries currently use a large portion of their limited water resources for crops that they export to developed nations. Thus, the problem of embedded water raises many additional questions about how to really impact water conservation, both at home and abroad.

17. The author would least likely agree with which of these conclusions?
    A. The UK's water conservation schemes are inadequate.
    B. Conserving water is not as difficult as people might think.
    C. Current efforts to conserve water in the UK are sufficient.
    D. More effective water conservation will require further measures.

18. Most water in England and Wales is used in:
    A. toilets, baths and showers.
    B. milk production.
    C. making food and drink.
    D. gardens, lawns and farms.

19. The passage includes examples of embedded water that involve all of the following except:
    A. alcoholic and non-alcoholic drinks
    B. agricultural exports
    C. livestock
    D. clothing

20. Water use a half-century ago in England and Wales must have been:
    A. one-half of current levels.
    B. two-thirds of current levels.
    C. 30% less than today.
    D. 50% more than today.

The International Table Tennis Federation (ITTF) has recently changed some of the key rules of competitive table tennis, also known as ping-pong. Starting in 2000, the ITTF increased the diameter of table tennis balls from 38 mm to 40 mm. While this difference in diameter may seem a minor issue, the resulting reduction in speed and spin gave an advantage to players who favoured a slower style of play. The change in ball size was challenged unsuccessfully by the Chinese National Team, whose players led the world table tennis rankings before the change, and who were known at the time for a playing style marked by smashes and quick attacks. ITTF-sanctioned balls must be white or orange, and are printed with three stars, which indicate the quality of the ball; lesser quality balls might be printed with only one or two stars. The stars on ITTF-approved balls may be printed in certain possible colours: most balls have black or blue stars, though the stars on some will feature a second colour (red, green or purple). Balls of these colours are thought to be easiest to see on tables with a green or blue surface, the only two colours of table surface that are approved for ITTF competition.

A year after their decision changing the size of table tennis balls, the ITTF adjusted the scoring system for competitive table tennis, so that the first player to score 11 points wins a game, unless both are tied on 10, in which case the first player to score a 2-point lead is the winner. Prior to this, a game was won by the first player to reach 21 points. The ITTF felt the change in scoring was necessary to make games more exciting, and to shorten the length of matches, so these would be more engaging to television audiences. (A match consists of an odd number of games, and a player must win a majority of games to win the match; matches in competitive table tennis consist of five or seven games.) Whether the scoring change succeeded in meeting this goal is an open question, but matches finish much more quickly, since nearly half as many points are now required to win most games (except, of course, in the case of a 10–10 tie). In spite of this, amateur players often play a game until someone scores 21 (or wins by at least 2 points), either because they are nostalgic for the old scoring system or because they are unaware of the ITTF's decision.

21. The author would most likely agree that non-professional players:

    A. do not always know of rule changes in professional sport.
    B. always abide by the current rules of sporting associations.
    C. do not have an opinion on the actions of sporting associations.
    D. always prefer to play a sport under the rules they first learned.

22. Under current ITTF rules, a table tennis game could be won by a score of:

    A. 11–10
    B. 12–11
    C. 13–11
    D. 21–20

23. It must be false that the Chinese National Team:

    A. were known for a faster style of play.
    B. campaigned against the increase in ball size.
    C. did better with smaller balls, as they had more spin.
    D. prefer the larger ball size.

24. The stars on table tennis balls sanctioned for ITTF play may include any of these colours except:

    A. black
    B. green
    C. orange
    D. purple

In the mid-nineteenth century, the French novelist Emile Zola announced to his publisher that he was embarking on a cycle of novels in the style of Balzac that would explore various aspects of life in France during the Second Empire. Unlike *La Comedie Humaine*, though, Zola's cycle would focus its attentions on one family, allowing Zola to explore his strong interests in heredity, evolution and genealogy at the same time as he offered a literary account of the Second Empire. What resulted was Zola's twenty-novel cycle, collectively known as *Les Rougon-Macquart* and subtitled *Histoire naturelle et sociale d'une famille sons le Second Empire* ('Natural and social history of a family during the second empire'). Zola's work in these novels established his reputation as a pre-eminent proponent of naturalism, a literary movement that emphasised the harsh realities of life through a frank, if pessimistic, depiction of subject matter such as sexuality, corruption and disease that had previously been considered too sordid to be included in literature.

Almost all of the protagonists of the Rougon-Macquart family are introduced in Zola's first novel, *La Fortune des Rougon*. The family centres on Adelaide Fouque, a middle-class French woman from Provence with a slight mental deficiency, and her three children: Pierre Rougon, the legitimate child from her marriage to Rougon, and Antoine and Ursule Macquart, illegitimate children by her lover, the smuggler Macquart. With Adelaide at the centre-point, the novel explores the three strands of her family: the Rougons, who are upper class and well educated; the Macquarts, who are mostly blue-collar workers or soldiers; and the Mourets (the family of Adelaide's illegitimate daughter Ursule Macquart), who live a more middle-class and balanced life.

Zola traced each of his more than 300 characters carefully. Before even beginning to write *La Fortune des Rougon*, he set about creating an elaborate family tree that included each character's name, date of birth, properties of heredity (including their mental proclivities and physical likeness), details of their biography and death date. In each character, Zola traces the competing influences of blood and environment, set against the political, economic, cultural and artistic backdrop of France (and Paris, particularly) from 1852 to 1870. Even in closing this cycle of novels, Zola accounts for the fate of all of his characters. In his final novel, *Le Docteur Pascal*, Zola includes a long chapter that reconnects with all of his living characters, tying up loose ends in their narratives and finishing each of their stories. In this respect, Zola succeeded where Balzac failed; Balzac never finished *La Comedie Humaine*, consisting at the time of his death of more than 90 novels, short stories and essays that represented his only cycle of novels—and, indeed, the entire literary output of his adult life.

25. The Second Empire occurred in the 19th century.

   A. True
   B. False
   C. Can't tell

26. Zola was a notable naturalist.

   A. True
   B. False
   C. Can't tell

27. Zola's novels are set in Paris.

   A. True
   B. False
   C. Can't tell

28. Balzac wrote a cycle of twenty novels, featuring a number of different families.

   A. True
   B. False
   C. Can't tell

Single-sex education for both men and women is declining in the UK. Today, only about 11% of all boys and girls graduate from a single-sex secondary school, and the number of all-women's secondary schools is down to 400, from an historical UK high of about 2,500 in the 1960s. Nevertheless, a debate about the necessity, quality and advantages of single-sex education continues among academics and public officials.

The 1944 Education Act guaranteed free education for all students, regardless of gender, from primary to secondary school. Full access to all levels of education, however, was not fully instituted until the late 1980s, until which point many universities and grammar schools maintained strict quotas on the number of female students they would admit. The increased access women enjoy to all levels of education may explain some of the reasons why the country has seen a decline in the number of women'-only institutions; in fact, women now outnumber men in higher education in the UK. However, there still seem to be some benefits to single-sex education. All-girls schools regularly report highly competitive GCSEs and low dropout rates. Studies suggest that those pupils who are struggling most when they enter the single-sex educational environment are often the students most likely to benefit. Other studies, targeted at adults in their 40s, indicate that graduates of single-sex schools of either gender are less likely to have studied gender-stereotyped subjects in school. Women from this group who graduated from all-girls schools also have higher earnings on average than women who attended school with boys.

Some researchers suggest that the results from these studies, particularly test scores and graduation rates, may be skewed by the economic and class differences at work. Alan Smithers, Professor of Education at the University of Buckingham, argues that pupils in these schools succeed because of their ability and social background, and not the particular environment of the schools.

29. Women in the UK first had full and equal access to education at all levels in the:

    A. 1940s
    B. 1960s
    C. 1980s
    D. 1990s

30. The author seems open to the possibility that:

    A. no students would benefit from a single-sex school.
    B. single-sex schools do not benefit women students.
    C. student success depends only on student ability.
    D. student success is tied to socioeconomic factors.

31. It must be false that there are more men than women among UK:

    A. adults aged 40 to 49.
    B. professors of education.
    C. secondary school students.
    D. university students.

32. At their peak, secondary schools in the UK that enrolled only women students numbered:

    A. fewer than two thousand.
    B. more than two thousand.
    C. more than three thousand.
    D. fewer than five hundred.

In late 2006, scientists and beekeepers in North America noted an alarming number of incidents in which all the worker bees from a beehive previously thought to be well functioning and healthy suddenly disappeared. The sudden, sharp rise in this phenomenon, known as colony collapse disorder (CCD), is very worrying, due to the significant share of the world's diet that depends on pollination by bees. More than four-fifths of food crops worldwide that require pollination are pollinated by honey bees; thus, colony collapse disorder—which has now spread to Europe, Asia and South America—represents a serious threat to the food supply.

What, exactly, is causing the disappearance of the bees? Pesticides were the original suspect, and were known to have exterminated the entire population of bees in one Chinese province in the 1980s. Further research has shown that a combination of two infections—a virus and a fungus—is far deadlier for bees than either would be on its own. One hundred per cent of collapsed hives in the study were found to have traces of invertebrate iridescent viruses (IIVs); however, since these are often found in strong colonies, IIVs alone cannot be responsible for colony collapse. A variety of microbes that attack invertebrates were found in most of the collapsed colonies, but most could be eliminated as possible culprits, as they occurred in only a few collapsed hives. However, one fungus called Nosema, which consists of a single cell and targets bees specifically, was found in most of the collapsed colonies in the study. Scientists determined that Nosema is not likely to predict the likelihood of collapse when found in an otherwise healthy hive, absent any traces of IIVs; conversely, the presence of both Nosema and IIVs is a strong indicator of the likelihood of collapse, given the high correlation of the two in collapsed colonies in the study.

There is an added twist to this latest discovery, as tests that had earlier proven that pesticides commonly used on flowers and crops in the USA and Europe are not significantly harmful to bees were flawed; the USA's Environmental Protection Agency confirmed in a confidential report that was subsequently leaked to the press that clothianidin, a pesticide widely used on corn, can be 'highly toxic' and present a 'long-term risk' to bee colonies. Now that the paired infections are understood to cause colony collapse disorder, we must take great care to protect the health of the world's bees. The use of any pesticide thought to make bees more vulnerable to infection should be studied closely and, if found to make bees more likely to be infected by IIVs or Nosema, must be curtailed. The world's food supply faces a potentially catastrophic risk from the continued loss of bees, so any lesser course of action would be inadequate and irresponsible.

33. Which of the following statements about the world's food supply is best supported by the passage?
   A. Most of the world's crops depend on bees for pollination.
   B. Nosema infections are the greatest threat to the world's food supply.
   C. Pesticides are the greatest threat to the world's food supply.
   D. Most of the world's pollinated food crops depend on bees for pollination.

34. The writer of the passage would most likely find which of the following actions sufficient in its attempt to prevent the collapse of further colonies of bees?
   A. Any pesticides that are shown in tests to harm bees should be banned.
   B. Any pesticides that make bees more vulnerable to IIV infection should be banned.
   C. Any pesticides that are shown in tests to make bees more vulnerable to two particular types of infection should be banned.
   D. Any beehives found to contain traces of Nosema should be isolated and fumigated.

35. According to information in the passage, why do scientists believe that IIVs are not the sole cause of colony collapse disorder?
   A. They are found in 100 per cent of collapsed colonies.
   B. They occur in strong colonies as well as collapsed colonies.
   C. They are not found in colonies that are infected with Nosema.
   D. They are more likely to be found in hives that have been sprayed with clothianidin.

36. Which of the following findings, if true, would call into question the finding that paired infections are responsible for colony collapse disorder?

    A. A review of the study that linked IIV and Nosema infections as the joint cause of CCD determines that 75% of the colonies in the study were taken from areas where corn was the primary agricultural crop.

    B. A review of the study that linked IIV and Nosema infections as the joint cause of CCD determines that Nosema infected the colonies in the study that had both infections only after the worker bees had disappeared or died due to IIV infection.

    C. A review of the study that linked IIV and Nosema infections as the joint cause of CCD determines that 75% of the colonies in the study were taken from areas where the crops had not been treated with clothianidin.

    D. A review of the study that linked IIV and Nosema infections as the joint cause of CCD determines that Nosema infection led to IIV infection in the colonies in the study that were infected by both.

In November 1936, Crystal Palace, relocated since the Great Exhibition of 1851 to Sydenham Hill, burned to the ground. The enormous glass and cast iron construction had by that time fallen into disrepair, though in recent years it had seen a revival under the leadership of Sir Henry Buckland and his board of trustees. What started as a small office fire took off quickly, and 89 fire engines and 400 firemen could not stop the blaze. 10,000 people came out to Sydenham Hill to watch the palace as it burned to the ground.

The building that was destroyed in 1936 was very different from that erected in Hyde Park for the Great Exhibition over eighty years earlier. Though all the construction materials had been moved south of London after the six months of the exhibition, what was erected on Sydenham Hill was really a Beaux Arts form, and not the greenhouse-like construction designed by Chatsworth House gardener Joseph Paxton. Some of the same features—public toilets, for example—that had debuted at Crystal Palace during the Great Exhibition were installed in the new site as well. But, the structure had been modified and enlarged, so much so that it exceeded the bounds of the new park designed for its construction.

The relocation of Crystal Palace was an expensive feat, costing £1.3 million (£96.5 million today), over a £1 million more than it had taken to build the original structure. The relocation put Crystal Palace in debt from which it never recovered. Although two separate train stations were built to serve the permanent exhibition, by the 1890s the structure had seriously deteriorated. The palace was used in World War I as a naval training establishment and was later the site of the first Imperial War Museum. Buckland's leadership in the 1920s and 30s improved the gardens and brought visitors back to the palace for the exhibitions and regular fireworks shows, but the 1936 fire prevented him from fully realising the palace's old glory. Nevertheless, as Buckland predicted, Crystal Palace is not forgotten today. In fact, the area of Penge Common and Sydenham Hill, where the structure was relocated over 150 years ago, is now known as Crystal Palace.

37. The Imperial War Museum is located at Crystal Palace.

    A. True

    B. False

    C. Can't tell

38. The Great Exhibition of 1851 featured the first public toilets.

    A. True

    B. False

    C. Can't tell

39. Crystal Palace was originally in Hyde Park.

    A. True

    B. False

    C. Can't tell

40. A fireworks display started the fire that destroyed Crystal Palace.

    A. True

    B. False

    C. Can't tell

At the end of 2010, the Bank of England announced plans to increase the number of £5 notes in circulation in the UK. At that time, there was a total of 1.5 billion £20 notes, 640 million £10 notes and 250 million £5 notes in circulation, leading to much frustration among businesses and customers alike. The dearth of £5 notes in the country often requires businesses to give change using £1 and £2 coins, and results in the stock of circulating £5 notes wearing out more quickly than any other UK banknote. The £5 note can only circulate for a year before becoming too damaged for further use. By contrast, the £50 note has the longest lifespan of any British note, lasting five years before having to be replaced. But, then, £50 notes are not dispensed at cash points.

The Bank of England's plan involves a massive rise in the number of £5 notes in circulation—to include 400 million more £5 notes by 2012—and to increase the share of £5 notes in cash withdrawn from cash machines from 0.2% to 1.2%. To reach this target, the Bank of England has encouraged high street banks to make £5 notes available at more cash machines, as the vast majority give out only £10 and £20 notes. Of the 63,268 cash machines in the UK network in 2010, only 1,435 dispense £5 notes. Most high street banks have made £5 notes available more widely at cash machines, but have not added enough capacity to reach the Bank of England's targets. The reticence to make £5 notes more available at UK cash machines is likely due to banks' decision to follow the model of American ATMs (or 'automated teller machines', as they are known) before cash machines exploded in popularity in this country. (There were only 20,000 cash machines on the UK network in 1990.) Most American cash machines give out only $20 bills, as this is thought to be simpler for banks and customers. It's no wonder, then, that the £20 note is the king of the UK cash machine, and that the £5 note continues to struggle to get into our wallets.

41. The bank note you are least likely to withdraw from a UK cash machine is the:

    A. £5 note
    B. £10 note
    C. £20 note
    D. £50 note

42. It is correct to infer that, over two decades:

    A. the number of UK high street banks has doubled.
    B. the number of £5 notes in circulation has dropped.
    C. the number of UK cash machines has more than trebled.
    D. the lifespan of £5 notes has increased.

43. In 2010, the Bank of England had a 2-year plan to increase:

    A. the inventory of cashpoints that dispense £10 notes.
    B. the number of £5 notes by 60%.
    C. the inventory of £5 notes circulating by 160%.
    D. the number of £5 notes taken from cashpoints by 1%.

44. It must be false that:

    A. the £5 note lasts longer than the £10 note.
    B. the £10 note lasts longer than the £5 note.
    C. the £20 note lasts longer than the £10 note.
    D. the £50 note lasts longer than the £20 note.

STOP. IF YOU FINISH BEFORE TIME IS UP, CHECK ANY QUESTIONS YOU HAVE MARKED FOR REVIEW. YOU MAY GO BACK TO QUESTIONS IN THIS SECTION ONLY.

This section contains 9 sets of data, each of which is followed by four questions. Each question will have five answer choices. Your task is to select the best option based on the data provided.

Answer all 36 questions in Section 2, selecting one of the possible answers and circling the letter corresponding to the appropriate answer in your test booklet.

When you are finished with this section, you may use any remaining time to review your work in this section only. Once you proceed to the next section, you may not return to this section.

You will have 22 minutes to answer the questions. It is in your best interest to select an answer for every item as there is no penalty for wrong answers.

You may use a calculator to answer the questions in this section. On Test Day, you will be provided with an onscreen calculator that can perform the four basic operations (addition, subtraction, multiplication and division) along with only a few extra features (percentage, reciprocal, square root and memory buttons). You should not use any functions beyond these on the calculator used for this Kaplan UKCAT Mock Test.

Set your timer for 22 minutes, turn the page and begin the section.

The graph below shows the annual sales of Spiral Enterprises in different parts of the country.

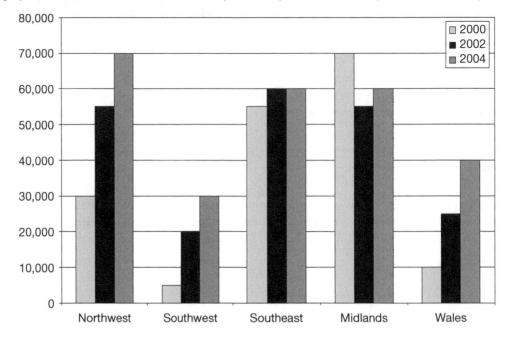

1. Which region had the highest average sales for the 3 years shown?
    A. Northwest
    B. Southwest
    C. Southeast
    D. Midlands
    E. Wales

2. Which region had the highest sales in 2004?
    A. Northwest
    B. Southeast
    C. Midlands
    D. Northwest and Midlands
    E. Southwest and Midlands

3. Which region experienced the greatest growth percentage in sales from 2002 to 2004?
    A. Northwest
    B. Southwest
    C. Southeast
    D. Midlands
    E. Wales

4. What were the total sales for all five regions in the year with the highest total sales?
    A. 170,000
    B. 215,000
    C. 260,000
    D. 270,000
    E. Can't tell

The diagram below shows the floor plan of a new suite of offices for a small company.

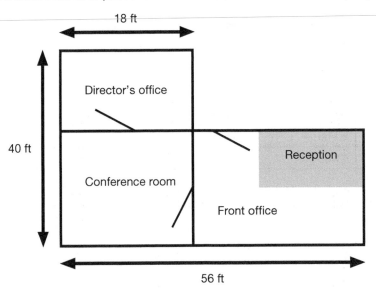

+ The reception area (shaded in the diagram above) is 35% of the area of the combined reception/front office room. This is shown as an approximation, and is not to scale.

+ The floors of the offices can be covered with carpeting, at a cost of £2.99 per square foot, or with laminate flooring, at a cost of £4.45 per square foot.

5. The director's office is 108 square feet smaller than the conference room. What is the area of the conference room, in square feet?

    A. 306
    B. 414
    C. 684
    D. 720
    E. 874

6. What is the total area of the reception/front office room?

    A. 306 ft^2
    B. 484 ft^2
    C. 568 ft^2
    D. 874 ft^2
    E. Can't tell

7. What are the dimensions of the reception area?

    A. 17 ft × 18 ft
    B. 15 ft × 20.4 ft
    C. 19 ft × 30 ft
    D. 20 ft × 24.2 ft
    E. Can't tell

8. What is the total cost of carpeting the entire suite of offices, except for the reception area?

    A. £3,851.42
    B. £4,766.06
    C. £5,732.05
    D. £7,093.30
    E. Can't tell

Below is a table showing the exam scores for a group of friends.

	English	Maths	Science	French
Derek	44/60	39/80	84/100	80/100
Zack	48/60	64/80	78/100	65/100
Amanda	29/60	74/80	54/100	42/100
David	4/60	75/80	47/100	18/100
Emily	58/60	76/80	89/100	100/100
Joel	41/60	28/80	96/100	74/100

9. Which of the six friends scored the highest in Science?

    A. Amanda

    B. David

    C. Derek

    D. Emily

    E. Joel

10. Who scored the best across all subjects?

    A. Amanda

    B. Derek

    C. Emily

    D. Joel

    E. Zack

11. David resits his English exam, and scores 36/60. What is the percentage rise in his English score?

    A. 60%

    B. 80%

    C. 600%

    D. 800%

    E. Can't tell

12. What is the mean score of all the Science marks of all six friends to the nearest integer?

    A. 69/100

    B. 75/100

    C. 79/100

    D. 84/100

    E. 88/100

Below are the profits Equinox Holdings made from their different businesses across sectors including Retail, Leisure, Commercial and Industrial in the past three years.

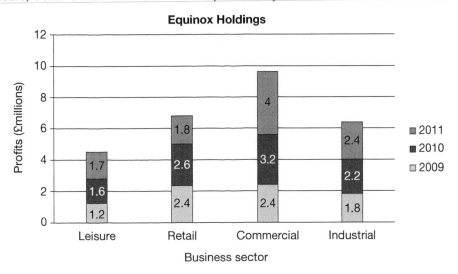

Profit figures above are given in millions of pounds, e.g. 2.2 refers to £2,200,000.

13. How much profit did businesses in the Retail sector make in 2010?
    A. £2,400,000
    B. £2,600,000
    C. £2,800,000
    D. £24,000,000
    E. £26,000,000

14. How much profit did businesses in the Leisure sector make in 2011?
    A. £1,200,000
    B. £1,600,000
    C. £1,700,000
    D. £16,000,000
    E. £17,000,000

15. The profits of the Commercial sector increased by what percentage from 2009 to 2010?
    A. 20%
    B. 25%
    C. 30%
    D. 33%
    E. 37%

16. What was the total profit across all business sectors in 2010?
    A. £7.8 million
    B. £8.6 million
    C. £9.6 million
    D. £9.9 million
    E. £10.3 million

A medical school surveyed its 336 first-year students, and asked them to pick their favourite module from the year. All students selected one option only, as illustrated in the table.

Module	Number of students selecting this as their favourite module
Cellular Biology	45
Genetics	68
Immunology	67
Pathology	44
Pharmacology	81
Ethics	22
Other	9

Among 'Other' modules, only Physiology and Patient Safety (2 votes each) received more than a single vote.

17. According to the survey, what is the most preferred module?

    A. Cellular Biology

    B. Genetics

    C. Immunology

    D. Patient Safety

    E. Pharmacology

18. What proportion of students chose one of the three most popular modules as their favourite?

    A. 1:4

    B. 3:7

    C. 4:9

    D. 9:14

    E. 11:17

19. What percentage of students chose Physiology as their favourite module?

    A. 1%

    B. 2%

    C. 5%

    D. 6%

    E. 7%

20. Which module was selected as the favourite by the fewest students?

    A. Ethics

    B. Pathology

    C. Patient Safety

    D. Physiology

    E. Can't tell

Whilst holidaying in Majorca, Christos and Vasilis enjoy spending time on the water, riding in a motorboat and on jet skis with a top speed of 60 miles per hour.

21. Christos rides a jet ski for 1 hour, 12 minutes, at an average speed of 45 miles per hour. How far does Christos travel on his jet ski?

    A. 48 miles
    B. 50 miles
    C. 52 miles
    D. 54 miles
    E. 56 miles

22. Vasilis starts out on his jet ski at the same time as Christos, but Vasilis travels 16 miles further than Christos, in a total time of 75 minutes. What is Vasilis's average speed, in miles per hour?

    A. 46
    B. 47
    C. 56
    D. 57
    E. 58

23. How many minutes will it take Christos to catch up to Vasilis, if he travels at top speed?

    A. 16
    B. 21
    C. 25
    D. 26
    E. Can't tell

24. The next day, Vasilis covers the same distance at a more leisurely pace, completing his jet ski ride in 2 hours. By what percentage has his journey time increased?

    A. 40%
    B. 60%
    C. 64%
    D. 67%
    E. 167%

Mr Johnston has a circular area in his garden that he wishes to renovate. The radius of this area is 5 metres. He has two options for the ground work in the garden and the cost of purchasing the materials for these is listed in the table below.

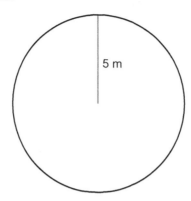

5 m

	Materials cost (£/m²)	Labour cost (£/m²)
Lawn turf	£2.00	£3.00
Paving slabs	£6.00	£2.00

25. If Mr Johnston uses lawn turf on the entire circular garden, how much will the materials cost?
   A. £78.50
   B. £95.50
   C. £157.00
   D. £314.00
   E. £412.50

26. If Mr Johnston uses paving slabs on the entire circular garden, how much will the materials cost?
   A. £235.50
   B. £471.00
   C. £612.00
   D. £720.50
   E. £760.00

27. Mr Johnston has a budget of £750 for the renovation project. If he uses paving slabs across the entire garden, how much money will he have left in his budget after considering material and labour costs?
   A. £14.00
   B. £43.50
   C. £122.00
   D. £174.50
   E. £279.00

28. Mr Johnston decides to put a new circular garden fountain with a diameter of 2 m in the middle of the garden. What is the area of the garden that is not covered by the new fountain?
   A. 56.2 m
   B. 65.9 m
   C. 67.2 m
   D. 68.4 m
   E. 75.4 m

The trend in gold and silver prices per ounce for the past 10 years is shown below. Gold and silver are both traded in US dollars.

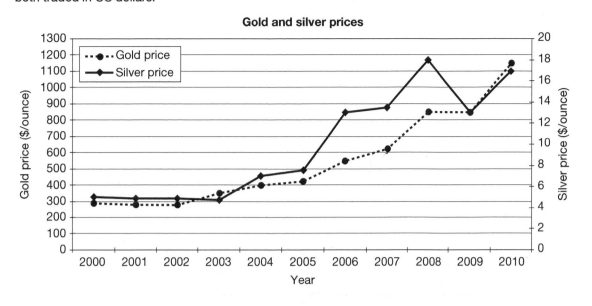

29. Approximately what was the price of gold in dollars per ounce in 2007?

    A. 850
    B. 860
    C. 890
    D. 920
    E. Can't tell

30. Which year recorded the greatest difference between gold and silver, in price per ounce?

    A. 2002
    B. 2003
    C. 2006
    D. 2008
    E. 2010

31. By what percentage did silver increase in price per ounce from 2000 to 2010?

    A. 183%
    B. 240%
    C. 260%
    D. 325%
    E. 350%

32. At 2010 prices, how many ounces of silver could you buy for the value of 100 ounces of gold?

    A. 104
    B. 620
    C. 6,197
    D. 6,765
    E. 7,500

Mohsin is training for the London Marathon and as part of his preparation he runs daily for 42 kilometres. His fastest time to complete 42 km is 3 hours, 25 minutes.

33. What was Mohsin's average speed in kilometres per hour (km/h), when he ran his fastest run of 42 km?
    A. 12.1
    B. 12.3
    C. 12.5
    D. 12.7
    E. 12.9

34. If Mohsin runs for 21 km at a speed of 13 km/h, which of the following is the minimum average speed in kilometres per hour he needs to run to achieve a new fastest time?
    A. 11.1
    B. 11.4
    C. 11.7
    D. 12.3
    E. 12.6

35. Last Saturday, Mohsin decided to take a new route and did not record the distance he travelled. If he spent 3 hours, 45 minutes running and his average speed was 12 km/h, what distance did he run?
    A. 45 km
    B. 46 km
    C. 47 km
    D. 48 km
    E. 49 km

36. Mohsin has set a target of 3 hours, 15 minutes for the London Marathon; to ensure he achieves this target, he must train at a speed such that his time is 5% quicker than his target. At what speed must he train?
    A. 12.9
    B. 13.1
    C. 13.3
    D. 13.6
    E. 13.8

STOP. IF YOU FINISH BEFORE TIME IS UP, CHECK ANY QUESTIONS YOU HAVE MARKED FOR REVIEW. YOU MAY GO BACK TO QUESTIONS IN THIS SECTION ONLY.

This section contains 55 questions, in one or two of the following question types:

- Type 1 questions will include a total of 5 test shapes, along with a Set A in which all the items are similar to each other and a Set B in which all the items are similar to each other. Your task is to determine in what way the shapes in each set are similar and to decide whether each test shape fits into Set A, Set B or neither set.

- Type 2 questions will include a progression of four boxes in a single row. Your task is to select the test shape that comes next in the progression.

- Type 3 questions will include a statement, with two boxes in the top row and two boxes in the bottom row. There is some progression from the first box to the second box in the top row, and the second box in the bottom row is blank. Your task is to select the test shape that fills the blank box, so that the progression in the bottom row is the same as the progression in the top row.

- Type 4 questions will include a Set A in which all the items are similar to each other and a Set B in which all the items are similar to each other. Your task is to choose the test shape that belongs to the set mentioned in the question.

Answer all 55 questions in Section 3, selecting one of the possible answers and circling the letter corresponding to the appropriate answer in your test booklet.

When you are finished with this section, you may use any remaining time to review your work in this section only. Once you proceed to the next section, you may not return to this section.

You will have 13 minutes to answer the questions. It is in your best interest to select an answer for every item as there is no penalty for wrong answers.

Set your timer for 13 minutes, turn the page and begin the section.

Set A

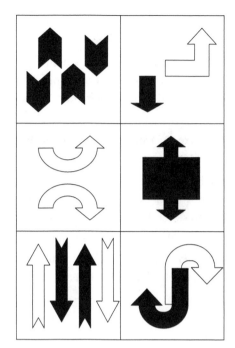

Set B

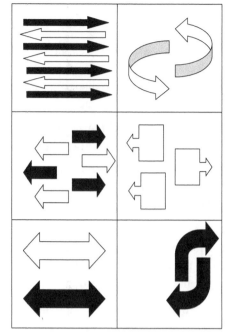

Test Shapes

1	2	3	4	5

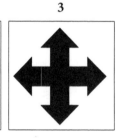 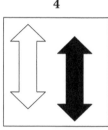 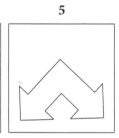

1
A. Set A
B. Set B
C. Neither *(circled)*

2
A. Set A
B. Set B *(circled)*
C. Neither

3
A. Set A *(circled)*
B. Set B
C. Neither

4
A. Set A
B. Set B *(circled)*
C. Neither

5
A. Set A
B. Set B
C. Neither *(circled)*

Set A	Set B

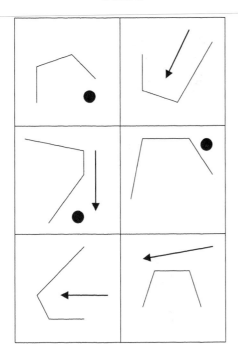 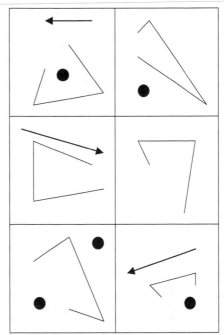

Test Shapes

6	7	8	9	10

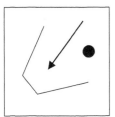 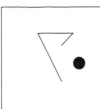 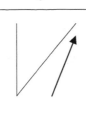 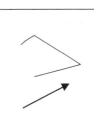 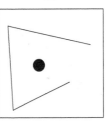

A. Set A	A. Set A	A. Set A	A. Set A	A. Set A
B. Set B	B. Set B	B. Set B	B. Set B	B. Set B
C. Neither	C. Neither	C. Neither	C. Neither	C. Neither

Set A   **Set B**

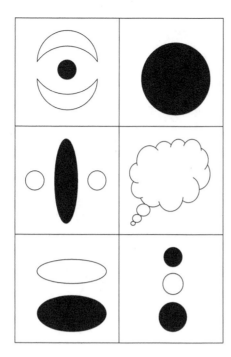
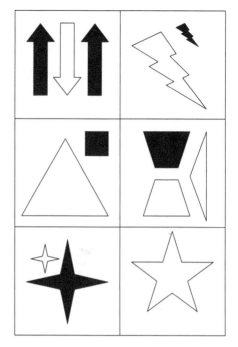

Test Shapes

11	12	13	14	15

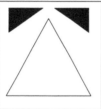
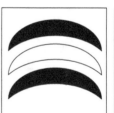

11	12	13	14	15
A. Set A	A. Set A	A. Set A	A. Set A	A. Set A
B. Set B	B. Set B	B. Set B	B. Set B	B. Set B
C. Neither	C. Neither	C. Neither	C. Neither	C. Neither

11. B. Set B
12. B. Set B
13. C. Neither
14. A. Set A
15. C. Neither

Set A   **Set B**

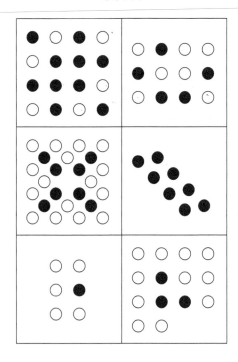
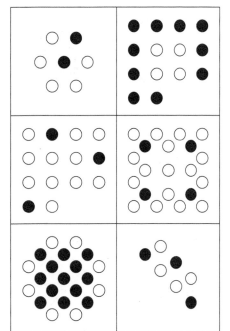

Test Shapes

16	17	18	19	20

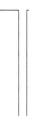 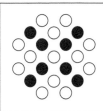 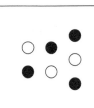 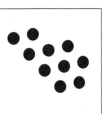 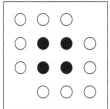

16	17	18	19	20
A. Set A	A. Set A	A. Set A	A. Set A	A. Set A
B. Set B	B. Set B	B. Set B	B. Set B	B. Set B
C. Neither	C. Neither	C. Neither	C. Neither	C. Neither

Set A   **Set B**

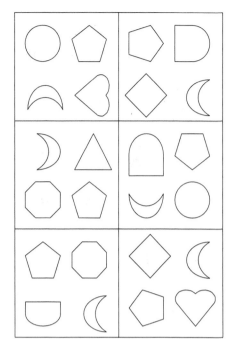 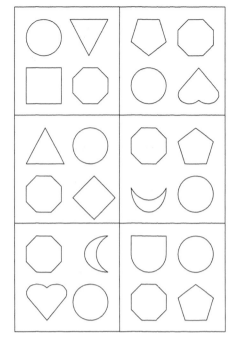

Test Shapes

21	22	23	24	25

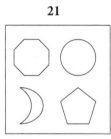 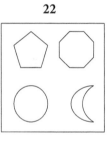 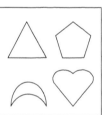 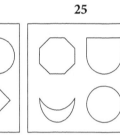

A. Set A   A. Set A   A. Set A   A. Set A   A. Set A

B. Set B   B. Set B   B. Set B   B. Set B   B. Set B

C. Neither   C. Neither   C. Neither   C. Neither   C. Neither

Set A	Set B

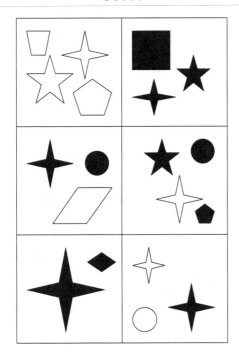 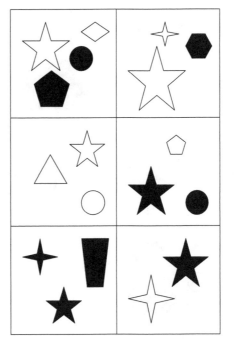

Test Shapes

26	27	28	29	30

 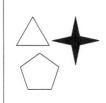 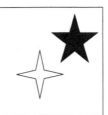 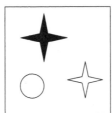 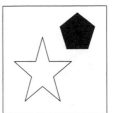

26	27	28	29	30
A. Set A	A. Set A	A. Set A	A. Set A	A. Set A
B. Set B	B. Set B	B. Set B	B. Set B	B. Set B
C. Neither	C. Neither	C. Neither	C. Neither	C. Neither

Set A   **Set B**

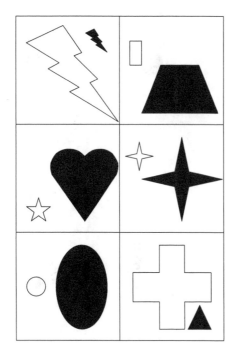
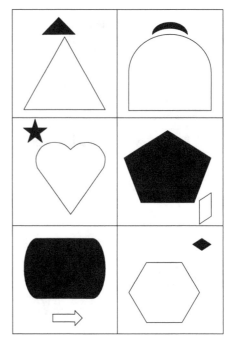

Test Shapes

31	32	33	34	35

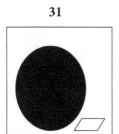  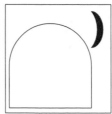 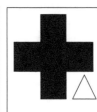

31	32	33	34	35
A. Set A	A. Set A	A. Set A	A. Set A	A. Set A
B. Set B	B. Set B	B. Set B	B. Set B	B. Set B
C. Neither	C. Neither	C. Neither	C. Neither	C. Neither

Set A   **Set B**

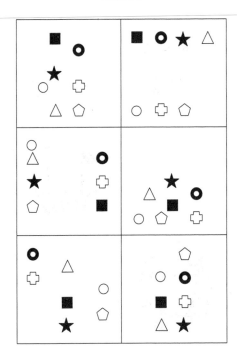
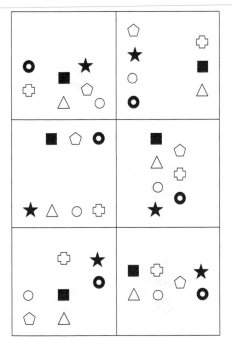

Test Shapes

36	37	38	39	40

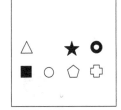
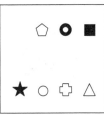
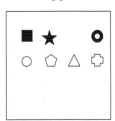
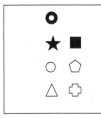
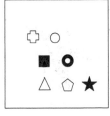

A. Set A	A. Set A	A. Set A	A. Set A	A. Set A
B. Set B	B. Set B	B. Set B	B. Set B	B. Set B
C. Neither	C. Neither	C. Neither	C. Neither	C. Neither

Set A

Set B

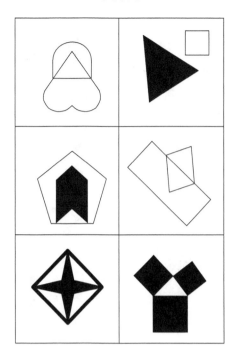
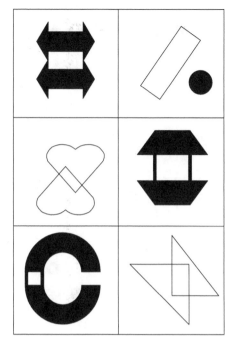

Test Shapes

41	42	43	44	45

 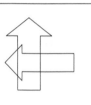 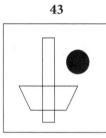  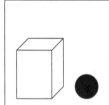

41	42	43	44	45
A. Set A	A. Set A	A. Set A	A. Set A	A. Set A
B. Set B	B. Set B	B. Set B	B. Set B	B. Set B
C. Neither	C. Neither	C. Neither	C. Neither	C. Neither

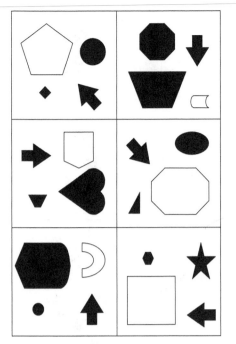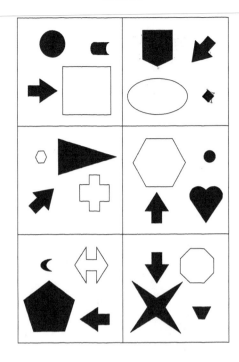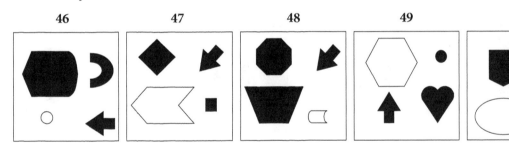

Set A   **Set B**

Test Shapes

46	47	48	49	50

46
A. Set A
B. Set B
C. Neither

47
A. Set A
B. Set B
C. Neither

48
A. Set A
B. Set B
C. Neither

49
A. Set A
B. Set B
C. Neither

50
A. Set A
B. Set B
C. Neither

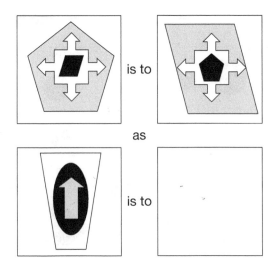

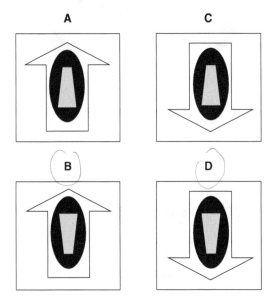

51. Which figure completes the statement?

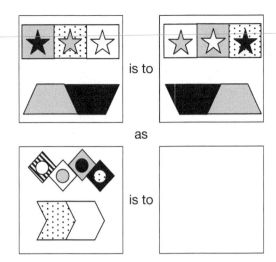

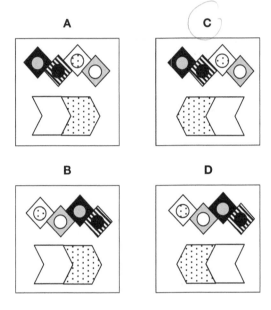

52. Which figure completes the statement?

A   C

B   D

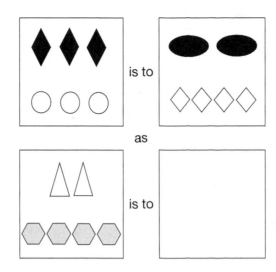

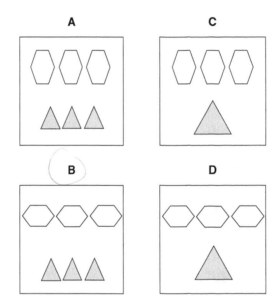

53. Which figure completes the statement?

| A | C |
| B | D |

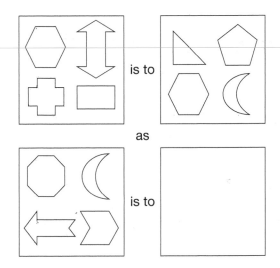

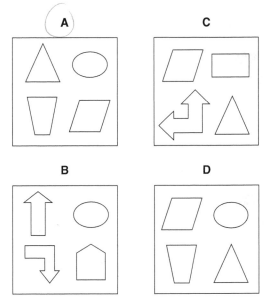

54. Which figure completes the statement?

A

C

B

D

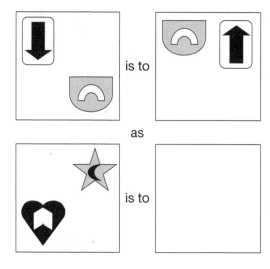

is to

as

is to

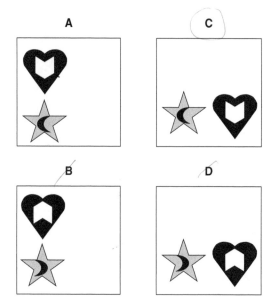

55. Which figure completes the statement?

A

C

B

D

STOP. IF YOU FINISH BEFORE TIME IS UP, CHECK ANY QUESTIONS YOU HAVE MARKED FOR REVIEW. YOU MAY GO BACK TO QUESTIONS IN THIS SECTION ONLY.

This section contains information relating to a scenario. Your task is to answer a number of questions based on your interpretation of the information provided. Additional information will be presented after you have completed some of the questions. This new information will apply to subsequent questions.

Answer all 28 questions in Section 4, selecting one of the possible answers and circling the letter corresponding to the appropriate answer in your test booklet. A few questions will require you to select two answers from the options given, as two correct answers must be chosen in order to answer such questions correctly.

When you are finished with this section, you may use any remaining time to review your work in this section only. Once you proceed to the next section, you may not return to this section.

You will have 33 minutes to answer the questions. It is in your best interest to select an answer for every item as there is no penalty for wrong answers.

Set your timer for 33 minutes, turn the page and begin the section.

Astronaut Code

On afternoons when you don't have lectures, you volunteer as a tour guide at the Science Museum. At the end of a tour, a small child runs down a corridor that you were told not to enter. You give chase, and find the child has entered a secret room that contains an electronic panel with a series of switches and lights corresponding to letters and numbers. The meaning of the letters and numbers are given in a table of codes posted on the wall above the panel, along with a series of messages written in code. You instantly recognise the electronic panel from photographs you have seen of an early prototype of the space shuttle, and the messages seem to relate the adventures, experiences and personal thoughts and insights of astronauts. After taking the child back to his parents, you return to the secret room and attempt to determine the code's exact logical workings.

Some of the information will be strange or incomplete but all of the messages contain some logic. You will therefore need to make assessments based on the codes rather than what seems like the most predictable translation. Every code has a best answer that makes the most sense based on all the information presented, but remember that this test requires you to make judgements rather than simply apply logic and rules.

Table of Codes

Operators & General Rules	Specific Information Basic Codes
A = big	1 = star
B = negative	2 = moon
C = fast	3 = human
D = up	4 = them
E = beyond	5 = home
F = opposite	6 = ship
G = one	7 = journey
H = fix	8 = burn
J = grow	9 = stop
K = new	10 = head
	11 = today
	12 = air
	13 = tank
	14 = fuel
	15 = cold
	16 = plant
	17 = waste

Example 1

What is the best interpretation of the coded message: A1, 14, 16J

- A. Plant fuel makes the star grow big. *(recombines elements from the message)*
- B. One sun fuels the growing plants. *(one is in the table, but not in the message)*
- C. The sun is fuel for plant creatures. *(creatures is not a good representation of grow)*
- D. Growing plants are fuel for the star. *(omits a representation of big)*
- E. The sun fuels plant growth. *(CORRECT)*

Example 2

What is the best interpretation of the coded message: 5(F2), A(A7)

- A. Earth is not very far away. *(negative is in the table, but not in the message)*
- B. Earth is very far away. *(CORRECT)*
- C. The home planet is not far away. *(negative is in the table, but not in the message)*
- D. Their home planet is very far away. *(them is in the table, but not in the message)*
- E. Our home planet is a very long journey from here. *(no representation of our in the message)*

1. What is the best interpretation of the coded message: 2D, 3, 9, 10(7)
   A. The human stopped the leader of the moon voyage.
   B. Humans stop the journey leader on the moon.
   C. Humans on the moon stop the head ship.
   D. Humans go on a head-trip at night.
   E. At night, humans stop thinking.

2. What is the best interpretation of the coded message: F4, 12(7), F2, A7, F2
   A. The distance between planets was too far to travel.
   B. We flew a great distance between planets.
   C. The distance between suns was too far for us to travel.
   D. We flew from a planet to a distant moon.
   E. The distance from planet to sun is too far for them to fly.

3. What would be the best way to encode the following message?
   Message: The aliens don't eat plants.
   A. G16, B14, 4(F5)
   B. 16, 14, 4(F3)
   C. G16, B, 4(F5)
   D. 16, B14, 4(F5)
   E. G16, 14, 4(F3)

4. What is the best interpretation of the coded message: F4, F9, 5, 16(BJ)
   A. We stopped opposite the house with no plants.
   B. We went to the house with no plants.
   C. We left home because plants couldn't grow.
   D. We left Earth because there were no plants.
   E. No plants grow on Earth, so we have a new home.

5. What is the best interpretation of the coded message: J3, 12(13), FJ(JC)
   A. Growing humans use up more air from the tank.
   B. More humans will use up the air tanks.
   C. More humans empty the air tank more quickly.
   D. A growing human's air tank slowly shrinks.
   E. Humanity's air tank is not growing.

6. What would be the best way to encode the following message?
   Message: A new planet with plants is our new home.
   A. K(F2, 16), K(5, F4)
   B. K(F2), J16, K5, J(F4)
   C. K(F2), JA16, K5, F4
   D. F2, K16, K5, F4
   E. F2, K16, K(5, F4)

Table of Codes

Operators & General Rules	Specific Information Basic Codes
A = big	1 = star
B = negative	2 = moon
C = fast	3 = human
D = up	4 = them
E = beyond	5 = home
F = opposite	6 = ship
G = one	7 = journey
H = fix	8 = burn
J = grow	9 = stop
K = new	10 = head
	11 = today
	12 = air
	13 = tank
	14 = fuel
	15 = cold
	16 = plant
	17 = waste

7. What is the best interpretation of the coded message: 6(A8(14), AC(7D)), E11

    A. In future, the rocket ship will journey into space.

    B. Tomorrow, the ship burns the rockets.

    C. In future, the rocket ship will fly past the sun.

    D. Tomorrow, we will launch the ship into space.

    E. The rocket ship launches tomorrow.

8. What is the best interpretation of the coded message: F2, J(15, C), B, F4(3)

    A. A fast-freezing planet is not for us humans.

    B. We humans cannot live on a fast-freezing planet.

    C. We humans can't stay on a fast-freezing planet.

    D. A quickly cooling sun is no place for humans or aliens.

    E. A quickly cooling sun is alien to us.

9. What would be the best way to encode the following message?

Message: In the distant future, the sun will shrink and become cold.

    A. A(AE11), A1, FJ, 9(8)

    B. E11, A1, FJ, JC

    C. A(AE11), A1, FJ, JC

    D. E11, A1, BJ, 9(8)

    E. A(F11), A1, BJ, JC

10. What would be the best way to encode the following message?

Message: One night, many stars fell around us.

    A. 2D, J1, 7(FD), FE, F4

    B. G(2D), F(G1), 7(FD), FE, F4

    C. G(2D), A(A1), 7(FD), FE, 4

    D. 2D, A(A1), F9, FD, 4

    E. G(2D), F(G1), F9, FD, 4

11. What is the best interpretation of the coded message: 4(F5), B9, 6(F4), 8B

    A. The aliens burned our ship, but didn't stop us.

    B. We stopped the aliens from burning our ship.

    C. The broken laser on our ship allowed the aliens to escape.

    D. The aliens didn't stop our ship with the evil laser.

    E. We didn't stop the alien ship because the laser failed.

After doing your preliminary research, you discover the code is in fact much more complex than you originally thought. The additional codes and information complete the table as follows:

Table of Codes—Complete Code

Operators & General Rules	Specific Information Basic Codes	Complex Information Additional Information	Reactions/Outcomes Emotions
A = big	1 = star	101 = launch	201 = panic
B = negative	2 = moon	102 = time	202 = love
C = fast	3 = human	103 = orange	203 = sorrow
D = up	4 = them	104 = fight	204 = easy
E = beyond	5 = home	105 = army	205 = hopeful
F = opposite	6 = ship	106 = money	206 = different
G = one	7 = journey	107 = sail	207 = worry
H = fix	8 = burn	108 = search	
J = grow	9 = stop	109 = scratch	
K = new	10 = head	110 = rock	
L = give	11 = today	111 = find	
M = special	12 = air	112 = learn	
	13 = tank		
	14 = fuel		
	15 = cold		
	16 = plant		
	17 = waste		
	18 = heart		
	19 = send		

12. What is the best interpretation of the coded message: A1, BM, JA(J1, JA1, J2, JF2)
    A. The sun is not unique in the universe.
    B. The stars are not alone in our galaxy.
    C. The sun is unique in the galaxy.
    D. The galaxy is nothing without the sun.
    E. The universe is unique because of the sun.

13. What is the best interpretation of the coded message: 10(3), 9(6, 7), H(7, K1)
    A. The captain stopped the ship and realigned its path for a new star.
    B. The captain stopped the ship's progress and set course for a new star.
    C. After stopping the ship, the captain set course for a new star.
    D. The captain set course for a special star while the ship was stopped.
    E. The head ship's progress was stopped and changed from one star to another.

14. What is the best interpretation of the coded message: A(FL12, J, 202, 9(FL12)), E2, F204
    A. Life in space is unusual.
    B. Life in space is not easy.
    C. Life in space is hard.
    D. It's not easy to live in space.
    E. It's hard to live your whole life in space.

Table of Codes—Complete Code

Operators & General Rules	Specific Information Basic Codes	Complex Information Additional Information	Reactions/Outcomes Emotions
A = big	1 = star	101 = launch	201 = panic
B = negative	2 = moon	102 = time	202 = love
C = fast	3 = human	103 = orange	203 = sorrow
D = up	4 = them	104 = fight	204 = easy
E = beyond	5 = home	105 = army	205 = hopeful
F = opposite	6 = ship	106 = money	206 = different
G = one	7 = journey	107 = sail	207 = worry
H = fix	8 = burn	108 = search	
J = grow	9 = stop	109 = scratch	
K = new	10 = head	110 = rock	
L = give	11 = today	111 = find	
M = special	12 = air	112 = learn	
	13 = tank		
	14 = fuel		
	15 = cold		
	16 = plant		
	17 = waste		
	18 = heart		
	19 = send		

15. What would be the best way to encode the following message?

Message: A rich man will pay for a private space launch.

     A. 3(A106), L106, A101, E2

     B. 3(106), L106, 7D, E2

     C. 3(A106), L106, 7D, E2

     D. 3(106), L106, M101, 2

     E. 3(A106), L106, M101, E2

16. What is the best interpretation of the coded message: 3(107, 6), (108, B111), 103(2), 14(F9)

     A. The astronaut discovered a fuel source on the orange moon.

     B. The pilot explored the orange moon for a fuel source.

     C. The orange moon is a fuel source for the space shuttle Explorer.

     D. The space shuttle sought, but did not find, a fuel depot on the orange moon.

     E. The fuel depot on the orange moon was discovered by astronauts.

17. What is the best interpretation of the coded message: 105(E2), 9(104), K(FA105), B111, 105

     A. The reinforcements couldn't find the space army, so the army surrendered.

     B. The replacements found the space army, but the army did not stop fighting.

     C. The space army surrendered because the reinforcements couldn't find them.

     D. The fighting stopped when the new troops found the space army.

     E. One space army stopped fighting and sent new troops to find another army.

18. What is the best interpretation of the coded message: 3(107, 1), L, J(10, 18, FG), E102, 19(6)

     A. A ship sends an astronaut to a distant time and place.

     B. The astronaut sent the ship to give a body to his future self.

     C. A ship without an astronaut gives everything to the future.

     D. An astronaut gives his entire body and future to the mission.

     E. Astronauts give everything for a mission far, far away.

19. What is the best interpretation of the coded message: A110(107(E12), G102), B(F101), 5(F2)

     A. The asteroid fell down to Earth.

     B. The space rock failed to launch.

     C. We don't launch rockets at home, but one time we did.

     D. Home is no place to launch a rocket, but one time we went sailing.

     E. The comet fell to Earth.

Table of Codes—Complete Code

Operators & General Rules	Specific Information Basic Codes	Complex Information Additional Information	Reactions/Outcomes Emotions
A = big	1 = star	101 = launch	201 = panic
B = negative	2 = moon	102 = time	202 = love
C = fast	3 = human	103 = orange	203 = sorrow
D = up	4 = them	104 = fight	204 = easy
E = beyond	5 = home	105 = army	205 = hopeful
F = opposite	6 = ship	106 = money	206 = different
G = one	7 = journey	107 = sail	207 = worry
H = fix	8 = burn	108 = search	
J = grow	9 = stop	109 = scratch	
K = new	10 = head	110 = rock	
L = give	11 = today	111 = find	
M = special	12 = air	112 = learn	
	13 = tank		
	14 = fuel		
	15 = cold		
	16 = plant		
	17 = waste		
	18 = heart		
	19 = send		

20. What is the best interpretation of the coded message: B16(J3), A207

    A. No plants grow humans; it's not a concern.

    B. No plants can grow humans, so don't worry.

    C. The lack of food is a serious concern.

    D. It's not a big concern that plants can't grow humans.

    E. The absence of edible plants is not a big problem.

21. What is the best interpretation of the coded message: A103(12), J206, 3(10, 205)

    A. The orange gas cloud expands differently than a person would expect.

    B. The orange gas grows just as you would hope.

    C. The orange gas sample grows differently than you would hope.

    D. The orange gas expands in the tank differently than expected.

    E. A person would hope the orange gas expanded, but it didn't.

22. What would be the best way to encode the following message?

Message: I seek a planet where all beings are equal.

    A. G(F4), 109, F2, AJ(3, 4(F5)), B206

    B. F4, 111, F2, AJ3, F206

    C. G(F4), 108, F2, AJ(201, 202, 203, 204), B206

    D. F4, 108, F2, AJ3, F206

    E. G(F4), 108, F2, AJ(3, 4(F5)), B206

23. What is the best interpretation of the coded message: 102(FD), 101, L(F4), J(207, B201)

    A. Countdown to launch makes me emotional.

    B. Countdown to launch can play on our nerves.

    C. We worry but don't panic when countdown begins.

    D. We worry but don't panic when they begin the countdown to launch.

    E. Countdown is worrying, but don't panic while we launch.

24. What is the best interpretation of the coded message: A7, H, JA(F202, 203, 104, F205), FE(18, FH)

    A. Travel is the solution for an aching and sentimental heart.

    B. Space travel helps the emotional and heavy-hearted.

    C. Distance heals all the bad feelings within a broken heart.

    D. Time is the furthest distance from trouble to a clean heart.

    E. A great journey fixes all your problems and your heart.

25. What would be the best way to encode the following message?

Message: An astronaut expands knowledge, not conflict.

    A. 3(107, 1), J(FE10), BJ105

    B. 3(107, 1), J(A112), BJ104

    C. 3(107, 1), J10, BJ105

    D. 3(107, 6), J(A112), BJ105

    E. 3(107, 6), J10, BJ104

26. Which of the following would be the most useful and second most useful additions to the codes in order to convey the message accurately?

Message: Poison ivy makes skin red and itchy.

    A. poison

    B. ivy

    C. skin

    D. red

    E. itch

27. Which of the following would be the most useful and second most useful additions to the codes in order to convey the message accurately?

Message: We changed the tank to finish the soldier's blood transfusion.

    A. change

    B. finish

    C. soldier

    D. blood

    E. transfusion

28. Which of the following would be the most useful and second most useful additions to the codes in order to convey the message accurately?

Message: Drop rubbish in a bin, not into space.

    A. command

    B. drop

    C. rubbish

    D. bin

    E. space

STOP. IF YOU FINISH BEFORE TIME IS UP, CHECK ANY QUESTIONS YOU HAVE MARKED FOR REVIEW. YOU MAY GO BACK TO QUESTIONS IN THIS SECTION ONLY.

This section contains 17 theoretical scenarios, each involving a medical or dental professional, or a student preparing for a career in medicine or dentistry. Your task is to read the scenario carefully, and then make a series of judgements about possible options for responding to the situation in the scenario. There are two types of scenarios in this section:

Appropriateness: These scenarios will ask you to rate whether possible responses to the scenario are appropriate or inappropriate.

Importance: These scenarios will ask you to rate whether certain factors are important or not important to consider when responding to the scenario.

The first part of the section will contain Appropriateness scenarios; the final part of the section will contain Importance scenarios. Be sure to answer based on the appropriateness or importance of the response/factor to the person who is named in the question under the scenario. Evaluate the responses/factors independently of each other; do not assume that there will be a response/factor corresponding to each answer choice for each scenario.

Answer all 71 items in Section 5, selecting one of the possible answers and circling the letter corresponding to the appropriate answer in your test book.

When you are finished with this section, you may use any remaining time to review your work in this section only. Once you complete this section, you are finished with the Mock Test. You may then assess your results using the scoring tables that follow.

You will have 26 minutes to answer the questions. It is in your best interest to select an answer for every item as there is no penalty for wrong answers.

Set your timer for 26 minutes, turn the page and begin the section.

Adam is a second-year medical student who must attend anatomy and dissection classes as part of his preclinical training. During his first session he felt very queasy, but manages to make it through the class without vomiting. He is thus very nervous about his second session. He decides to attend; however, before even starting the dissection, he began to feel very sick. His friend, Bella, says that he looks very pale.

How **appropriate** are each of the following responses by **Adam** in this situation?

1. Tell Bella he feels sick, ask her to inform the tutor, and leave the class

    A. A very appropriate thing to do

    B. Appropriate, but not ideal

    C. Inappropriate, but not awful

    D. A very inappropriate thing to do

2. Walk out immediately so as not to disrupt his peers and avoid being sick in the classroom

    A. A very appropriate thing to do

    B. Appropriate, but not ideal

    C. Inappropriate, but not awful

    D. A very inappropriate thing to do

3. Finish the session and afterwards write to the medical school to explain he is unable to continue with anatomy and dissection due to ill health and will instead learn from anatomy books at home

    A. A very appropriate thing to do

    B. Appropriate, but not ideal

    C. Inappropriate, but not awful

    D. A very inappropriate thing to do

4. Tell the instructor he feels unwell, leave the class and catch up on what has been missed later

    A. A very appropriate thing to do

    B. Appropriate, but not ideal

    C. Inappropriate, but not awful

    D. A very inappropriate thing to do

5. Finish this session, and in future pretend to be ill during anatomy sessions

    A. A very appropriate thing to do

    B. Appropriate, but not ideal

    C. Inappropriate, but not awful

    D. A very inappropriate thing to do

Umar is a junior doctor working on a busy hospital ward. He enters the supply cupboard, turns on the light and discovers another junior doctor, Darryl, sat on the floor, crying and drinking from a bottle of whisky. Darryl says that his wife has just left him for another man, and there is no point in going on.

How **appropriate** are each of the following responses by **<u>Umar</u>** in this situation?

6. Express support for Darryl, whilst reminding him that this is not the time or place to drown his sorrows
    A. A very appropriate thing to do
    B. Appropriate, but not ideal
    C. Inappropriate, but not awful
    D. A very inappropriate thing to do

7. Ask Darryl if he would like to chat about what is going on
    A. A very appropriate thing to do
    B. Appropriate, but not ideal
    C. Inappropriate, but not awful
    D. A very inappropriate thing to do

8. Ask Darryl if he is seeing patients today
    A. A very appropriate thing to do
    B. Appropriate, but not ideal
    C. Inappropriate, but not awful
    D. A very inappropriate thing to do

9. Contact the hospital anonymously through their website to report that a doctor has a drinking problem
    A. A very appropriate thing to do
    B. Appropriate, but not ideal
    C. Inappropriate, but not awful
    D. A very inappropriate thing to do

10. Offer to help Darryl get a taxi to take him home
    A. A very appropriate thing to do
    B. Appropriate, but not ideal
    C. Inappropriate, but not awful
    D. A very inappropriate thing to do

11. Encourage Darryl to let his consultant know that he is having a hard time
    A. A very appropriate thing to do
    B. Appropriate, but not ideal
    C. Inappropriate, but not awful
    D. A very inappropriate thing to do

Saba is a junior doctor on the surgical ward. She is well liked by the patients, who say she is always friendly and cheerful. One morning Saba receives a message from a social networking site from a man who she recognises as being a former patient. The patient has requested to add Saba as a contact on the social networking site; Saba can accept, deny or ignore his request.

How **appropriate** are each of the following responses by **Saba** in this situation?

12. Report the patient to the police
    - A. A very appropriate thing to do
    - B. Appropriate, but not ideal
    - C. Inappropriate, but not awful
    - D. A very inappropriate thing to do

13. Deny the man's request
    - A. A very appropriate thing to do
    - B. Appropriate, but not ideal
    - C. Inappropriate, but not awful
    - D. A very inappropriate thing to do

14. Accept the man's request temporarily, so that she can email him to explain why they cannot socialise
    - A. A very appropriate thing to do
    - B. Appropriate, but not ideal
    - C. Inappropriate, but not awful
    - D. A very inappropriate thing to do

15. Ignore the man's request
    - A. A very appropriate thing to do
    - B. Appropriate, but not ideal
    - C. Inappropriate, but not awful
    - D. A very inappropriate thing to do

Dr Davies approaches the nurse's station to make an urgent enquiry regarding a patient. The two nurses at the nurse's station continue to gossip about whether or not an attractive doctor has a girlfriend, without acknowledging Dr Davies.

How **appropriate** are each of the following responses by **Dr Davies** in this situation?

16. Instruct the nurses that they are behaving unprofessionally
    A. A very appropriate thing to do
    B. Appropriate, but not ideal
    C. Inappropriate, but not awful
    D. A very inappropriate thing to do

17. Apologise for interrupting the nurses, and request the information she requires
    A. A very appropriate thing to do
    B. Appropriate, but not ideal
    C. Inappropriate, but not awful
    D. A very inappropriate thing to do

18. Clear her throat several times
    A. A very appropriate thing to do
    B. Appropriate, but not ideal
    C. Inappropriate, but not awful
    D. A very inappropriate thing to do

19. Ask the nurses if one of them could assist with her urgent enquiry regarding a patient
    A. A very appropriate thing to do
    B. Appropriate, but not ideal
    C. Inappropriate, but not awful
    D. A very inappropriate thing to do

Ian is seated directly behind his best friend, Ben, in a written examination. During the examination, Ian notices that Ben has notes written on his arm, hidden by the sleeve of his hoodie, and Ben keeps referring to them. Ian has never witnessed Ben cheating before and knows he would not normally do so, but Ian knows that recently Ben has been very upset over the divorce of his parents, and so may not have had time to prepare adequately for this exam.

How **appropriate** are each of the following responses by <u>Ian</u> in this situation?

20. Tell Ben afterwards that he should not cheat next time
   A. A very appropriate thing to do
   B. Appropriate, but not ideal
   C. Inappropriate, but not awful
   D. A very inappropriate thing to do

21. Raise his hand and discreetly tell an invigilator about Ben
   A. A very appropriate thing to do
   B. Appropriate, but not ideal
   C. Inappropriate, but not awful
   D. A very inappropriate thing to do

22. Wait until the end of the examination to tell an invigilator
   A. A very appropriate thing to do
   B. Appropriate, but not ideal
   C. Inappropriate, but not awful
   D. A very inappropriate thing to do

23. Talk to Ben afterwards about how he is coping with the divorce and whether there is anything Ian can do to support him
   A. A very appropriate thing to do
   B. Appropriate, but not ideal
   C. Inappropriate, but not awful
   D. A very inappropriate thing to do

24. Contact the medical school anonymously explaining what has been witnessed in the exam
   A. A very appropriate thing to do
   B. Appropriate, but not ideal
   C. Inappropriate, but not awful
   D. A very inappropriate thing to do

A junior doctor, Arissa, is attempting to obtain consent for treatment from a patient, but the patient does not respond to any of her questions. The patient appears to listen to what Arissa is saying, but says nothing in response.

How **appropriate** are each of the following responses by **<u>Arissa</u>** in this situation?

25. Check the patient's name to see if she is foreign
    - A. A very appropriate thing to do
    - B. Appropriate, but not ideal
    - C. Inappropriate, but not awful
    - D. A very inappropriate thing to do

26. Proceed with the treatment, explaining each step calmly and clearly
    - A. A very appropriate thing to do
    - B. Appropriate, but not ideal
    - C. Inappropriate, but not awful
    - D. A very inappropriate thing to do

27. Seek advice from a senior colleague
    - A. A very appropriate thing to do
    - B. Appropriate, but not ideal
    - C. Inappropriate, but not awful
    - D. A very inappropriate thing to do

Joanna and Freddie are the two new junior doctors on the wards. Joanna decides to spend most afternoons teaching the medical students, leaving Freddie to do the boring paperwork.

How **appropriate** are each of the following responses by **<u>Freddie</u>** in this situation?

28. Tell their consultant that Joanna is not doing her fair share of the work
    - A. A very appropriate thing to do
    - B. Appropriate, but not ideal
    - C. Inappropriate, but not awful
    - D. A very inappropriate thing to do

29. Talk to Joanna about taking it in turns to teach the medical students
    - A. A very appropriate thing to do
    - B. Appropriate, but not ideal
    - C. Inappropriate, but not awful
    - D. A very inappropriate thing to do

30. Tell the medical students to leave the junior doctors alone as they have work to do
    - A. A very appropriate thing to do
    - B. Appropriate, but not ideal
    - C. Inappropriate, but not awful
    - D. A very inappropriate thing to do

31. Tell Joanna he does not want to do all the paperwork himself
    - A. A very appropriate thing to do
    - B. Appropriate, but not ideal
    - C. Inappropriate, but not awful
    - D. A very inappropriate thing to do

Olubayo is a dentist who is about to perform a procedure on a patient that requires the use of several different electrical instruments that must be plugged into the mains. There have been severe storms throughout the day, and the power to the dentist's surgery has gone out twice. The back-up generator failed the second time the power went out. Olubayo hears thunder in the distance, and is certain that another severe storm is approaching. The lights in the surgery begin to flicker.

How **appropriate** are each of the following responses by **Olubayo** in this situation?

32. Ask if the patient is comfortable with going ahead with the procedure

      A. A very appropriate thing to do
      B. Appropriate, but not ideal
      C. Inappropriate, but not awful
      D. A very inappropriate thing to do

33. Notify the patient that it is unsafe to proceed due to inclement weather

      A. A very appropriate thing to do
      B. Appropriate, but not ideal
      C. Inappropriate, but not awful
      D. A very inappropriate thing to do

34. Close the surgery for the rest of the day, and reschedule patients for the earliest available appointments

      A. A very appropriate thing to do
      B. Appropriate, but not ideal
      C. Inappropriate, but not awful
      D. A very inappropriate thing to do

Whilst Eoghan, a medical student, is taking a history from a patient, the patient asks if the consultant will be here to see him as he has some questions to ask about his operation which is taking place tomorrow. Eoghan knows that the consultant does not get back from holiday until tomorrow.

How **appropriate** are each of the following responses by <u>**Eoghan**</u> in this situation?

35. Tell the patient that the consultant is on holiday
    - A. A very appropriate thing to do
    - B. Appropriate, but not ideal
    - C. Inappropriate, but not awful
    - D. A very inappropriate thing to do

36. Offer to get a doctor to come and talk to the patient
    - A. A very appropriate thing to do
    - B. Appropriate, but not ideal
    - C. Inappropriate, but not awful
    - D. A very inappropriate thing to do

37. Reassure the patient that he can answer all the patient's questions himself
    - A. A very appropriate thing to do
    - B. Appropriate, but not ideal
    - C. Inappropriate, but not awful
    - D. A very inappropriate thing to do

38. Try and answer any simple questions himself, then get a doctor to come and talk to the patient
    - A. A very appropriate thing to do
    - B. Appropriate, but not ideal
    - C. Inappropriate, but not awful
    - D. A very inappropriate thing to do

Hannah, a paediatrician, is examining a patient, Alfie, who is aged seven and has a headache and a sore throat. Whilst listening to Alfie's breathing, Hannah notices several bruises in various stages of healing on Alfie's chest, all of which are concealed by his shirt. Alfie's carer is not in the examination room; she has stepped outside to have a cigarette. Alfie seems shy and withdrawn, and tries to pull away when he sees that Hannah has noticed the bruises on his chest.

How **appropriate** are each of the following responses by __Hannah__ in this situation?

39. Ask Alfie what happened
 A. A very appropriate thing to do
 B. Appropriate, but not ideal
 C. Inappropriate, but not awful
 D. A very inappropriate thing to do

40. Step outside and ask Alfie's carer for consent to examine the bruises on his chest
 A. A very appropriate thing to do
 B. Appropriate, but not ideal
 C. Inappropriate, but not awful
 D. A very inappropriate thing to do

41. Reassure Alfie that she wants to help him feel better
 A. A very appropriate thing to do
 B. Appropriate, but not ideal
 C. Inappropriate, but not awful
 D. A very inappropriate thing to do

42. Phone children's services at the local council immediately to report a suspected case of child abuse
 A. A very appropriate thing to do
 B. Appropriate, but not ideal
 C. Inappropriate, but not awful
 D. A very inappropriate thing to do

Nieve, a medical student, wakes up with a severe hangover after a late night party. She is scheduled to attend teaching this morning and help on a busy medical ward after the teaching has ended. Her friend, Leila, was at the same party and also has the same timetable as Nieve.

How **appropriate** are each of the following responses by <u>**Nieve**</u> in this situation?

43. Ask Leila to report Nieve is unwell without mentioning the party, while also emailing the medical school to report her absence and catch up on what has been missed the following day

    A. A very appropriate thing to do
    B. Appropriate, but not ideal
    C. Inappropriate, but not awful
    D. A very inappropriate thing to do

44. Attend the teaching session, but refuse to work afterwards due to ill health

    A. A very appropriate thing to do
    B. Appropriate, but not ideal
    C. Inappropriate, but not awful
    D. A very inappropriate thing to do

45. Tell Leila there was a family emergency and ask her to report this to the tutor before the start of the class

    A. A very appropriate thing to do
    B. Appropriate, but not ideal
    C. Inappropriate, but not awful
    D. A very inappropriate thing to do

46. Ask Leila not to say anything, then catch up on the missed work with Leila late

    A. A very appropriate thing to do
    B. Appropriate, but not ideal
    C. Inappropriate, but not awful
    D. A very inappropriate thing to do

47. Attend the teaching and work on the ward despite the feelings of nausea and not having had time to shower beforehand

    A. A very appropriate thing to do
    B. Appropriate, but not ideal
    C. Inappropriate, but not awful
    D. A very inappropriate thing to do

Dr Miller, a junior doctor, has just finished ward rounds when a woman approaches him in the corridor. She says that she is the niece of a patient that Dr Miller is looking after in the Intensive Care Unit. She wants to know everything about her uncle and how long it will be until he is well enough to go home. Dr Miller's consultant will be busy in clinic all day, and Dr Miller knows that the patient is very sick, with only days to live; the patient asked the consultant to inform the family of this himself.

How **appropriate** are each of the following responses by **Dr Miller** in this situation?

48. Tell the woman that he is too busy to talk to her

    A. A very appropriate thing to do

    B. Appropriate, but not ideal

    C. Inappropriate, but not awful

    D. A very inappropriate thing to do

49. Tell the woman that he cannot tell her anything regarding a patient

    A. A very appropriate thing to do

    B. Appropriate, but not ideal

    C. Inappropriate, but not awful

    D. A very inappropriate thing to do

50. Suggest that the woman wait for the consultant in the relatives' room

    A. A very appropriate thing to do

    B. Appropriate, but not ideal

    C. Inappropriate, but not awful

    D. A very inappropriate thing to do

51. Confirm the relationship to the patient, take the woman to the relatives' room, and ask if there are any questions he can answer while she waits for the consultant

    A. A very appropriate thing to do

    B. Appropriate, but not ideal

    C. Inappropriate, but not awful

    D. A very inappropriate thing to do

Jackson and Zakariyah are medical students. Upon walking into the supply cupboard one day, Zakariyah sees Jackson filling a rucksack with bags of intravenous fluid and equipment for inserting drips. He asks Zakariyah not to tell the nurse in charge or their consultant.

How **important** to take into account are the following considerations for **Zakariyah** when deciding how to respond to the situation?

52. Jackson says that he is sending the supplies to a charity hospital in Cambodia
    A. Very important
    B. Important
    C. Of minor importance
    D. Not important at all

53. Zakariyah has heard Jackson discussing putting up drips on himself and his friends when they have been out drinking
    A. Very important
    B. Important
    C. Of minor importance
    D. Not important at all

54. The intravenous fluid bags are past their expiry dates
    A. Very important
    B. Important
    C. Of minor importance
    D. Not important at all

55. Zakariyah knows that Jackson is on his final warning in terms of appropriate behaviour whilst at medical school
    A. Very important
    B. Important
    C. Of minor importance
    D. Not important at all

Liam, a junior doctor, approaches Conor, another junior doctor, and asks Conor to take over the case of a patient he has just been assigned, Mr Abdul. Conor asks why, and Liam explains he cannot deal with 'another one of those people'. Conor asks Liam to explain himself, and Liam says that Conor knows all about 'all these outsiders' coming to the UK so they can 'go on benefits' and 'impose their religion' on this country.

How **important** to take into account are the following considerations for **Conor** when deciding how to respond to the situation?

56. Liam's brother was injured in the war in Afghanistan
    A. Very important
    B. Important
    C. Of minor importance
    D. Not important at all

57. Conor's girlfriend is from another country
    A. Very important
    B. Important
    C. Of minor importance
    D. Not important at all

58. Whether there are any patients or staff nearby
    A. Very important
    B. Important
    C. Of minor importance
    D. Not important at all

59. Liam has not made comments of this nature to Conor before
    A. Very important
    B. Important
    C. Of minor importance
    D. Not important at all

60. Conor and Liam are supervised by the same consultant
    A. Very important
    B. Important
    C. Of minor importance
    D. Not important at all

61. Liam recently helped Conor when his mother was seriously ill
    A. Very important
    B. Important
    C. Of minor importance
    D. Not important at all

The medical team decides that a patient should have a non-urgent chest X-ray before he goes home, but that this would not alter his treatment whilst in hospital. A junior doctor, Dr O'Keefe, is asked by the team to organise the X-ray. The next day, however, Dr O'Keefe admits to Dr Bates, a senior doctor on the medical team, that she has forgotten to organise the X-ray.

How **important** to take into account are the following considerations for **Dr Bates** when deciding how to respond to the situation

62. The consultant had specifically asked for the X-ray to be completed in the next 24 hours
    - A. Very important
    - B. Important
    - C. Of minor importance
    - D. Not important at all

63. Dr O'Keefe was dealing with a very sick patient all of the previous afternoon
    - A. Very important
    - B. Important
    - C. Of minor importance
    - D. Not important at all

64. The patient is not scheduled to go home until next week
    - A. Very important
    - B. Important
    - C. Of minor importance
    - D. Not important at all

65. Dr O'Keefe had some bad news about her grandmother's cancer diagnosis a few days ago
    - A. Very important
    - B. Important
    - C. Of minor importance
    - D. Not important at all

A group of medical students have been assigned to prepare and give a presentation; they will be assessed jointly for their work. At the first group meeting, they select Maisie as group leader. A few minutes before the second group meeting, Maisie receives a text message from Catriona, another group member, stating that she has car trouble and cannot come to the meeting; Catriona asks Maisie to cover for her.

How **important** to take into account are the following considerations for **Maisie** when deciding how to respond to the situation?

66. There is a private spot near the meeting room, where Maisie could ring Catriona

    A. Very important
    B. Important
    C. Of minor importance
    D. Not important at all

67. Whether Catriona lives near enough to the meeting venue that she could walk or take public transport

    A. Very important
    B. Important
    C. Of minor importance
    D. Not important at all

68. The assignment clearly requires them to prepare and give the presentation as a group

    A. Very important
    B. Important
    C. Of minor importance
    D. Not important at all

Two junior doctors, Addison and Petra, are called to a meeting with a hospital administrator to discuss what happened during a procedure that caused serious health problems for the patient, leading to a formal complaint from the patient and the threat of a lawsuit. When asked to explain what she did during the procedure, Petra omits to mention a minor error she made that Addison remembers noticing at the time.

How **important** to take into account are the following considerations for **Addison** when deciding how to respond to the situation?

69. Petra's error may be directly responsible for the patient's health problems that resulted frrm the procedure
    A. Very important
    B. Important
    C. Of minor importance
    D. Not important at all

70. The administrator does not ask Addison directly about the error made by Petra
    A. Very important
    B. Important
    C. Of minor importance
    D. Not important at all

71. Other staff present at the time may have noticed Petra's error
    A. Very important
    B. Important
    C. Of minor importance
    D. Not important at all

STOP. IF YOU FINISH BEFORE TIME IS UP, CHECK ANY QUESTIONS YOU HAVE MARKED FOR REVIEW. YOU MAY GO BACK TO QUESTIONS IN THIS SECTION ONLY

Verbal Reasoning

1. B
2. D
3. B
4. A
5. C
6. A
7. B
8. C
9. D
10. C
11. A
12. A
13. A
14. B
15. C
16. B
17. C
18. A
19. C
20. B
21. A
22. C
23. D
24. C
25. A
26. A
27. C
28. B
29. C
30. D
31. D
32. B
33. D
34. C
35. B
36. B
37. C
38. A
39. A
40. B
41. D
42. C
43. C
44. A

Quantitative Reasoning

1. D
2. A
3. E
4. C
5. B
6. D
7. E
8. A
9. E
10. C
11. D
12. B
13. B
14. C
15. D
16. C
17. E
18. D
19. A
20. E
21. D
22. C
23. A
24. B
25. C
26. B
27. C
28. E
29. C
30. E
31. B
32. D
33. B
34. C
35. A
36. D

Abstract Reasoning

1. C
2. B
3. C
4. A
5. C
6. A
7. B
8. C
9. C
10. B
11. B
12. B
13. C
14. A
15. C
16. C
17. B
18. B
19. A
20. C
21. C
22. C
23. A
24. C
25. B
26. C
27. A
28. A
29. C
30. B
31. B
32. A
33. C
34. B
35. C
36. A
37. C
38. A
39. C
40. B
41. C
42. C
43. B
44. A

Abstract Reasoning (continued)

45. B
46. B
47. C
48. A
49. C
50. C
51. D
52. A
53. B
54. D
55. C

Decision Analysis

1. E
2. B
3. D
4. C
5. C
6. A
7. E
8. A
9. C
10. B
11. D
12. A
13. B
14. C
15. E
16. B
17. A
18. D
19. E
20. C
21. A
22. E
23. B
24. C
25. B
26. C and D
27. A and D
28. A and B

Kaplan UKCAT Mock Test Scoring Table: Sections 1–4

1. Count up your number of correct answers in each scored section.

2. Find your approximate score for each section in the table below.

	Number Correct	Approximate UKCAT Score
Verbal Reasoning	_____	_____
Quantitative Reasoning	_____	_____
Abstract Reasoning	_____	_____
Decision Analysis	_____	_____

3. Add your section scores to find your total score: _____

Approximate UKCAT Score	Number of Questions Answered Correctly			
	Verbal Reasoning	**Quantitative Reasoning**	**Abstract Reasoning**	**Decision Analysis**
300	0–5	0–3	0–6	0–2
330	6	4–5	7–8	3
350	7	6	9–10	4
370	8	7	11–12	5
400	9–10	8	13–14	6
430	11–12	9	15–16	7
450	13–14	10	17–18	8
470	15	11	19–20	9
500	16	12	21–22	10
530	17–18	13	23–24	11
550	19–20	14–15	25–26	12
570	21–22	16–17	27–29	13
600	23–24	18–19	30–32	14–15
630	25–26	20–21	33–34	16
650	27–28	22–23	35–36	17
670	29–30	24	37	18
700	31	25	38–39	19
730	32	26	40–41	20
750	33	27	42–43	21
770	34	28	44–45	22
800	35–36	29	46–47	23
830	37–38	30	48–49	24
850	39–40	31–32	50–51	25
890	41–42	33–34	52–53	26
900	43–44	35–36	54–55	27–28

NB These scores are for approximation purposes only. Scores on the UKCAT are given in 10-point intervals, so actual scores will vary slightly from this scheme. This table is designed to err on the side of caution, so in most cases a similar performance on the UKCAT would result in a slightly higher score.

Situational Judgement

1. C
2. C
3. D
4. A
5. D
6. C
7. A
8. A
9. D
10. A
11. A
12. D
13. C
14. D
15. A
16. C

17. A
18. C
19. A
20. D
21. A
22. C
23. A
24. D
25. D
26. D
27. A
28. D
29. A
30. D
31. C
32. D
33. A
34. A
35. D

36. A
37. D
38. D
39. A
40. A
41. A
42. D
43. A
44. B
45. D
46. D
47. D
48. D
49. D
50. A
51. B
52. D
53. B
54. D

55. D
56. D
57. C
58. A
59. D
60. A
61. C
62. A
63. A
64. B
65. D
66. A
67. B
68. A
69. A
70. D
71. C

Kaplan UKCAT Mock Test Scoring Table: Section 5

1. Count up your number of correct answers in this section.

2. Find your approximate scoring band for this section in the table below.

	Number Correct	Approximate UKCAT Score
Situational Judgement	_____	_____

Approximate UKCAT Scoring Band	Number of Questions Answered Correctly
Band 4	0–17
Band 3	18–35
Band 2	36–53
Band 1	54–71

Getting Ready for Test Day Success

You are nearly ready for Test Day. You have completed two full-length Kaplan UKCAT practice tests, and learned and practised Kaplan's top tips for each section of the UKCAT. Hopefully, the top tips helped you improve your performance from the Kaplan UKCAT Diagnostic Test to the Kaplan UKCAT Mock Test. You will most likely have made some mistakes on the Mock Test, and these mistakes are to your advantage: any mistake you make while practising is one you can learn from, and avoid on Test Day. Be sure to review the worked answers for the Mock Test in full, so you can learn from your mistakes. You should also review the explanations for the questions you got right, to ensure that you got them right for the right reasons.

When athletes prepare for a major match or competition, they visualise success: a boxer imagines the series of punches and jabs that will defeat his opponent; a runner sees herself breaking away and crossing the finish line ahead of her rivals. When faced with an important and challenging exam such as the UKCAT, you must also get ready for success by visualising it. Imagine yourself working through each section of the test, applying the Kaplan top tips, keeping an eye on the clock while you work at a good pace, eliminating answers and moving on rather than fretting about a difficult question, maximising your marks section by section, and then the moment when you finish and are handed your result: it will be a happy moment indeed!

The remaining tips in this chapter are designed to help you get ready for Test Day, so you can get ready for success. Some of these tips may seem a bit obvious, or a bit unusual, but they have been tried and tested by thousands of students. Getting ready for Test Day is not simply about revising and practising, but also about preparing yourself, in body, mind and spirit.

Kaplan Top Tips for Getting Ready for Test Day

1. Make a study plan for the final days/weeks, and stick to it

Count up the number of weeks and days from now to Test Day, and work out exactly what you are going to do in that time to finish getting ready. If you have only a few days from now until Test Day, then keep it simple: review the Kaplan top tips and practice questions (and explanations) in this book. You should also download the free practice tests from the UKCAT website (www.ukcat.ac.uk), and sit one of these. If you have a week until Test Day, then you should complete the online practice questions, and be sure to allow time afterwards for a full review of the worked answers. If you have more than a week, then you should try and take one or two practice tests per week. These could include the free practice tests from the UKCAT website, and also the free practice test from the Kaplan website (www.kaptest.co.uk/ukcattest). If you have taken the Kaplan UKCAT preparation course and thus have access to further Kaplan practice tests, then you would do well to plan to take one or two of these a week, always reviewing the full worked answers very soon after completing a practice test. Be cautious about using any practice tests from other sources, as these are likely to diverge significantly from the format, timing or style of the UKCAT. Don't negate all your hard work by studying with flawed materials.

Be sure to check the Online Resource Centre that accompanies this book, along with the UKCAT website, so that you are aware of any changes to the test format (including number of questions and timing for each section) in the year that you sit the UKCAT. The UKCAT website is normally updated in late April with the basic details of the exam format for the current year; the practice tests on this website may be updated again in late June or early July, just before testing begins, to reflect the proportion of question types in each section in the current year. We will post any related updates in the Online Resource Centre, once the information on the UKCAT website has changed—so be sure to plan to check online in the weeks ahead of Test Day. See page ix.

2. Stress is normal—expect it, and manage it

Everyone feels anxious and pressurised about doing well on the UKCAT. Feelings of stress are to be expected when an exam is so important to your future. The best way to deal with stress is to understand it, acknowledge it, and limit its impact on your Test Day performance. By 'stress', we mean any factor that can keep you from doing your best on Test Day. Stress can include your own anxieties, comments from family and friends, and any problems that arise on Test Day. Feeling stress does not mean that you are unprepared, or stupid, or weak, or any other negative thing that might come to mind; feeling stress means that you're human. By acknowledging stress, you can then proceed to manage it, depending on its source:

Stress about the test itself. As we've seen through the course of this book, the UKCAT is a challenging and very tightly timed exam. This is its very nature, so the UKCAT is objectively stressful for everyone. However, consider the fact that most test-takers do very little to prepare for the UKCAT. Some even believe that it is impossible to prepare, so they do nothing at all. Most test-takers will look over a few practice questions, and perhaps try a full mock test. But relatively few among the UKCAT cohort will take the time to learn the Kaplan top tips, practise them so they become second nature, and practise as well for pacing. You are among the select few who are very well positioned for success on Test Day. Sure, the UKCAT is challenging and fast-paced; but you're prepared to work fast, and to meet its challenges. This gives you a huge advantage, and should also give you confidence.

Stress from family and friends. It is natural for family and friends to ask about how you're getting on with your UKCAT revision, and for them to want you to do well on the exam. Sometimes, though, comments from parents or friends that are meant to be supportive and encouraging have the unintended result of increasing stress. Such added pressure is more likely to result when comments are frequent—for instance, if your parents check in on your progress at least once a day. To limit stress from such friendly sources, you might mention to your parents (or friends, or whoever's the source) that you are getting on very well with your UKCAT preparation, and that it will help you do even better on Test Day if you can clear your head when you're not revising. They can help you succeed by keeping your mind on other things when you're not revising—even the most talented and brilliant among us need a break!

Stress about Test Day. The procedures on Test Day can be a source of anxiety and uncertainty. You should read through the information about what to expect on Test Day on the UKCAT website, and review their simulation of the Pearson testing centre. Sitting the official UKCAT practice tests will also help you to familiarise yourself with the format of the test interface that you will use on Test Day. You will also want to ensure you review the route from home to the test centre a day or two before the test. Be sure to plan for an alternate route to the test centre, whether you're driving or taking public transport; this will ensure that transport problems do not keep you from making it to the test centre in time.

3. Wind down your preparations in the last day or two before Test Day

Many students assume that it's best to keep on revising right up until the minute they walk into the exam room. In fact, such last-minute preparations are unhelpful for the UKCAT, because it's not a content-based exam. The skills you need for UKCAT success are developed through practice; they can't be 'crammed' for. Following the guidance in this book, and coming up with a study plan to incorporate any practice tests you can reasonably fit in between now and Test Day, is the best way to revise for the UKCAT.

In the last day or two before the UKCAT, however, you need to finish your revision efforts and make more time to relax in a 'test-free zone'. It is okay to finish looking over the worked answers from your final practice test, but don't assume that cramming in one more practice test will make you more prepared.

You would do better to look back over the Kaplan top tips from each chapter of this book, to make sure that these are 'fresh', but otherwise to spend time taking your mind off the UKCAT. Returning to basics and relaxing in a 'test-free zone' is the best way to build confidence, reduce stress and make the most of your time just before Test Day.

You will also want to ensure that you get a good night's sleep each night in the week before Test Day. Don't stay up very late studying and then sleep late, as you will be sitting the exam during the day, and will want to be rested and fully awake. Getting into a regular sleep cycle will ensure that you do not feel tired while sitting the UKCAT.

Once you get ready for Test Day, the only thing that remains is to sit the UKCAT. Our final set of Kaplan top tips will help you make the most of the Test Day experience.

Kaplan Top Tips for Test Day

1. Warm up your body and brain before the test

Allow yourself plenty of time for a pre-test ritual, and ensure that you wake up early enough to do so. Eat a decent breakfast, with servings of protein and carbohydrates, so you are fully energised and don't get hungry during the test. Spend some time before the test reading something stimulating, to 'activate' your brain for the level of thinking and speed required on the UKCAT. You could read during breakfast or on the journey to the test centre. Just be sure not to go into the exam with an empty stomach, or without 'jump-starting' your brain. Students who do so usually have difficulty with the first section, which usually results in a far lower than expected Verbal Reasoning score. Warm up properly, so you can attack the Verbal section with the full force of your awesome UKCAT skills arsenal!

2. Make sure everything's in your bag

Before you leave home, check (and then double-check) that you have a copy of your UKCAT registration and an approved photo ID. You will also want to be prepared to put everything else except your clothes and your photo ID into your bag, which you will have to put in a locker before entering the exam room. You will only be allowed to take your photo ID and the locker key (and whatever clothes you didn't leave in the locker) into the exam room. Any jewellery and anything in your pockets—including your phone, wallet, watch and tissues—must be left in the locker. This is a rule that cannot be waived, so make sure everything is in your bag.

3. Ask for an extra noteboard

Just before you enter the exam room, the invigilator will give you a wet-erase pen and a 'noteboard', which is a plasticised sheet of A4 paper. You can write on both sides of the noteboard, but you can't rub it out without a moist cloth. You are welcome to ask for an additional noteboard during the exam—and should do so by raising your hand, ideally just before the end of a section, so you'll have a new noteboard at the start of the next section. However, there's no harm in asking for an extra noteboard before starting the exam. The invigilator may say no—but they may just as well say yes.

4. Take control of your testing station

Once you enter the exam room, you will be assigned to a testing station, consisting of a desktop computer, with mouse and keyboard, and a chair. Most testing stations will be separated by partitions; you must ensure that you do not get out of the chair without first getting the invigilator's permission, and you must take special care to make sure your eyes do not look anywhere other than inside your testing station during the exam. Even so, you can take control of your testing station before starting the exam. If the chair is a swivel chair, adjust the seat to an appropriate and comfortable height. You might also move the keyboard out of the way, and set up your noteboard and mouse so you can use them easily and quickly. Just be sure to bring the keyboard out for the Quantitative section, as you'll work much more quickly by typing the figures into the onscreen calculator than by using the mouse.

5. Take 'mini-breaks' between the sections

Remember, you have one minute to read the instructions for each section. However, the instructions are always the same. At Kaplan we find that many of our students like to take a 'mini-break' during the minute for instructions. A mini-break might involve stretching in your seat—extending your arms and legs, and shaking them a bit to get the blood flowing; you might do the same with your head, neck and shoulders, but just be careful not to look outside your partition! You might also try blinking rapidly for several seconds, or closing and opening your eyes at 10-second intervals, to alleviate any eyestrain and freshen your eyes for the next section. You should not take a toilet break during the exam, as this will cost valuable time for answering questions. Most students find it helpful to use the toilet just before entering the exam room, as this will minimise the likelihood of any disruptive emergencies—so you can focus on building a great UKCAT score.

6. One question at a time

This is the simplest tip, and perhaps the most important. On Test Day, keep your focus on the question at hand. You will get through each section by answering the questions one at a time; great results are built on success in individual questions. Remember to follow the tips about maximising marks, and don't waste time on questions that are especially difficult or time-consuming. There won't be very many of these questions, and they will be difficult or time-consuming for all test-takers. Only the prepared test-taker will have the foresight and confidence to expect such questions, and to deal with them quickly and efficiently, marking an answer, marking for review, and moving on to quicker, easier marks.

7. Don't think about your score during the exam

You will get your result as soon as you finish. So don't think about how well you're doing, or whether the questions seem generally easy or difficult. Just focus on answering the questions one by one, and keep an eye on the clock so that you pace yourself and mark an answer for all the questions in each section.

8. Answer every question

There's no negative marking, so there is no reason not to mark an answer for every question. The computer cannot tell whether you got a question correct because you worked it out, because you eliminated the wrong answers, or because you guessed blindly. The computer only knows that you got the question correct, and so you get the mark. You do have to work very quickly on the UKCAT, and will almost certainly have to make your best guess after partial elimination on at least a few questions in each section. Expect this, embrace it, mark your best answers confidently, and keep moving. Students who don't understand how to pace themselves on the UKCAT and how to eliminate and guess strategically leave lots of questions unanswered—ensuring they get low scores. Answering all the questions will help you secure a top score.

Now that you have learned the Kaplan top tips for UKCAT success, all that remains is to follow through on your study plan, and put the top tips into practice on Test Day. We at Kaplan are honoured to have helped you prepare for the UKCAT, and wish you all the very best, on Test Day and in your future medical practice. Hard work makes great doctors—you are on your way!

Appendix A

Kaplan Top Tips for Test-Takers with Learning Difficulties

The UKCAT Consortium offers a second standardised version of the exam, UKCATSEN, or UKCAT Special Educational Needs, for candidates with learning difficulties. You can sign up for UKCATSEN through the UKCAT website, and this version of the exam allows approximately 25% extra time in each section. This extra time is intended to help candidates with common learning difficulties, such as dyslexia, dysgraphia or working memory deficit.

Candidates should only register for UKCATSEN if they normally receive extra time on exams, and should ensure that they will be able to provide clinical evidence of the relevant learning difficulty, in the form of a written diagnosis in an approved format. This evidence is not required until later in the admissions process, and must be given directly to the universities; candidates who sit the UKCATSEN and are subsequently unable to furnish the required evidence will have their test results voided. So you should only sit UKCATSEN if you have a diagnosed learning difficulty. Check the UKCAT website for the latest details on timing for UKCATSEN, and follow up directly with the UKCAT Consortium with any questions about required evidence, as this can vary from country to country.

Kaplan Top Tips for Test-Takers with Learning Difficulties

1. Determine which sections require a different approach

Depending on the exact nature of your learning difficulty, you may need to take a slightly different approach in one or more sections. Some common adjustments include:

Verbal Reasoning: If you have trouble scanning for keywords, try reading the first statement, then reading through the passage quickly, in about a minute. Then, use your knowledge of the passage to evaluate the statements. If you find the answer to the first statement while reading the passage, mark it, read the next statement, and continue reading the passage. This is a slower approach overall, but dyslexic test-takers may find it more useful than scanning for keywords.

Quantitative Reasoning: If you have trouble thinking through how to solve the questions quickly, try skipping to the end of each question, rather than reading through from the beginning. Most of the time, the last few words of the question will describe what you must solve for—reading this first can help you to focus, and can save time and limit confusion as you set up and solve.

Abstract Reasoning: If you have trouble keeping the patterns in Set A and Set B distinct in your mind, then jot down a few notes on each on your noteboard. This can be especially helpful when there are multiple features, but test-takers with working memory deficit might want to make brief notes on the patterns in each set, to save time and avoid frustration.

Decision Analysis: If you have trouble remembering what the codes mean, or how they are combined, then try writing out the literal translation completely for each message—but practise doing so as efficiently and accurately as possible. If you have trouble copying out the translation accurately, then try keeping track of it in your head—this approach tends to work best for test-takers with dysgraphia.

Situational Judgement: The challenges in this section are very similar to those in Verbal Reasoning. Test-takers with dyslexia will want to allow a bit of extra time to read through each scenario before evaluating the related responses; if you read quickly, it is very easy to miss out a word or two that could be the key to the central issue in the scenario. Practise for this as you revise, to build your confidence and work out the best balance of time between scenario vs responses for you. You may find that it works better to spend more like 45 seconds or a minute per scenario, rather than the standard 30 seconds, so you can be certain of identifying the key issues.

2. Practise your different approach, for speed and accuracy as well as for timing

While you will be able to spend 25% more time in each section of the UKCAT, this is not a huge amount of extra time. You will still want to ensure you can answer the questions as efficiently as possible, and should practise for this through your remaining UKCAT practice tests, and in any questions in this book you have not yet attempted. Practising your different approach for any sections requiring one will build your speed, accuracy and confidence, and will help you to answer the most possible questions correctly in the time allotted. You will also need to think about how many minutes/seconds to spend per set and per question. Your ability to pace yourself, even in sections that are especially challenging, is essential.

3. Prepare for all sections of the test

Due to the varied nature of the sections on the UKCAT, your learning difficulty may affect your approach to one or more sections, but may not affect your approach to all sections. For example, a test-taker with dyslexia will not experience any extra challenges in Abstract Reasoning. Such a test-taker should follow the Kaplan top tips for Abstract Reasoning, and should see that section as a special opportunity to maximise marks. If you put in extra effort in a section that does not present extra challenges, and earn a score that is well above average, then you will make yourself truly stand out from the competition. An especially high result in such a section will also counterbalance a less than stellar performance in a section that is more challenging. So you should use the varied nature of the test to your advantage.

4. Remember—the UKCAT is objectively difficult for everyone

The final tip may seem a bit obvious, and perhaps not so helpful. But it's essential to remember that the UKCAT is designed to be challenging for students who are among the best in their year at school, and who will be competitive for admission to the top medical schools in the UK. The UKCAT is not an easy test, in terms of the question formats or the timing, which is brutal. If you have a learning difficulty, one or more sections of the UKCAT may seem like an almost impossible challenge. But it's important to keep in mind that the same section seems just as horrifying to all your fellow test-takers. This is the nature of the exam, and a major source of stress that causes many test-takers to cave under pressure each year. Follow the Kaplan top tips in this book, practise thoroughly and smartly, and be confident in the fact that you have a major advantage over the competition. Keep positive, work efficiently and calmly, and visualise success—you are on your way to a great result and an amazing future.

Appendix B

Chapter 2 Kaplan UKCAT Diagnostic Test Explanations

Verbal Reasoning

1. (B)

The final sentence of the second paragraph states that brown bears live in a forest and eat a diet that includes meat, plants and berries. Thus, (B) cannot be true and is the correct answer.

2. (B)

The ancestry of today's polar bears is explained in the first paragraph. Today's polar bears have the same mitochondrial DNA as prehistoric brown bears that were found in Ireland. Answer (B) is therefore correct.

3. (D)

Iceland is never mentioned in the passage, so there is no basis in the passage for inferring anything that must be true about Iceland. Eliminate (A) and (C). The first sentence of the final paragraph states that Ireland's climate cooled considerably during the Ice Age; the correct answer is (D).

4. (A)

The passage never states directly that some bears survived the Ice Age. However, it is correct to infer this, based on the fact that today's polar bears share mitochondrial DNA with prehistoric brown bears that lived during the Ice Age. If some bears had not survived the Ice Age, then today's polar bears would not continue to carry the mitochondrial DNA of their Ice Age ancestors. Answer (A) is correct.

5. (A)

This is a negative question; the three wrong answers will be supported by the passage, and the one correct answer won't be. Bernhardt's career is discussed throughout the passage, so look for a keyword from each answer choice. Films are mentioned in the passage's first and penultimate sentences, which make clear that Bernhardt appeared in films. (A) contradicts the passage, so it is false—and the correct answer.

6. (C)

The keywords 'The Three Musketeers' appear (in very helpful italics) midway through the second paragraph. The Three Musketeers was written by the novelist Alexandre Dumas, son of the author Alexandre Dumas (who wrote Kean). Scanning the answers quickly, you will likely notice that (C) is clearly correct. **NB** Wrong answer trap (A), as the passage does not say that Dumas the father was a novelist or that Kean was a novel.

7. (C)

The keywords 'personal history' are a bit hard to scan for; hopefully, you were able to find the reference to her 'biography and early life' midway through the second paragraph. This part of the passage states that little is known about Bernhardt's personal history, and that her past is largely inscrutable. These details are paraphrased in (C), which is therefore correct. If you were tempted by the other answers, note that Bernhardt's history was not entirely fabricated, and it is relevant to her reputation (given all the rumours about her). Rumours that she was a vampire are not mentioned.

8. (D)

The keywords 'French' and 'government' appear together in the passage's second sentence, which says that the French Conservatoire was a Government-sponsored school of acting that Bernhardt attended in the mid-1800s. Thus, the correct answer is (D).

9. (B)

The Town and Country Planning Act is mentioned throughout the passage, so check for keywords from each answer. (A) is contradicted by the third paragraph, which states that the Act was revised 59 years after it became law. The first sentence explains that the Act was passed in 1947, so you can determine that it was revised in 2006. (B) is correct.

10. (C)

This is a negative question, asking for something that must be false. Thus, the correct answer must contradict the passage; any answers that are supported by the passage will be incorrect. Listed buildings are mentioned in the second paragraph; owners of such buildings are legally required to keep them in good repair, and must get special consent before making any alterations that affect the building's character or appearance. From this, you can infer that listed buildings can be repaired (once consent is obtained). (C) contradicts the passage on this point, so (C) must be false—and is therefore the correct answer.

11. (A)

Work on a previous question revealed that the Town and Country Planning Act was revised in 2006, and this detail was found in the final paragraph—so check that paragraph for details about the requirements of a UK planning application today. The third sentence of this paragraph indicates what must be included in such an application, such as the extent of public engagement. Thus, (A) is correct.

12. (B)

It is safe to infer that the author would agree with anything that is not described negatively in the passage. The question also contains the keywords 'town planning', and the accomplishments of town planning are mentioned in the second paragraph. These include the government achieving objectives for climate control, reduction of carbon emissions and housing access. The only answer that fits these details is (B), which is therefore correct.

13. (B)

The second paragraph states that testimony transcribed in Arabic can only be summarised into French at head office, due to a shortage of Arabic–French translators in the field. From this, it is safe to infer that some translators at head office translate Arabic. On this point, the statement contradicts the passage, so the statement is false.

14. (A)

The first paragraph says that testimony must be transcribed in the language in which it is given, and that testimony can be taken in English. Thus, testimony could be taken and transcribed in English. The second paragraph states that testimony must also be summarised in English or French. Thus, testimony could be taken, transcribed and initially summarised entirely in English. The answer is (A).

15. (B)

The passage's first sentence says that testimony must be transcribed in the language in which it is given, and that testimony may be given in a tribal language. Hence, it is safe to infer that testimony given in a tribal language must be transcribed in the same tribal language. This statement says otherwise; as such, the statement contradicts the passage, and is false.

16. (C)

Strasbourg is mentioned in the second paragraph as the location of the commission's head office; the same paragraph also states that testimony taken and transcribed in Arabic can only be summarised into French at head office. However, the passage does not specify that testimony taken in Arabic can only be summarised into English (the other permissible language for summaries) at head office. The passage likewise does not say that Arabic-language testimony can be summarised into English in the field. Based on information in the passage, there isn't enough information to answer; the correct answer is therefore (C).

17. (B)

The second paragraph states that there are 28 World Heritage Sites in the UK and its overseas territories, with 17 in England, 4 in Scotland and 3 in Wales. These add up to 24, so the proportion is 24:28, which reduces to 6:7, or six-sevenths. Answer (B) is correct.

18. (C)

The costs to the UK of preserving UNESCO sites are given in the final paragraph. The UK spends £130,000 per year on sites in developing countries, and £150,000 per year on the UK's sites. Thus, the UK's total annual cost is £280,000. The correct answer is (C).

19. (D)

The keywords 'UNESCO' and 'priority' appear in the second sentence of the first paragraph. UNESCO wants to give priority to land and sea habitats in need of protection. Answer (D) paraphrases this detail from the passage, so it is correct.

20. (D)

This is a negative question, asking for something that is false; the correct answer will contradict the passage. The keywords 'cultural landmarks' appear in two answers, and also at the end of the first paragraph: the vast majority of current World Heritage Sites are cultural landmarks. Thus, (A) and (C) are supported by the passage, and cannot be correct. This same sentence of the passage, and the sentence before, mention sites of natural importance as the other type of World Heritage Sites (other than cultural landmarks), so it is correct to infer that a minority of World Heritage Sites are ecological areas. It must therefore be false that no World Heritage Sites are ecological areas; (D) is the correct answer.

21. (C)

This is a negative question asking for something the author would be least likely to agree with; thus, any answer that the author would agree with will be incorrect, and the correct answer will most likely contradict the passage. The keyword 'blizzard' appears in inverted commas in the first paragraph; the author uses this term to describe snowfall of 5 to 8 inches in 24 hours, so you can infer that the author thinks that snowfall of 5 inches in 24 hours is not technically a blizzard. Eliminate (A). (B) is supported by the details in the first two sentences of the passage, so eliminate (B). (C) makes a claim that directly contradicts (A), and thus contradicts the author's opinion; (C) is therefore correct.

22. (D)

The keywords 'gritting salt' lead to the fourth sentence of the first paragraph, which states the circumstances in which gritting salt is not effective. The previous sentence says that gritting lorries are sufficient for snowfalls of 3 inches or less. Answer (D) is thus supported by the passage, and is correct.

23. (B)

Heathrow is mentioned near the end of the passage; a blizzard in 2010 resulted in hundreds of planes at Heathrow having to be dug out by hand, as there was no equipment at Heathrow that could undertake this task. The previous sentence explains that airports in the USA and Canada have mechanised equipment that can do this. Thus, it is correct to infer that Heathrow does not have all the same equipment as Canadian airports, as Heathrow does not have all the same snow-clearing equipment. The correct answer is (B).

24. (C)

This question asks about the passage as a whole, so you must check each answer choice to see if it is mentioned as a consequence of heavy snow in the UK, and then compare those that are to see which is the most severe. The passage states that children sometimes miss a week of school or more, so (A) is less severe than the actual detail in the passage. Slippery pavements are not mentioned in the passage. Financial losses are mentioned in the final sentence, and the detail here is a paraphrase of (C). The passage says nothing about Heathrow hiring American equipment. Answer (C) is therefore correct.

25. (C)

'Chekhov' is mentioned in the second paragraph as a writer who strongly influenced Mansfield, and to whose work she was introduced when she was living in Germany. The sentence that mentions this specifies that Chekhov is 'late', or deceased, so it is not a basis for inferring that Mansfield met Chekhov in Germany, or that he lived there when she became aware of his work in that country. The passage never says whether Chekhov lived in Germany for a time, or if he lived exclusively elsewhere (e.g. his native Russia). The answer is Can't tell.

26. (B)

The first paragraph states that Mansfield studied cello at Queen's College, but that she was best known for her short stories; her writing continues to be taught today. Thus, it is safe to infer that Mansfield is best known for her achievement in writing, not in music. This statement contradicts the passage, so the statement is false.

27. (C)

The last paragraph gives information about Mansfield's publications; she published more than a dozen short stories in a socialist magazine, *The New Age*. This is the passage's only reference to socialism; no information is provided about Mansfield's political views, so it is impossible to determine on the basis of the passage whether or not she was a socialist. The answer is (C).

28. (A)

Virginia Woolf is mentioned in the second paragraph, which explains that Mansfield was close to many important members of London's literary community in the early twentieth century, including Woolf. This statement is a close paraphrase of the passage, so it is true.

29. (D)

This question is a bit tricky, as teachers are not explicitly mentioned in the passage. There is a reference in the first paragraph to everyone learning about pi as schoolchildren, and that pi has been without controversy until now, when a dissenting group of mathematicians and scientists are advocating for tau, which is double the value of pi. The final sentence of the passage states that pi requires unnecessary factors of 2 in most cases beyond the maths classroom. From this information, it is safe to infer that teachers do not support replacing pi with tau, as pi is easier to use in the maths classroom. The answer that fits this best is (D), which is correct. If you were stuck, note that the wrong answers include things that are not mentioned in the passage: there is no reference to a vote by mathematicians, an international conference, or teachers wanting to replace pi with tau.

30. (A)

The definition of pi is given in the first paragraph as the ratio of a circle's circumference to its diameter. Answer (A) is a paraphrase of this same concept, so it is correct.

31. (A)

The keywords 'unnecessary factor of 2' lead to the passage's final sentence, which states that pi requires such factors in most cases beyond the maths classroom. From this information, it is safe to infer that calculations by teachers would not involve unnecessary factors of 2, as these would be the calculations in the maths classroom. If you did not see this inference, then you could also answer by checking against the real-life applications mentioned earlier in the sentence; the only one not mentioned is teaching, so the answer is (A).

32. (B)

The passage explains the relationship of a circle's radius to its circumference in the first paragraph, and to its area and to the area of the base of a cylinder in the second paragraph. There is no relationship mentioned between a circle's radius and the height of a cylinder, so (B) is correct.

33. (C)

Television is mentioned in the passage's first sentence as part of BAFTA's name, but the rest of the passage deals only with BAFTA's film awards. It is not clear from the passage whether or not BAFTA also gives awards for television. Therefore, the answer is Can't tell.

34. (B)

The final sentence of the first paragraph states that BAFTA awards are open to nominees of all nationalities, like the Oscars. From this, it is safe to infer that Oscar nominations are not limited to a single nationality such as Americans. On this point, the statement contradicts the passage, so the answer is (B).

35. (B)

2004 is mentioned in the second paragraph as the year when Mary Selway, in whose memory the Rising Star Award is given, passed away. However, the next sentence mentions that James McAvoy was given the first Rising Star Award in 2006. The statement contradicts the passage, and is false.

36. (A)

The next-to-last sentence of the passage states that James McAvoy won the Rising Star Award in 2006. The previous sentence explains that the Rising Star Award winner is the only BAFTA winner chosen by the public. Thus, James McAvoy is a BAFTA winner; the statement is true.

37. (A)

The passage includes a description of a sixth-form disco, which involves food (crisps) and music (one student's cassettes), and which was held to celebrate the end of exams. The current-day equivalent is an American-style 'prom', with catering and a hired DJ updating the food and music to a much more costly standard, but still for the same purpose of celebrating the end of exams. The writer of the passage refers to the earlier disco as a 'tradition', so there is enough information in the passage to support this statement. The answer is (A).

38. (B)

The second paragraph says that American-style proms did not exist (in the UK, anyway) 10 years ago. From this, it is safe to infer that American-style proms existed in America, which ultimately led to their prevalence in the UK. The statement contradicts the passage on this point, so the statement is false.

39. (C)

According to the second paragraph, girls must buy a formal dress for an American-style prom, and many girls spend hundreds of pounds on one. 'Many' (which means some number more than one, and is often understood to mean a large number) is not necessarily the same as 'most' (which means a majority). The passage gives no information to determine whether the 'many' girls who spend hundreds of pounds on prom dresses actually constitute a majority—or that they don't—so the answer is (C).

40. (C)

The figure of '£10,000 or more' is suggested as a possible total for the cost to the school in paying for catering, decorating and hiring a DJ. The passage does not specify the possible charge for hiring a DJ as independent of the other costs, or as a relative share of the total, so it is impossible to say based on the passage whether or not some schools spend £10,000 on a DJ. The answer is Can't tell.

41. (B)

The figures on lengths of commutes are given in the first paragraph. A majority is more than 50%, so add up the percentages for the different answers until you find the one that is more than 50%. The percentage of people in London with commutes of 30 minutes or less is 18% + 26% = 44%. Eliminate (A). 20% of Londoners have a commute of 31–45 minutes, so adding in this group to the 44% with commutes of 30 minutes or less would constitute a majority. (B) is therefore correct.

42. (D)

This question is very wordy, but it is asking for a relatively straightforward detail in the second paragraph. In the rest of the UK, 76% of people commute by driving. The correct answer is (D).

43. (A)

Anything that contradicts the information in the passage is something that the author would be unlikely to agree with; any answers supported by the passage will be incorrect. The work on previous questions has shown that there are significant differences in commutes in London and the rest of the UK, so (A) contradicts the passage. (A) is correct. **NB** If you weren't confident about this, you could check the other answers, and you would have found that they all describe the information in the passage accurately.

44. (B)

This is a negative question, so the correct answer must be false—it must contradict the passage. (A) is a statement about 'most people', but the passage only discusses people commuting in the UK; there is no basis for the claim in (A) to be supported or to contradict the passage. (B) deals with people in the UK, so it can be compared to the passage. The start of the final paragraph states that 71% of UK workers drive a car to work, so most people in the UK do not commute by public transport. (B) must be false, and is thus correct.

Quantitative Reasoning

1. (A)

A total of 4768 crimes were committed locally, and 283 of those were thefts of a motor vehicle. Divide to find the percentage: $283 \div 4768 = 0.059$, or 6%, answer (A).

2. (E)

The table shows that there were 4768 total crimes in Lincoln in 2005–2006, and that Lincoln had a population of 86,547. Divide to find the rate of crimes per person: $4768 \div 86,547 = 0.055$. Since this is more than 1:20 (which equals 0.05), test the two answer choices that are larger in your calculator. $1 \div 19 = 0.0526$, and $1 \div 18 = 0.0556$; the correct answer is (E).

3. (C)

The national crime rates are given in figures per 1000 population, so divide the national population by 1000 before multiplying by the rate of violent crimes against a person rate: $60,200,000 \div 1000 = 60,200$. The national rate of violent crimes against a person was 19.97 per 1000 population, so the total national number of violent crimes against a person was $19.97 \times 60,200 = 1,202,194$, or approximately 1.2 million. The answer is (C).

4. (B)

The total number of burglaries in the 2005–2006 table is given as 552. 10% of this is 55.2, or approximately 55. Therefore the total number in the 2006–2007 table will be $552 + 55 = 607$. The correct answer is (B).

5. (C)

This question requires you to simply look at the chart and find the smallest segment. The smallest segment is the one with 10% of the total share, and represents Mathematics. The correct answer is (C).

6. (B)

There are three steps to finding the answer to this question. First, find the proportion of total student visitors from the Faculty of Medicine. The chart shows this to be 20%, or 1/5. To get from 20% to 100%, or 1/5 to 1, multiply by 5; thus, multiplying the number of student visitors from the Faculty of Medicine by 5 will give the total number of student visitors. $800 \times 5 = 4000$. The correct answer is therefore (B).

7. (A)

To solve, find the number of Law student visitors, then work out 25% of that number to find the answer. The question gives the number of Mathematics student visitors, and the chart shows that for every 10 Mathematics student visitors, there were 30 Law students visitors; hence, a ratio of 1:3. Thus, multiplying the number of student visitors in Mathematics by 3 will give the number of Law student visitors: $400 \times 3 = 1200$. The correct answer is 25% of this total, or 300. The correct answer is (A).

8. (B)

To solve, simply subtract the Humanities and the Law percentages from the total (100%) given in the chart. 100 – 25 – 30 = 45. The correct answer is (B).

9. (D)

To solve, add up all the prices of the items in the table: 185 + 45 + 75 + 32 + 19 = 356. The correct answer is (D).

10. (B)

The sales target is 300 tickets at £1.50 each. If Omar hits the sales target exactly, he will make 300 × £1.50 = £450 in income. Subtract the cost of the raffle—the total cost of the prizes—to determine Omar's profit: £450 – £356 = £94. The correct answer is (B).

11. (C)

According to the final bulleted item, there are two electrical prizes in the raffle: the MP3 player and the hair dryer. They have a total cost of £75 + £19 = £94. If they were on sale for 50% off, Omar would save 0.5 × £94 = £47. The correct answer is (C).

12. (C)

To make a profit of £300, Omar will need to make £300 plus the cost of the prizes, which was £356. This total will equal the cost of a ticket (£1.50) times the number of tickets, which is unknown. Substitute x for the unknown number of tickets, and set up an algebraic equation: £300 + £356 = £1.50(x). Add the total on the left: £300 + £356 = £656 = £1.50(x). Then, divide by £1.50 to solve for x: x = £656 ÷ £1.50 = 437.33. Thus, Omar must sell 438 tickets to make a profit of £300. The correct answer is (C).

13. (C)

The total unshaded area is 18 m². Multiply the cost per m² (£70) by the unshaded area to find the total cost: 18 m² × £70 = £1,260. The answer is therefore (C).

14. (D)

Russell's vegetable patch is half of the unshaded area, and half of 18 m² is 9 m². 1 m = 100 cm, so 1 m² = 1 m × 1 m = 100 cm × 100 cm = 10,000 cm². Thus, the area of Russell's patch in cm² is 9 m² × 10,000 cm² = 90,000 cm². The answer is (D).

15. (B)

The total area of shaded land is 8 m × 10 m = 80 m². Pauline buys 30% of the total area of the shaded land, or 0.3 × 80 m² = 24 m². She pays £114 per m², so the total cost is 24 × £114 = £2,736. The correct answer is (B).

16. (C)

Pauline started with half of the unshaded area, or 9 m². She then bought 30% of the shaded area, which was found to be 24 m² in the work for the previous question. Finally, she buys half of Russell's patch, for a further 4.5 m². The total area of Pauline's patch after all these additions is 9 + 24 + 4.5 = 37.5 m². Answer (C) is correct.

17. (B)

To calculate how many miles a car can drive on one gallon of fuel, find that particular model on the graph and check for motorway or city driving, as appropriate. In this case, the motorway driving bar on the graph for the Denver car corresponds to 55 miles, so the answer is (B).

18. (E)

There are three steps to answering this question. First, read the graph to find the fuel economy of the Satola car in the city, which is 30 miles per gallon; this means that a 30-mile city journey will use up a gallon of fuel. Next, check the conversion factor under the graph to find that 1 gallon = 4.5 litres. Finally, multiply the price of the fuel to find the cost for 4.5 litres of fuel: £1.10 × 4.5 = £4.95. The correct answer is (E).

19. (C)

The simplest way to tackle this question is by glancing at the graph to see which car provides the best fuel economy. A quick glance shows that Ecogo has the best fuel economy for both motorway and city driving. The correct answer is therefore (C).

20. (D)

First, check how many miles one gallon of fuel allows you to travel on the motorway in a Cruiser. This value is 45 miles, according to the graph. Next, divide 45 by the total miles in the journey to determine how many gallons are required: $405 \div 45 = 9$. The answer is (D).

21. (C)

The exchange rate for pounds to dollars is £1:$1.60760. Multiply the sum in pounds to find the equivalent in dollars: £540 × ($1.60760/£1) = $868.104. The answer is therefore (C).

22. (E)

The answer to the previous question gave Peter's starting sum in US dollars as $868.10. If he returns with $38, then he spent $868.10 − $38 = $830.10 on his holidays. This means that he spent $830.10 \div 868.10 = 0.956$, or approximately 96% of his original money. The correct answer is (E).

23. (A)

First, convert £108 into euros. The exchange rate for pounds to euros is £1:€1.16667, so multiply to find the sum in euros: £108 × (€1.16667/£1) = €126.00. Divide by €2 to find the number of €2 coins required for this total amount: €126 ÷ €2 = 63 coins. The answer is (A).

24. (D)

The table does not give a rate to convert Japanese yen directly into New Zealand dollars, so convert yen first into US dollars, euros or pounds, then convert that total into NZ dollars. The table shows that US$1 = 81.91 yen, so divide by 81.91 to find the equivalent value of the yen in US dollars: 1000 yen ÷ 81.91 = US$12.2085. The table also shows that US$1 = NZ$1.34644; multiply to find the value in NZ$:US$12.2085 × 1.34644 = NZ $16.438, so the correct answer is (D).

25. (C)

Arabella rode Truffles a total of 11 miles, in a ride that took 1 hour, 14 minutes, or 74 minutes. Convert this to hours: 74/60 hours = 1.233 hours. Use the speed formula to find the average trotting speed: Speed = Distance ÷ Time = 11 miles ÷ 1.233 hours = 8.92 mph. The answer is therefore (C).

26. (B)

To find Jack of Hearts's average speed on the total ride, find the total distance and total time, and then use the speed formula: Speed = Distance ÷ Time. The total distance is 11 miles × 2 = 22 miles. The time for the first part of the journey is 44 minutes, 44/60 hours = 0.733 hours. Since the speed on the first part of the journey is twice the speed on the second part, use the speed formula to find the speed for the first part of the journey: Speed = 11 miles ÷ 0.733 hours = 15 mph. The speed on the second part of the journey is half of this, or 7.5 mph. Thus, the time on the second part of the journey must be twice the time on the first part of the journey (since the distance is the same—if unsure, you could confirm this with the speed formula). The time on the second part of the journey is 44 minutes × 2 = 88 minutes, so the total time is 44 + 88 = 132 minutes, or 132/60 hours = 2.2 hours. Use the speed formula one more time, to calculate the average trotting speed for the total ride: Speed = 22 miles ÷ 2.2 hours = 10 mph. The correct answer is (B).

27. (D)

Use the speed formula to find Peppermint's trotting speed: Speed = Distance ÷ Time. The distance is the length of the trail and back again, or 22 miles. The time is 2 hours, 39 minutes, or 159 minutes = 159/60 hours = 2.65 hours. Plug these figures into the speed formula to solve: Speed = 22 miles ÷ 2.65 hours = 8.3 mph. The answer is therefore (D).

28. (A)

The work required to solve the previous three questions gave average trotting speeds for three horses: Truffles's trotting speed was 8.9 mph, Jack of Hearts's was 7.5 mph and Peppermint's was 8.3 mph. The previous question stated that Dazzle's average trotting speed was 1.4 mph faster than Peppermint's, so calculate: 8.3 + 1.4 = 9.7 mph. Thus, Dazzle has an average trotting speed that is faster than any of Arabella's other horses—and also faster than Galaxy, her brother's horse, whose average trotting speed is given at the top of the page as 9.2 mph. The correct answer is (A).

29. (D)

The first pie chart, representing Joe's viewing for May, shows that approximately one-third of his TV hours were spent watching comedies. The answer is therefore (D).

30. (E)

In June, romantic programmes were just over a quarter of Joe's TV viewing hours. Since he spent 234 hours watching TV, divide by 4 to approximate the hours spent watching romantic programmes: 234 hours ÷ 4 = 58.5 hours. Remember, romantic programmes were slightly more than a quarter of the total, so the correct answer must be 60 hours, answer (E).

31. (C)

In May, the first pie chart, documentary and adventure programmes add up to one-quarter of the total viewing hours, or 25% of the total. The correct answer is (C).

32. (B)

Joe spent one-third of his TV viewing time watching comedies in May; divide the total hours by 3 to find the number of comedy hours: 150 ÷ 3 = 50 hours in May. Joe spent just over half of his viewing hours watching comedies in June, so divide the total by 2 to find the number of comedy hours: 234 ÷ 2 = 117. The difference in comedy hours from May to June is 117 − 50 = 67. Percentage change equals difference divided by original, so divide to find percentage change: 67 ÷ 50 = 1.34, or 134%. Remember, the comedy hours for June were slightly more than half of the total, but the calculation used 50% rather than the larger percentage. The correct answer is therefore slightly larger than 134%. Thus, answer (B) must be correct.

33. (A)

Because percentage change equals difference divided by original, the band with the greatest percentage rise from Week 2 to Week 3 will have the steepest increase in the slope of the line connecting those two points on the graph; that is, it will have a relatively large difference compared to its original value in Week 2. The two bands with the steepest increases from Week 2 to Week 3 are Toxic Shock and Cambridge Town Vocal Choir, so compare their figures using the percentage change formula. Toxic Shock has an original value of 15,000 in Week 2 and a final value of 50,000 in Week 3, for a difference of 50,000 – 15,000 = 35,000. The percentage change is 35,000 ÷ 15,000 = 2.33, or 233%. Cambridge Town Vocal Choir has an original value of 2,000 and a final value of 10,000, for a difference of 10,000 – 2,000 = 8,000. The percentage change is 8,000 ÷ 2,000 = 4, or 400%. The answer is therefore (A).

34. (C)

The week with the greatest total sales will have the highest combined values for all five bands, and would likely have the highest sales of any week for some of the bands. The highest individual sales for any band (by 10,000) are the sales for Toxic Shock in Week 3; Cambridge Town Vocal Choir also had their best sales by a significant margin in that week; even though these are the lowest for Week 3, the total of 10,000 is about 8,000 more than the worst-selling band in any other week. The high margin of success for these two bands in Week 3 is more than enough to make up for the difference in the figures for the other three bands, who had their second or third best weeks in Week 3, but by a much narrower margin. Thus, a quick visual estimate shows that the answer must be (C).

35. (E)

Proceed carefully, as this question is not asking for a percentage decrease, but a simple numerical decrease. The biggest drop in sales from one week to the next is the line on the graph with the sharpest decline, which represents the sales for Toxic Shock from Week 3 (50,000) to Week 4 (3,000). None of the other bands recorded sales in excess of 40,000 in a single week, so no other band could have a greater decrease from one week to the next than Toxic Shock. The answer is (E).

36. (D)

MC Einstein's single sold 35,000 in Week 5, and the total sales were approximately 35,000 + 30,500 + 9,000 + 100 + 100 = 74,700. Divide to find the percentage: 35,000 ÷ 74,700 = 0.4685, or 47%. The correct answer is (D). Note that there is a slight shortcut here: once you determine the total, you might have noticed that MC Einstein's sales were not 50% of the total (as this would have required a total of 70,000), but are only slightly less than half of the total. If you were in a rush, this would have been sufficient justification for marking (D).

Abstract Reasoning

1. (C)

This pattern involves features of shapes, and also arrangement. In Set A, the arrows are arranged to point at the two shapes that have the same number of sides. In Set B, the arrows are arranged to point at the two shapes that have the same shading. The arrows in the first test shape point at two shapes with 5 sides each, which fits the pattern for Set A. However, the two pentagons are both shaded black, so the test shape also fits the pattern for Set B. Since the test shape can belong to both sets, it fits exclusively into neither. The answer is (C).

2. (C)

The arrows in this test shape point at a triangle and a lightning shape, with 11 sides. Since the two shapes do not have the same number of sides, the test shape does not belong to Set A. The triangle is grey and the lightning is white, so the test shape does not belong to Set B. The answer is therefore (C).

3. (B)

This test shape has arrows pointing at the two white shapes, a hexagon and a circle. This fits the pattern for Set B.

4. (A)

This test shape includes arrows pointing at two quadrilaterals, one white and one grey. This fits the pattern for Set A.

5. (C)

The test shape contains a two-headed arrow, which points at two identical grey crosses. Since the crosses have the same number of sides, the test shape belongs to Set A. Since the crosses have identical shading, the test shape belongs to Set B. Since the test shape can belong to both sets, it belongs exclusively to neither. The answer is therefore (C).

6. (C)

This pattern involves type of shape. Each box in Set A contains a diamond. Each box in Set B contains a hexagon. The first test shape contains a pentagon, a star and a heart, so it does not fit the pattern for either set. The answer is (C).

7. (A)

This test shape includes a diamond, so it fits the pattern for Set A.

8. (B)

There is a hexagon in this test shape, so it belongs to Set B.

9. (C)

This test shape includes a diamond, so it belongs to Set A. However, it also includes a hexagon, so it also belongs to Set B. Since the test shape can belong to both sets, it belongs exclusively to neither. The answer is therefore (C).

10. (B)

The final test shape contains a hexagon, so it belongs to Set B.

11. (B)

This pattern involves a feature of the shapes in each box, which appear to form a 'clock' figure, with a short hand and long hand. In Set A, the smaller angle formed by the hands of the clock measures less than 90°; in Set B, the smaller angle formed by the hands of the clock measures larger than 90°. In the first test shape, the smaller angle formed by the hands of the clock is greater than 90°; the test shape therefore belongs to Set B.

12. (C)

The hands on the clock in this test shape form an angle of exactly 90°, meaning that the test shape cannot belong to either set. The answer is (C).

13. (C)

The clock in this test shape has two short hands, rather than a short hand and a long hand. This fits the pattern for neither set. The answer is therefore (C).

14. (A)

The angle formed by the hands of the clock in this test shape measures less than 90°, so the test shape fits into Set A.

15. (B)

This test shape features a clock with hands forming a smaller angle of just under 180°. This angle is larger than 90°, so the test shape fits the pattern for Set B.

16. (C)

This pattern involves two features of shapes: size and colour. Each box in both sets contains a grey shape. In Set A, the grey shape is the largest shape in each box; in Set B, the grey shape is the smallest shape in each box. The first test shape does not include a grey shape, so it belongs to neither set.

17. (A)

The largest shape in this test shape is grey, so it fits the pattern for Set A.

18. (B)

The smallest shape in this test shape is grey, so it fits the pattern for Set B.

19. (B)

This test shape includes more individual shapes than any box in either set; remember, however, that the overall number of shapes in the box is not relevant to the pattern. The smallest shape is grey, so the test shape belongs to Set B.

20. (C)

The grey shape included in this test shape is neither the smallest nor the largest, so it fits into neither set.

21. (C)

This pattern involves arrangement of the shapes in each box. In Set A, each box includes two shapes that 'cross over', or overlap, each other; in Set B, each box includes three shapes that cross over each other. Any shapes that do not overlap are irrelevant to the pattern. The first test shape includes a total of four overlapping shapes, so it belongs to neither set.

22. (B)

This test shape includes a total of three overlapping shapes, so the answer is (B).

23. (C)

The test shape contains a total of seven shapes, but none of them crosses over any of the others. This does not fit the pattern for either set. The answer is therefore (C).

24. (A)

This test shape includes a diamond overlapping an octagon, and thus fits the pattern for Set A.

25. (A)

The test shape contains two shapes that cross over, so the answer is (A).

26. (B)

This pattern involves a feature of the shapes in each box: the number of sides. In Set A, the shapes in each box have a total of 12 sides. In Set B, the shapes in each box have a total of 8 sides. The first test shape has two rainbow shapes with 4 sides each, for a total of 8 sides; as such, it belongs to Set B.

27. (B)

The pentagon and triangle in this test shape have a total of 8 sides, so the answer is (B).

28. (C)

The two triangles and diamond in this test shape have a total of 10 sides. Since this does not fit the pattern for either set, the answer is (C).

29. (C)

This double-headed arrow has a total of 10 sides, so it fits into neither set.

30. (A)

The test shape contains an octagon and a diamond, with a total of 12 sides; as such, the test shape belongs to Set A.

31. (A)

This pattern involves a particular type of shape in each set. In Set A, each box contains an isosceles triangle (a triangle in which two of the sides are of equal length). In Set B, each box contains a right triangle. The triangle in the first test shape has two equal sides, so it fits the pattern for Set A.

32. (C)

The triangle in this test shape has three sides of equal length, so it does not fit the pattern for Set A. Because it is an equilateral triangle, all its angles measure 60°; as such, it does not fit the pattern for Set B. Thus, the test shape belongs to neither set, and the answer is (C).

33. (C)

The test shape contains a triangle with two sides of equal length, so it belongs to Set A. However, the triangle also features a right angle, so it also belongs to Set B. Since the test shape can fit into both sets, it belongs exclusively to neither. The answer is therefore (C).

34. (A)

This test shape includes a triangle with two equal sides and no right angle. Thus, the test shape fits into Set A.

35. (B)

The final test shape contains a triangle with a right angle and sides of varying length. As such, the test shape belongs to Set B.

36. (A)

This pattern involves the relative arrangement of the two shapes within each box. In Set A, the two shapes are identical, but one is rotated 90° from the position of the other. In Set B, the two shapes are identical, but one is rotated 90° and reflected across a horizontal axis of symmetry (or 'flipped' horizontally). The first test shape includes two identical shapes, one of which is rotated 90° to the right from the position of the other. As such, the test shape belongs to Set A.

37. (B)

This test shape has two identical shapes, with one rotated 90° to the right and then 'flipped' horizontally from the position of the other. This fits the pattern for Set B.

38. (C)

The two shapes in this test shape are identical, except that one has been flipped horizontally from the position of the other. Since the shape has not also been rotated 90° to the right, the test shape belongs to neither set.

39. (B)

This test shape includes two identical shapes, one of which has been rotated 90° to the right and then flipped horizontally. The test shape therefore belongs to Set B.

40. (C)

The two shapes in this test shape are identical, except that one has been flipped vertically from the position of the other. This does not match the pattern for either set. The answer is therefore (C).

41. (C)

The boxes in these sets each appear to contain a letter, which has been broken down into the line segments that make up the letter. In Set A, each box contains a total of three line segments. In Set B, each box contains a total of two line segments. The first test shape contains four line segments, so it does not fit into the pattern for either set. The answer is therefore (C).

42. (A)

This test shape include three line segments, so it fits the pattern for Set A.

43. (C)

The test shape consists of a single line segment, forming an 'O'. As such, it belongs to neither set.

44. (B)

Two line segments make up this test shape, which therefore fits the pattern for Set B.

45. (A)

The final test shape includes a total of three line segments, so it belongs to Set A.

46. (A)

All boxes in both sets contain a star and a circle with an arc around it. The difference in the patterns involves the arrangement of the star and the arc. In Set A, if the star is below the circle, the arc opens downwards; if the star is above the circle, then the arc opens upwards. This conditional pattern is reversed in Set B: if the star is below the circle, the arc opens upwards; if the star is above the circle, the arc opens down. In the first test shape, the star is below the circle, and the arc opens downwards. This fits the pattern for Set A.

47. (C)

There is no star in this test shape, so it belongs to neither set.

48. (B)

The star is above the circle and the arc opens downwards, so this test shape belongs to Set B.

49. (C)

The test shape includes a circle, a star and an arc, but the circle isn't arranged within the arc. As such, the test shape fits the pattern for neither set.

50. (B)

The star is below the circle, and the arc opens upwards; thus, this test shape belongs to Set B.

51. (C)

The circles in each column are arranged in three columns. These are coloured white, black, grey, in the first box; the colours shift one position to the left (with the leftmost coming round to the rightmost position) in each subsequent box in the progression. The order in the fourth box is white, black, grey, so the order in the correct answer must be black, grey, white. Eliminate (A) and (B). There is a further element to the progression: in the first box, the top circle in the rightmost column is dotted; this shifts to the top circle in the middle column in the second box, then back to the top of the rightmost column in the third box. Thus, the final item in the sequence will have the top circle in the rightmost column dotted. The correct answer is (C).

52. (D)

The first box includes a small triangle atop a medium-sized diamond atop a large square. In the second box, each shape has moved down the stack—and thus increased in size—except for the large square, which is now the topmost, smallest shape. The triangle also flips vertically with each subsequent box, so that it points up, then down, then up, then down. Thus, the triangle must be pointing up in the final shape; eliminate (A) and (B). The stack of shapes is the same in (C) and (D), so check the shading. In the original boxes, the large shape always has vertical stripes, and the smallest shape has horizontal stripes. Thus, answer (D) must be correct.

53. (B)

It can be very hard to see the progression when the type of shape changes with each subsequent box, so see if there are other elements that will help you eliminate quickly. The colour of the shapes changes between white and black, so the correct answer will have white shapes; eliminate (C) and (D). The key to the pattern is the total number of sides in each box, which doubles with each subsequent box. Thus, the first box has a total of 3 sides, the second a total of 6 sides, followed by boxes with totals of 12 and 24 sides. The final box will therefore have a total of 48 sides; the correct answer is (B).

54. (A)

Check each shape to see how many rotations it makes in the first four boxes. The white arrow rotates through four positions, and the black arrow rotates through three positions. Thus, in the correct answer, the white arrow will be in the first position and the black arrow will be in the second position. Answer (A) is therefore correct.

55. (C)

The parallelogram progresses through three types of shading: white, grey and striped. It is white in the fourth box, so it will be grey in the correct answer; eliminate (B) and (D). The grey triangle is in the same position in the remaining answers, so it will not help in determining which is correct. The black triangle alternates between two positions, adjacent and outside the parallelogram, or just inside the upper left corner. It is inside in the fourth box, so it must be outside in the correct answer. (C) is therefore correct.

Decision Analysis

1. (D)

The literal translation is *woman(guard, temple), kill(increase(snake))*. The first part of the message combines woman, guard and temple into a single concept; eliminate (E), which groups woman with snake, rather than the first part of the message. The second part of the message does not include L, big, or F, past, so eliminate (A) and (C). Of the remaining answers, (B) does not include a representation of increase, while (D) uses increase to modify snake, forming the plural, snakes. Because (B) omits a code that is included in the message, it cannot be correct. The answer is therefore (D).

2. (A)

The literal translation is *Egypt, increase(pharaoh), sleep(under, triangle(place))*. The first two answers are a good fit for the first two parts of the message; answers (C) and (E) make Egyptians plural, but this would require extra elements of the code (such as woman) to include the concept of Egyptian people rather than Egypt as a place, so eliminate (C) and (E). (D) interprets increase(pharaoh) as big pharaoh; however, big is L in the table but is not included in the message; eliminate (D). The final term is interpreted in the remaining answers with either sleep or buried. The table seems to require past, F, to form the past tense, and 'bury' is a more poetical interpretation of sleep, both of which make (B) a weaker answer. (A) does not have any weaknesses, and matches the meaning of the codes in the message very closely. For these reasons, (A) is correct.

3. (C)

The literal translation is *river, big(wash)(opposite(under)), big(big(place))*. The first three answers interpret the second part of the message as 'flood', which is literally a big washing over. Eliminate (D) and (E), which only include 'washing over', omitting a representation of big with the second part of the message. The only difference among the remaining answers is in their varied interpretations of the final part of the message. A building, a city and a pyramid could all be a 'big big place'; however, build is 4 in the table but is not included in the message, so the answer cannot be (A). Similarly, the correct answer to the previous question interpreted triangle(place) as pyramid; triangle is not included in the message, so pyramid is not a good interpretation of 'big big place'. The only remaining option is (C), which must be correct.

4. (E)

The answer choices give two different ways of encoding the concept of 'don't sleep': E(G10) is command(negative(sleep)) and G10 is negative(sleep). 'Don't sleep' is a command, so E is required to encode the message. Eliminate (A), (B) and (D), which omit E. The only difference between the remaining answers is within the brackets of the final element: (C) has L17, big(camel), and (E) has C17, pharaoh(camel). Pharaoh is required to encode the message, so the answer is (E).

5. (C)

The literal translation is *big(big(old)), increase(woman), past(opposite(leave), kill), god(river)*. The second part of the message must mean something like 'women'; eliminate (B) and (E), which wrongly broaden women to people. Of the remaining answers, two interpret the first part of the message as 'in olden times', and one gives it as 'in very ancient times'. 'Big old' could mean something like 'olden times', but the correct interpretation must include the second big modifying 'big old'. Thus, the only option for the first part of the message is 'in very ancient times', and the correct answer must be (C).

6. (B)

The literal translation is *increase(Egypt)(woman, opposite(woman)), past(build), big(triangle(place))*. The first part of the message could mean 'Egyptians', but does not include old, A, so it could not mean 'ancient Egyptians'; eliminate (A) and (D). Eliminate (E) as well, because (E) omits to include 'increase' with the first part of the message. The 'big triangle place' in the final part of the message could mean 'Great Pyramid', but cannot mean 'big building', as build is 4 in the table and is not included in the final part of the message; the 4 in the message is already represented in 'built' in both remaining answers. The answer is therefore (B).

7. (A)

The answers encode the first part of the message as E16, command(wash), or 16, wash. Because the message is a command, the first part of the coded message must include E. Eliminate (C) and (E), which don't. The final parts of the remaining answers start with E9, command(leave), or 9, leave. Since the final part of the message is a second command, the coded message must include a second E to modify leave. Thus, the answer is (A).

8. (D)

The literal translation is *wheat, increase(big), river(triangle)*. Answers (A) and (B) include flood and wash, respectively, which would require a further element from the table (such as 16) that is not in the message, so eliminate (A) and (B). (C) modifies wheat with increase, but increase modifies big; eliminate (C). The remaining answers are very similar, but there are two problems with (E): 'three rivers' is not a good interpretation of river(triangle), and the verb, was, is in the past tense; F, past, does not appear in the message. (D) is a good fit for the elements in the message, and does not include any other elements from the table of codes; (D) is correct.

9. (B)

The answers give two options for the first part of the message, new man: MA(M2) or BA(M2). M2 is opposite(woman), or man; MA is opposite(old), or new; BA is increase(old), or older. Eliminate (D) and (E). The verb in the message, lost, is in the past tense, so the second part of the message must include F; eliminate (C), which doesn't. The only difference between the remaining answers is in the final part of the message: D8 is under(river) and 8 is river. The man did not lose the camels under the river, so including D with 8 would change the meaning of the message. The answer is therefore (B).

10. (E)

The literal translation is *big(snake, snake), guard, temple, god(woman)(increase(wheat))*. The first part of the message seems to mean 'two big snakes', but could possibly mean 'big snakes', as there is more than one snake encoded in the message; eliminate (C) and (D), which omit 'big' in representing the snakes. (A) includes 'left' as the main verb, but this would require 9, leave, and F, past, neither of which is in the message; eliminate (A). The final part of the message combines woman and god into a single element, but (B) separates the woman and the god into separate concepts and different parts of the sentence. (E), however, represents these together as 'goddess', and is therefore correct.

11. (A)

The literal translation is *pharaoh, big(sleep), guard, opposite(big(sleep))*. Eliminate (E), which interprets the sleeping in the past tense, as the message does not include F, past. The second part of the message could be a good fit for 'long sleep', in answer (A), as long is a good representation for big. (B) and (D) interpret 'big' as 'well' and 'good', respectively, which would be a good representation for opposite(negative), but not for big. Eliminate (B) and (D); also, eliminate (C), which omits a representation of big. The answer must be (A).

12. (C)

The literal translation is *opposite(big)(woman), past(find), jar(perfume), wash(place)*. The first part of the message could mean 'girl' or 'small woman', but eliminate (D), which omits opposite(big). (B) omits a representation of past, giving 'finds' in the present tense, so eliminate (B). (E) includes perfume but omits jar, so eliminate (E). The final part of the message, wash(place), could mean bathroom; (A), however, omits place, and is therefore wrong. The correct answer is (C).

13. (B)

The literal translation is *guard(opposite(kill)), past(lead), pharaoh(woman), increase(tear)*. All the answers interpret the first part of the message as 'guard's death' or 'guard died'; however, died would require F, past, which is not combined with the first part of the message. Eliminate (A), (D) and (E). The most obvious difference between the remaining answers is whether to interpret C2 as 'queen' or 'pharaoh's wife'. There are two problems with (C): 'pharaoh's wife' would seem to require marry, which is 109 in the table but is not included in the message, and make is included in (C) and in the table as P, but is not part of the coded message. Thus, (C) cannot be correct. The answer must be (B).

14. (D)

The message is a command, so the first part of the coded message should start with E105, command(wrap). Eliminate (C) and (E). The remaining answers give three different ways to encode eyes: L104, big(eye); B104, increase(eye); (104, 104), (eye, eye). Eliminate (A), as big(eye) would mean a big eye, rather than two eyes; (B) and (D) could both mean 'eyes'. The only difference between (B) and (D) is in the final part of the message: 107(108) or 107(F108), robe(tear) or robe(past(tear)). Since torn is the past form of tear, the correct answer must include F108. The answer is therefore (D).

15. (C)

The literal translation is *hippopotamus, kill(boat), ride(opposite(under)), river*. The message does not include F, past, so the correct answer must have a main verb in the present tense. Eliminate (A), (B) and (E), which incorrectly use the past tense. The second part of the message, kill(boat), could mean 'destroying a boat'; however, it could not mean 'sailors', as sailors would require some further element beyond the concept of boat. Eliminate (D); the answer is (C).

16. (E)

The literal translation is *crocodile(fearful), snake(increase(cruel), big(increase)(kill))*. All the answers interpret the first part of the message in ways that could be correct. The second part of the message seems to make a distinction that the snake is more deadly than it is cruel; both are increased, but kill has a big increase. Eliminate (A), which modifies cruel with 'deadly' but does not modify 'kills' with anything stronger; also, eliminate (D), which modifies cruel and deadly with the same 'very highly'. (B) combines cruel, kill and the two varying levels of increase into 'very dangerous', but this obscures the difference between the two levels of increase; eliminate (B). (C) interprets cruel as 'nasty' and kill as 'venomous', which might seem to fit, except that 'nasty' does not include a representation of increase. Eliminate (C). (E) includes a good representation of increase(cruel) and big(increase)(kill), so it is correct.

17. (A)

The literal translation is *pharaoh, opposite(past)(ride), gold(boat), opposite(under), place(sun, leave(under))*. Answers (B), (C) and (E) give the second part of the message in the past tense, but the message has opposite(past), which must mean something like future. Eliminate (B), (C) and (E). The final part of the message literally means something like 'the place where the sun goes under'. The phrasing is a bit awkward, but a good representation of the concept of the horizon. The answer is therefore (A).

18. (B)

All the answers start with 201, lucky. The second part of the message is either 15, find, or F15, past(find). Since the message has 'found', which is the past of find, the answer must include F15; eliminate (D) and (E). The remaining answers include three versions of the third part of the message, so only one can be a good fit: 2 is woman; ML is opposite(big), or small; BL is increase(big), or bigger; MA is opposite(old), or young; BA is increase(old), or older. A smaller, new woman is the only logical fit for the young girl in the message; the answer must be (B).

19. (E)

The literal translation is *blue(hippopotamus), woman(fertile)*. The answers are very similar, so check to see whether any include codes from the table that are not in the message, or whether any recombine elements from the message into different groupings. (A) includes make, which is P in the table but not in the message; eliminate (A). (B) omits woman, so it cannot be correct. (C) includes 'see', which is not represented by any term in the message; it's not clear how 'see' would be represented in the table—perhaps with eye, 104—but it would require an element that is not in the message, in any case; eliminate (C). (D) includes only elements that are in the message; however, (D) recombines fertile with hippopotamus, whereas woman modifies fertile in the message. (E) includes only the elements in the message, in the correct groupings, so (E) is the correct answer.

20. (A)

The literal translation is *god(sun), make(fire)(lead), make(gold)(chair)*. The first part of the message could mean 'sun god' or 'god of the sun'; eliminate (D) and (E), which separate god and sun into separate concepts. The second part of the message could mean 'burns lead', as make(fire) could mean 'burn'; however, it could not mean 'makes fire sit', as sit does not make sense as a representation of lead, and it could not mean 'leads fire', which omits a representation of make. Eliminate (B) and (C); answer (A) is correct.

21. (D)

The literal translation is *opposite(wash)(robe), opposite(false)(eye), negative(lucky)(woman, lead, temple)*. The table of codes includes both negative and opposite, and it's important to be aware that these are not necessarily interchangeable. Thus, in the first element of the message, it is potentially significant that we have opposite(wash) rather than negative(wash). The latter would mean something like 'not washed' or 'unwashed'; the former means something like 'dirty'; on this basis, eliminate (A), (B) and (E). The second element literally means 'true eye'; this is given as 'sees too late' in (C) and as 'true sight' in (D). There is nothing in the message that could mean 'too late', so (D) must be correct. **NB** If you were not sure about negative versus opposite in the first element, you could have also eliminated (B) and (E) based on the second element, and (A) based on the final element.

22. (B)

The literal translation is *increase(big)(opposite(fearful)), opposite(past), increase(boat)(ride), opposite, increase(guard)(cruel, increase(kill))*. The first element includes the opposite of fearful, which means something like courageous or brave. However, this is modified by increase(big), which must be represented in the message; eliminate (C) and (D), which have bravery and courage but omit the modification. The second element is given as 'will' in all the remaining answers. The third element appears as navy and ride/carry in the remaining answers, so nothing can be eliminated. The fourth element, opposite, appears as 'against' in (A) and (B); eliminate (E), which instead has 'over'. The final element includes cruel in combination with increase(kill) in describing the guards or 'army'; eliminate (A), which omits increase(kill). The correct answer is (B).

23. (C)

All the answers encode the first two parts of the message, 'Egyptology' and 'finds', identically. There are five options for the third part of the message, 'truths': M206 is opposite(rare), or common; eliminate (A). 206 also appears in (D), as increase(common), and (E), increase(rare); eliminate (D) and (E). M208 is opposite(false), or true; thus, B(M208) is increase(true). Since this code seems to use increase to make nouns plural, the correct answer must be (C).

24. (E)

The literal translation is *increase(crocodile), past(kill)(hippopotamus), increase(opposite(woman)), past(kill)(increase(crocodile))*. The first two parts of the message seem to mean something like 'crocodiles killed a hippopotamus'; eliminate (B), (C) and (D), which incorrectly interpret hippopotamus as plural, as hippopotamus is not modified by increase in the message. The only difference between the remaining answers is that (E) links the details of the two killings with 'and', while (A) includes 'before'. Previous correct answers have included 'and' without requiring an element to represent it, but 'before' might need a further element. It is a bit unclear whether this is required, but (E) interprets the message without any such uncertainty; for this reason, (E) is correct.

25. (D)

The literal translation is guard, marry(woman), temple(opposite(under)(river)). Because the second part of the message modifies woman with marry, answer (A)—which regroups woman with guard—cannot be correct. The remaining answers are possible interpretations of the first two parts of the message, so eliminate based on the final part. Opposite(under) must mean something like 'over' or 'above'; eliminate (B) and (E), which omit opposite and thus interpret the final element incorrectly as 'underwater'. The difference between (C) and (D) is admittedly a subtle one, but across is not the opposite of under, so (C) cannot be correct. The correct answer is (D).

26. (C) and (E)

All the words are included in the message, so eliminate any words that can be formed with existing elements in the table of codes. Slaughter could be encoded as big(kill), LK, so eliminate (A). Fright could be used to encode scary, but it could be encoded with existing codes as make(fearful), P203; eliminate (B). Dark could be encoded as negative(sun) or negative(fire), G6 or G110; eliminate (D). Nothing in the table corresponds to the concept of dirt or smell, so the most useful new words are answers (C) and (E), which are correct.

27. (A) and (D)

All the words in the answers are included in the message, so check the answers against the existing table of codes. Book is 113, so eliminate (B). Library could be encoded as book(place), 113H; eliminate (E). Of the remaining answers, fashion is the easiest to encode: it could be represented as new(robe), MA(107). Eliminate (C), and the correct answers are (A) and (D), as tutor and culture cannot be represented with the existing table.

28. (B) and (D)

Again, all the answers are included in the message, so check against the table of codes. True appeared in the correct answer to a previous question as M208, opposite(false); eliminate (A). Common could be formed as M206, opposite(rare); eliminate (C). Legend could be encoded as big(book), L113, or big(history), L(FH); eliminate (E). There is no way to represent the concepts of life or love, so the answers must be (B) and (D).

1. (D)

This would be inappropriate, as Samia has not attempted a local solution to the problem by asking Hayley what has been going on. Also, Samia does not know for sure that Hayley has been lying.

2. (D)

Again, this would be inappropriate, as Samia has not approached Hayley first and also does not know for certain that Hayley is unwell.

3. (D)

This would be inappropriate as it does not offer Samia an opportunity to talk about what might be going on—she may be struggling with financial pressure and therefore feel that she has to skip medical school to work—a situation that could be eased with some advice and support.

4. (B)

Whilst this option is good in that it offers Hayley a chance to explain her actions, the wording is somewhat confrontational and may hinder a successful conversation about the problems that she may be having.

5. (A)

This open question allows Hayley to open up about the previous day without fear of condemnation or judgement. If she denies being out of the house, then Samia has a reason to challenge this and also a lead-in to doing so.

6. (A)

Since Shaun is Tameka's student and his remark was well out of order, it is very appropriate for Tameka to apologise to the patient on his behalf.

7. (A)

Since Shaun is Tameka's student and his remark was well out of order, it is very appropriate for Tameka to ask Shaun to apologise.

8. (A)

This response allows Tameka to address the patient's underlying concerns while also ensuring that the critical surgery can go ahead, so it is a highly appropriate response.

9. (B)

It is appropriate for Tameka to tell Shaun to keep his personal views to himself, and he will need to learn to do so if he is to have a career as a doctor. However, this response is not ideal, as it does not directly address why Shaun's views are inappropriate or the patient's underlying concern, which are the two main issues in this scenario.

10. (A)

As it seems highly likely that the coursework was meant for Lisa, this is a responsible and very appropriate course of action. She will likely need to complete the work by the same deadline to ensure she does not compromise any aspect of her training.

11. (B)

Whilst this is an acceptable course of action, it is not ideal, as Lisa may still be able to complete the coursework once she learns the details of the task involved. This would ensure there is no delay in her work. The most appropriate action would involve finding out the details of the coursework before requesting any extension if necessary, and enquiring if there have been any other emails she has not received and making sure she is on the correct mailing list for future emails.

12. (D)

Whilst her exams are extremely important, ignoring other pieces of work could compromise Lisa successfully qualifying from medical school. By ignoring the coursework, she would also be demonstrating lack of integrity, a trait paramount to students and doctors, who also have a responsibility for their own learning. Thus, this response is highly inappropriate.

13. (A)

Addressing the issue locally, immediately and discreetly is a very appropriate course of action, and would ensure Lisa has completed all the necessary coursework to qualify from medical school.

14. (D)

It is likely there has been a misunderstanding, mistake or perhaps no mistake in this situation; it is important to clarify with the administrator whether or not the email should have been sent to Lisa before escalating the case. This is a highly inappropriate course of action particularly as, at the moment, Lisa only has second-hand information from her peer and this solution is neither local, immediate nor discreet.

15. (C)

The consultant should respond to the patient, and he would be right to point out that there are standards of patient safety and medical professionalism at the hospital. This response, however, does not make these points quite so explicitly, and as such is inappropriate, but not awful.

16. (C)

While it is the job of a porter to assist patients in the hospital, this response is inappropriate as the patient seems extremely agitated and has directed his anger at the consultant, so a better response would be for the consultant to do something to help address the patient's agitation. However, this response is not awful, as a porter would have some role in helping a patient in this context.

17. (A)

This response would give the consultant a chance to understand the patient's exact concerns, and to do so immediately, discreetly and calmly. It is a very appropriate thing to do.

18. (A)

This is an immediate response, and a relatively calm and discreet one, so it is highly appropriate.

19. (A)

Doing a night shift in A&E is compulsory for this placement, so it is imperative Matthew undertakes this experience as part of his training. Swapping with another student, if possible, is an ideal course of action.

20. (D)

Not attending the shift is irresponsible as the team will be expecting Matthew's help; it also impacts negatively on Matthew's training. Furthermore, pretending to be ill is dishonest. This response is thus highly inappropriate.

21. (A)

Informing the team is appropriate, and also ensures that the night shift happens at a later date. Whilst Sunday night may initially seem an acceptable time to postpone the shift, it may be that a Saturday night is required because of the patients who may tend to present to A&E at this time. Offering to rearrange the shift to a Sunday or a Saturday is therefore sensible.

22. (D)

Not attending the shift as previously noted is inappropriate and impacts on Matthew's training. Asking a peer to lie, on top of this, is highly inappropriate.

23. (B)

Whilst this is appropriate for Matthew's training, as this is a weekend shift, the university would understand that occasionally important family events may occur at these times. So long as Matthew is able to rearrange his shift for another time that is convenient for the A&E team so he does not miss out on this part of his training, he would be able to attend the party. The ideal course of action would thus involve him rescheduling this weekend shift so he is able to attend the event.

24. (A)

This response is somewhat forceful, however it is highly appropriate, as Haroon can see that the receptionist is not working, and this is an immediate solution that will ensure the patients are attended to quickly while also avoiding any comments on the receptionist's professionalism in the presence of the patients.

25. (D)

The receptionist's behaviour is clearly unacceptable; however, addressing it in front of patients in this way is very inappropriate, particularly as the more pressing concerns are the ringing phone and the queue of patients waiting to speak to the receptionist.

26. (C)

This response is inappropriate, as the practice will not run more smoothly if Haroon helps the receptionist by answering the phone. However, this approach is not awful, as it does seem there are quite a lot of patients who need to be spoken to, and the patients will appreciate Haroon's intervention.

27. (A)

This is a very appropriate thing to do, as it will allow Haroon to address Mrs Rahman's concern discreetly, locally and immediately.

28. (D)

The patient has to come first in this situation and it would be very rude to keep the patient waiting, especially for that long. The patient would not even know where they were if they did not call the patient. The duo should go and see the patient together without Kyle and he should join them when he gets there.

29. (C)

This is not going to solve the current issue, which is that the students would be late to meet the patient. Whilst it is important that Kyle knows that he is letting the group down, telling him how the rest of the group feel is not going to get Kyle there any quicker. Thus, this response is inappropriate, but not awful.

30. (D)

This response will keep the patient waiting, and given the fact that the group has been late on all their previous visits, notifying the patient in advance of their tardiness will not reassure the patient. This response does not address the unprofessionalism of the group, and does nothing to avoid inconveniencing the patient, so it is highly inappropriate.

31. (A)

This option does not inconvenience the patient in any way, and the patient must be their first priority. It will also address the issue so that hopefully the situation will not happen again.

32. (C)

This is not ideal, as it does not involve working together as a group; they should both talk to Kyle, not just James, since the problem is affecting them both. However, it does not affect the patient, so it is not awful.

33. (D)

Katie's consultant appears to be a patient, and as such, he would expect a certain level of privacy and discretion. It would therefore be very inappropriate for Katie to ask him why he is here.

34. (A)

Given that it seems clear to Katie that the consultant is likely to be visiting the hospital as a patient, and that he does not seem to have seen her, it is best to pretend she didn't see him, unless he brings it up later.

35. (D)

If her consultant is attending the hospital as a patient, then asking if her friend who works there knows the consultant is highly inappropriate, as her friend is required to maintain patient confidentiality.

36. (A)

This is a very neutral question, and avoids the question of why Katie's consultant is at the hospital. As such, it is a highly appropriate thing to do.

37. (D)

This is not appropriate because it is not a local solution, and it does not deal with the situation immediately. Asking Tom to take off his watch would solve the problem quickly and prevent the spread of infection.

38. (D)

This action does not address the problem at all. In a hospital, it is everyone's responsibility to ensure that the whole team obeys the infection control rules in order to protect the patients from catching infections. Neha should say something to Tom, as it is in the best interests of the patients.

39. (D)

This does not address the issue straightaway, and therefore puts the patients at risk of catching infections. Since patient safety is of paramount importance, this is a very inappropriate response, even though it is a local solution.

40. (A)

This is an ideal solution, as it is local and addresses the problem immediately and discreetly.

41. (A)

This is a very appropriate response, as Emmanuel may need some support if the patient has said anything to make him feel uncomfortable. This will also inform Simone's decision as to whether to take over the patient's care.

42. (D)

This is a very inappropriate response, as there is no indication from what Emmanuel has said that he has behaved inappropriately towards the patient. Approaching the patient in this manner implies that Emmanuel may have done something wrong, which is not at all appropriate for Simone to do.

43. (B)

This response is appropriate, and Simone would be correct to remind Emmanuel of his duty to treat all patients, even when their beliefs differ from his own. However, this response is not ideal, as Emmanuel does seem unsettled by this patient; a more appropriate response would allow Simone to assess whether Emmanuel requires any support from her, and inform a decision as to whether to take over the care of this patient.

44. (B)

This is appropriate, as Esme would likely be endangering herself if she tried to drive to the hospital whilst feeling dizzy. However, it is not an ideal response, as it does not supply alternative sources of help for the junior colleague.

45. (D)

This option would ensure that Esme gets to the hospital safely without the risk of causing an accident. However, if she is too unwell to drive for even 5 minutes, then Esme should realise that she will not be able to give effective assistance to a patient in her condition. Reporting to the hospital to see patients in her current condition would thus be highly inappropriate.

46. (D)

This would not be appropriate as Esme is the consultant on call. If she does not feel able to complete her duties, then she should aim to find alternative cover, instead of leaving this to her junior colleague, who may well be busy with the unwell patient.

47. (A)

This is the best response to the problem. It allows Esme to take responsibility for finding appropriate cover when she is unable to fulfil her duties.

48. (D)

It would be highly inappropriate for Esme to endanger herself and other road users in this way.

49. (D)

This response is very inappropriate, as Luke does not actually know that the treatment is new; further-more, telling the patient that he does not know about the treatment will undermine patient confidence in the medical profession.

50. (A)

This is a very appropriate thing to do, as it maintains patient confidence in the profession and continuity of patient care, while also allowing Luke to take some time to look into the treatment and ensure he can provide the patient with the information requested.

51. (C)

This response is factually correct; however, it is inappropriate, as the fact that the prescribing doctor is away (and that Luke is unaware of the treatment) should not impact on patient care. However, this response is not awful, as it gives Luke an opening to provide the patient with the requested information.

52. (D)

Regardless of the reason that Rob is leaving, it is wrong to leave Jitesh to do his work for him, especially as Jitesh is only a medical student and is not being paid for his work.

53. (D)

Although Jitesh is doing tasks that are expected of him by his medical school, he is not there to replace the junior doctors. He is not qualified to do so, and he should not be doing the doctor's job for him.

54. (A)

This is very important, since Rob is not acting within the rules of the hospital trust where he works, which should be obeyed as part of his work contract with the hospital.

55. (B)

This is important, since this is the time when the ward is in most need of a junior doctor and by not being there Rob is putting his patients at risk. However, this is not of highest important to Jitesh in deciding how to respond because Rob should be there on the ward anyway, whether it is the busiest time or not.

56. (B)

This is an important factor to consider, as if there is a suitably private location for Lauren to change clothes, then her behaviour in the supply cupboard is highly unusual and must be addressed as such.

57. (D)

Nima's religious beliefs are entirely irrelevant to her response to Lauren's behaviour.

58. (A)

This is a very important factor, as it suggests that Lauren is not changing clothes, but undressing in the supply cupboard for some other reason, which must be addressed urgently.

59. (A)

This is extremely important, as it would mean that Lauren is lying about her reason for undressing in the supply cupboard, and thus it would be all the more urgent for Nima to address this with her.

60. (B)

This is an important factor, as it would indicate some other factor—such as an intoxicant or a psychiatric condition—that could play a role in Lauren's bizarre behaviour.

61. (D)

This is unimportant—he may have excellent hearing with his aids, or he may be able to lip read. Even if the elderly man cannot hear the junior doctors, it would be important to challenge the doctors to ensure that their behaviour is not repeated in front of an audience who can hear every word.

62. (C)

This mitigates the behaviour of the doctors slightly, but is mostly unimportant as the patient may be recognisable from other details. In addition, the public would not like to think of their own personal details being discussed in such a forum, even if they were not specifically mentioned by name.

63. (D)

This should not outweigh Abiola's responsibility to protect patient confidentiality and the public's opinion of the hospital and its staff. It is thus entirely unimportant.

64. (D)

This is unimportant, as the principles of medical professionalism and patient confidentiality must apply in all circumstances, regardless of whether the patient is known to others.

65. (A)

This is an important factor, as the tutor will expect Violet to behave professionally and notify him of the reason for her absence before the tutor group meets. If she has a phone number where she can reach the tutor, then she can be sure of having an opportunity to explain the situation with her grandmother, and make arrangements for making up anything she misses in the tutor group.

66. (C)

This factor is of minor importance, since Violet should only ask Uma to explain her absence as a last resort. She would do better to email or phone the tutor before the tutor group meets, so that she can explain her absence herself.

67. (A)

This is an important consideration, as if she will be able to email the tutor from the train, then she can proceed immediately to the train station and get to her grandmother as quickly as possible.

68. (A)

The fact that the medical school has made it clear that the students are expected to be presentable when on the wards is very important, as these are the rules that the students must obey. It reflects badly on the medical school and also on the hospital if the students are not smartly presented.

69. (D)

This is not at all important, as Adam needs to maintain a professional appearance in hospital, no matter what his situation is at home. It will reflect poorly on him, the hospital and the medical school if he appears scruffy and not smartly dressed.

70. (D)

This is not important, as you can still make yourself look presentable and not scruffy without spending money. If Adam was having financial difficulties that meant that he could not afford to buy suitable smart clothes for the wards, then he could approach his university for a hardship grant. Maintaining a professional appearance is important to help gain the respect and trust of patients.

71. (A)

The fact that Adam has signed an agreement means that he has no excuse for not knowing the rules and what is expected of him whilst in hospital. He has also agreed to follow those rules, especially if it is only his first week on the wards.

Chapter 8 Kaplan UKCAT Mock Test Explanations

Verbal Reasoning

1. (B)

A quick glance at the passage reveals that nearly all of it deals with the period prior to 2012, so scan for a keyword from each answer choice. The keyword 'BBC' appears towards the end of the final paragraph, which explains that Suu Kyi was unable to come to London to give lectures for the BBC in 2011, so these were recorded secretly in Myanmar, and her involvement was not announced until the BBC producers had safely left the country. Thus, (A) is incorrect, and (B) is a valid inference, as the BBC producers who visited in 2011 must have been in some danger if their participation could not be disclosed until they had 'safely' left the country. (B) is the correct answer.

2. (D)

This is a negative question, asking for something that cannot be true, so the correct answer will contradict the passage. The second paragraph mentions in brackets that the junta re-named Burma as Myanmar, so (A) is true and therefore incorrect. The final sentence states that Suu Kyi was elected to parliament in Myanmar in 2012, so (B) is also true, and also incorrect. The first sentence of the final paragraph says that Suu Kyi never became prime minister, so (C) is likewise true and incorrect. That same sentence clarifies that the Myanmar junta was dissolved in 2011, so Myanmar is not ruled by a junta. (D) is false, and thus the correct answer.

3. (B)

The keywords 'Nobel Peace Prize' appear in the final paragraph. Suu Kyi won the Nobel Peace Prize in 1991, but could not travel to Oslo to accept her award; she later went to Oslo to give her Nobel acceptance speech in 2012. Thus, (A) is incorrect—as Suu Kyi won, despite not being able to travel to Oslo in 1991—and (B) must be correct, as she won without being able to collect the award in person. If you were not sure about this, you could eliminate (C) as Suu Kyi was not a head of state or prime minister when she won the prize, and you could eliminate (D) as the other Nobel Prizes are not mentioned in the passage.

4. (A)

Military intervention in Burma in 1990 is mentioned midway through the passage; the military junta placed Suu Kyi under house arrest in 1989 and banned her involvement in the 1990 elections, so that she never became prime minister, despite her party winning 82% of the seats in Burma's parliament. Thus, it is correct to infer that the results of elections were not fulfilled; the answer is (A).

5. (C)

No references to 'most people in Hiddlesfield', or other numerical references to the support for or opposition against the planned supermarket, appear in the passage. The passage does mention a few individual opponents of the supermarket, such as the fishmonger and butcher; there's also the example of the county councillor who spoke in favour of the supermarket in the neighbouring village. None of this gives a basis to say whether or not a majority of people in Hiddlesfield oppose the supermarket, so the answer is Can't tell.

6. (A)

The keywords 'shops to close' lead to the second paragraph, and the example of the new supermarket in Aldersham, where half of the shops in the high street closed within six months of the supermarket's opening. This example from the passage involves a new supermarket causing some shops to close, so the statement is true.

7. (B)

The butcher is mentioned in the final paragraph, which states that she spoke forcefully against the supermarket. On this point, the statement contradicts the passage; the statement is therefore false.

8. (C)

The second paragraph includes a discussion of the new supermarket in Aldersham: the fishmonger uses it as an example of the damage caused to local shops by a new national supermarket; the county councillor suggests instead that the supermarket was a net positive for the village, in terms of new jobs and products. The passage does not state that one of these viewpoints is preferable to the other, and there is not enough information in the passage to decide whether or not the Aldersham supermarket was a success. The answer is (C).

9. (D)

This is a negative question, asking for something that must be false, so the correct answer will contradict the passage. The passage mentions that the Royal Court Theatre is a subsidised theatre in London, so (A) is true and thus incorrect. (B) is worded oddly and a bit hard to find in the passage, but it is supported by the detail in the final sentence of the second paragraph, which says that ticket sales represent a majority of revenue at UK theatres, even in the subsidised sector; (B) is thus true and incorrect. The passage gives examples of subsidised productions such as *Jerusalem* and *Clybourne Park* transferring to the West End, so (C) is also true and incorrect. (D) must therefore be the correct answer, and the details in the second paragraph reveal that the maximum figure for Lottery funding is 35%.

10. (C)

The keyword 'Broadway' appears in the passage's next to last sentence, which states that British plays that started at subsidised theatres and continue to play in the West End are a hit with critics and audiences on Broadway. *Jerusalem* started at the Royal Court Theatre and *War Horse* began at the National Theatre, so neither (A) nor (B) can be correct. (C) must be true, as both examples played in the West End. If you were not sure, you could check (D), which is not supported, as it is not clear that *Jerusalem* involved war or animals.

11. (A)

The keywords 'West End audiences' lead to the final sentence of the first paragraph; West End audiences in 2010 were down slightly from the total for 2009. The correct answer is (A).

12. (A)

The final paragraph begins with the claim that theatres would rightly argue that theatre involves a collective effort by artists with diverse skills, and could not succeed without all these various talents. (A) paraphrases this idea, so it is correct.

13. (A)

The keyword 'Durham' appears in the second paragraph, which states that students at Durham no longer had to pass a religious test for admissions after the 1871 Universities Test Act. From this information, you can infer that students at Durham did have to pass a religious admissions test before 1871; this statement is therefore supported by the passage. The answer is (A).

14. (B)

The keyword 'smallest' leads to the first paragraph, which states that Mansfield is Oxford's smallest college, except for Harris Manchester. This statement contradicts the passage, so it is false.

15. (C)

The keyword 'Chapel' occurs in the final paragraph, which explains that the Mansfield College Chapel continues to perform services and employ chaplains in the Nonconformist tradition. None of this indicates whether or not the chapel has been consecrated, so the answer is (C).

16. (B)

The keywords 'Oliver Cromwell' and '1662 dissenters' appear in the same sentence of the final paragraph. However, the first part of this sentence states that Cromwell died in 1658, four years before the dissenters separated from the Church of England. The answer is (B).

17. (C)

The author would least likely agree with the answer that contradicts the passage; any answer that is supported by the passage will be incorrect. The first sentence of the second paragraph states the author's opinion that the problem of water usage is much bigger than the current conservation efforts in the UK, which are detailed in the first paragraph. Thus, the author would agree with (A) and (D), and would disagree with (C). (C) is therefore correct.

18. (A)

The keywords 'England and Wales' appear in the passage's second sentence; the next sentence says that most water used daily by people in England and Wales is used in washing and toilet flushing. The correct answer is (A).

19. (C)

Examples of embedded water are given in the second paragraph. These include a pint of beer, a cup of coffee and a cotton T-shirt; there is also a mention of water used to grow crops that are exported to developed nations. There is, however, no example of livestock; the answer is (C).

20. (B)

The keywords 'a half-century ago' lead to the third sentence of the first paragraph; water use has increased by 50% in the last 50 years. Since there are no exact figures, it might be easier to think through the logic here algebraically. Call the water usage 50 years ago x. This amount increased by 50%, or $0.5x$, so that current water usage is $x + 0.5x = 1.5x$. Thus, water use 50 years ago was two-thirds of current levels. Answer (B) is correct.

21. (A)

The keywords 'non-professional players' lead to the end of the passage, where the final sentence explains that amateur players will often play a table tennis game under the old rules, either due to nostalgia or because they are unaware that the rules have changed. Answer (A) corresponds precisely with the second of these reasons, so it is correct.

22. (C)

Numbers make for great keywords, and scanning for 11 and 10 leads to the first sentence of the second paragraph, which explains that a player wins a game by scoring 11 points under ITTF rules, unless both are tied on 10, in which case a win requires a 2-point lead. Thus, a game could not be won by a score of 11–10 or 12–11, as, once both players have reached 10 points, the winner must have a margin of 2. The correct answer is (C).

23. (D)

This question asks for something that must be false, so the correct answer must contradict the passage regarding the Chinese National Team. The Chinese players are mentioned in the fourth sentence of the passage; they unsuccessfully challenged an increase in the diameter of table tennis balls, as the larger balls had less speed and spin, which were essential to the Chinese playing style. Thus, the first three answers are supported by the passage, and thus are incorrect; (D) contradicts the passage, and is correct.

24. (C)

The colours of stars on ITTF-sanctioned table tennis balls are indicated in the first paragraph. Stars may be black or blue, and may also include a second colour: red, green or purple. Orange is not mentioned as a possible colour for the stars, but rather as a possible colour of the ball itself; (C) is therefore the correct answer.

25. (A)

Scan for 'Second Empire', which is included in the title of Zola's cycle of novels set during that time period. The first paragraph does not specify the years of the Second Empire; however, the final paragraph indicates that Zola's cycle of novels were set in Paris from 1852 to 1870. Thus, it is safe to infer that the Second Empire took place during these years and therefore during the nineteenth century. The statement is true.

26. (A)

Scan for the keywords 'Zola' and 'naturalist'; these appear together in the last sentence of the first paragraph, which states that Zola's cycle of novels established his reputation as a pre-eminent proponent of the literary movement of naturalism. This statement is a close paraphrase of this detail from the passage, and is therefore true.

27. (C)

The keyword 'Paris' is found in brackets, midway through the final paragraph, indicating that Zola's novels in the cycle *Les Rougon-Macquart* are set in Paris. However, the passage does not clarify whether the novels in this cycle are the only novels that Zola wrote. If they are, the statement is true; if they are not, then the existence of any other novel he wrote that was not set in Paris would make it false. Since it is impossible to tell from the passage whether Zola wrote novels beyond this cycle, the answer is (C).

28. (B)

The keyword 'Balzac' appears in the first paragraph; the second sentence contrasts *La Comedie Humaine*, Balzac's cycle of novels, with Zola's cycle, which was to focus on a single family. Thus, it is safe to infer that Balzac's cycle involved more than one family. However, the passage does not indicate the exact number of novels in Balzac's cycle. The final sentence of the passage mentions that *La Comedie Humaine* included more than 90 works, some of which were novels, and represented the only cycle of novels that Balzac wrote. Thus, it is safe to infer from the passage that Balzac did not write a cycle of 20 novels; this statement says otherwise, so it is false.

29. (C)

The keywords 'full access to all levels of education' appear in the second paragraph, which states that women did not achieve this access in the UK until the late 1980s. The correct answer is (C).

30. (D)

This question is somewhat vaguely worded, but it's asking for something that the author would agree with. Scan for keywords from each answer, and eliminate those that are not supported by the passage. In the second paragraph, the author cites research that students who are struggling most when they start a single-sex school are most likely to benefit; (A) contradicts this point, so it is incorrect. The second paragraph lists several benefits to women students at single-sex schools, so (B) is incorrect. The final paragraph includes information that suggests that socioeconomic factors are tied to student performance in school. Hence, the author does not seem open to (C), and (D) is supported by the passage and thus correct.

31. (D)

This question asks for something that must be false, so the correct answer must contradict the passage. Scan for details about men outnumbering women in the UK, and you will find the information in the second paragraph that women outnumber men in higher education in the UK. Thus, there cannot be more men than women among UK university students. (D) is the correct answer.

32. (B)

The keywords 'at their peak' and 'secondary schools' lead to the first paragraph, where it is explained that there was a historical UK high of about 2,500 all-women's secondary schools in the 1960s. The answer is therefore (B).

33. (D)

Scanning for the keywords 'world's food supply' lead to the first paragraph, where the final sentence states that more than four-fifths of the world's food crops that require pollination are pollinated by honey bees. Answer (D) is a very close paraphrase of this detail from the passage, and is therefore correct. Hopefully, you weren't tempted by wrong answer (A), which is broader than the passage; there's no way to know from the passage whether most of the world's crops—which would include cotton, tobacco and other crops not grown for food—depend on bees for pollination.

34. (C)

This question asks about the writer's opinion on the most sufficient action to prevent further colonies of bees from collapsing; thus, scan for keywords related to further collapse and any that indicate the writer's opinion on that matter. The relevant details come near the end of the final paragraph: the writer says that any pesticides that might make bees more vulnerable to infection should be studied, and that those found to make bees more susceptible to IIV or Nosema infection should have their use curtailed. The answer that matches this detail from the passage is (C), as only (C) addresses the writer's proposal to ban pesticides that might make bees more vulnerable to IIV or Nosema infection.

35. (B)

The keywords 'IIV' and 'sole cause' lead to the second paragraph; the fourth sentence states that IIVs are found in 100% of collapsed hives in a study of CCD, but that IIVs are often found in strong colonies; as such, IIVs alone cannot be the cause of CCD. Answer (B) matches this detail from the passage, so it is correct.

36. (B)

The keywords 'paired infections' lead to the second paragraph, which explains the reason why scientists believe that hives infected with both IIVs and Nosema are likely to collapse. Since the study showed that both infections together correlate with CCD, and either infection on its own was not responsible, the answer that calls the study's finding about paired infections into question will likely suggest that something other than paired infections is responsible for CCD. The fact that most collapsed hives in the study came from areas where corn is the primary crop would not necessarily make it more likely that something other than paired infections led to CCD, as you cannot infer that the corn in these areas was treated with clothianidin; eliminate (A). If (B) is correct, and the worker bees had all disappeared or died due to IIV infection BEFORE Nosema infected the hive, then a paired infection cannot be responsible for CCD; scanning for worker bees leads to the first paragraph, where CCD is defined as the sudden disappearance of all the worker bees from a previously well-functioning and healthy hive. Thus, (B) would call the study's findings about paired infections causing CCD into question, as it would make it more likely that IIVs alone were responsible for CCD. The correct answer is (B). On Test Day, there would be no need to check the remaining answers—doing so would waste valuable time. For the purposes of revision, however, let's consider why (C) and (D) are wrong. The fact that most hives in the study came from areas where crops were not treated with clothianidin, as stated in (C), is not proof of anything, and would have no necessary effect on the results of the study. (D) suggests the possibility that Nosema infection led to IIV infection in the hives with both infections; however, this would have the effect of supporting the study's conclusion, not weakening it as this question asks you to do, because a hive with both infections would still have a paired infection. The answer is therefore (B).

37. (C)

The Imperial War Museum appears in the final paragraph, which states that the first Imperial War Museum was at Crystal Palace. The passage does not specify where the current Imperial War Museum is located, so there is no way of knowing based on the passage whether or not it is still at Crystal Palace. The answer is Can't tell.

38. (A)

Scanning the passage for information about the original Crystal Palace from the 1851 Great Exhibition should lead you to the second paragraph. This is also where you will find the passage's only mention of public toilets. The third sentence states that public toilets made their debut in the Crystal Palace during the Great Exhibition. This statement is true.

39. (A)

This statement may sound a bit unusual, but scanning for the keywords 'Hyde Park' leads to the first sentence of the second paragraph. The building destroyed in 1936, referred to in the previous paragraph sentence as Crystal Palace, was erected in Hyde Park for the Great Exhibition of 1851. This statement is supported by the passage, and is therefore true.

40. (B)

The fire that destroyed Crystal Palace is mentioned in both the first and the last paragraphs, but most of the key information is in the first paragraph. The final sentence gives us the details—the fire began as a small office fire and quickly expanded. Don't mix and match details. The final paragraph does state that the Crystal Palace was the site of regular fireworks shows in the early twentieth century, but these were not responsible for the fire. The answer is (B).

41. (D)

The UK banknotes dispensed from cash machines are discussed in both paragraphs, but the most relevant detail here comes at the end of the first paragraph. £50 notes are not dispensed at cash points, so this must be the banknote you are least likely to get from a UK cash machine. (D) is the correct answer.

42. (C)

The keywords 'two decades' do not appear in the passage, so check for other references to years and look for a gap of approximately 20 years. The third sentence of the second paragraph states that there were 63,000 cash machines on the UK network in 2010, and a subsequent sentence mentions that there were only 20,000 cash machines on this same network in 1990. Thus, the number of UK cash machines has more than trebled in 20 years. Answer (C) is correct.

43. (C)

The keywords '2010' and 'Bank of England' appear in the passage's first sentence. In 2010, the Bank of England planned to increase the number of £5 notes in circulation; at that time, there were 250 million £5 notes in circulation, and the start of the second paragraph specifies that the Bank planned to include 400 million more £5 notes by 2012. Percentage increase is difference divided by original, and 400 divided by 250 is 1.6, or 160%; the correct answer is (C).

44. (A)

The correct answer must contradict the passage. The lifespans of UK banknotes are discussed in the first paragraph. The £50 note lasts longer than any other British note, and the £5 note has the shortest lifespan; the lifespans of the £10 and £20 notes are not given. However, this is sufficient information to determine that (A) must be false, as the £10 note must last longer than the £5 note, which has the shortest lifespan. (A) is correct.

Quantitative Reasoning

1. (D)

To save time, avoid calculating the figures for all five regions by comparing data in the graph, using one figure as a benchmark against which you can assess the regions quickly. In this instance, the region with the highest average for all three years will be likely to have very high sales in all 3 years. Take 50,000 as the benchmark: two regions (Southwest and Wales) never sold 50,000 in a single year, but two regions (Southeast and Midlands) sold more than 50,000 in all three years. Thus, Southeast and Midlands are likely to have the highest averages, so check their figures a bit more closely. In fact, the first and second bars for Southeast are identical to the second and third bars for Midlands (55,000 and 60,000, respectively); the difference lies in the remaining bar, and the one for Midlands is higher than that for Southeast (70,000, as compared to 60,000). Thus, Midlands must have the highest average for the 3 years; the answer is therefore (D).

2. (A)

The region with the highest sales for 2004 is simply the region with the tallest rightmost bar in its set of 3 bars. Of these, the tallest is clearly that for Northwest, so the answer is (A).

3. (E)

To calculate the percentage growth in sales, use the sales figure for 2002 as the original, and divide the difference in sales from 2002 to 2004 by this original. When comparing percentages among all the answer choices, be sure to make a note of them on the noteboard; it may be easier to keep the notation in fraction form, as fractions can be faster to compare. Here are the notations for the percentages for the five regions, noted as fractions:

Northwest: $\dfrac{15}{55} = \dfrac{3}{11}$

Southwest: $\dfrac{10}{20} = \dfrac{1}{2}$

Southeast: Same sales total for 2002 and 2004, so no percentage growth.

Midlands: $\dfrac{5}{50} = \dfrac{1}{10}$

Wales: $\dfrac{15}{25} = \dfrac{3}{5}$

Of the four regions that had percentage growth in sales from 2002 to 2004, Wales recorded the greatest percentage growth (60%); the answer is therefore (E).

4. (C)

The graph shows that four regions had their highest sales in 2004; the region that didn't (Midlands) had its highest sales in 2000, when the sales for three of the regions were considerably lower—less than half their regional totals for 2004. Thus, 2004 must be the year with the highest sales. The sales for 2004 are $70,000 + 30,000 + 60,000 + 60,000 + 40,000 = 260,000$. The correct answer is (C).

5. (B)

The combined area of the director's office and conference room ($D + C$) has dimensions of 40 ft × 18 ft, so the combined area is $40 \times 18 = 720$ ft$^2 = D + C$. The area of the director's office equals the area of the conference room minus 108 square feet, or $D = C - 108$. Substitute this for the area of the director's office, and solve for the area of the conference room:

$C + C - 108 = 720$ ft^2

$2C - 108 = 720$ ft^2

$2C = 828$ ft^2

$C = 414$ ft^2

Thus, the area of the conference room is 414 ft^2, and the answer is (B).

6. (D)

Divide the conference room's area by its known dimension (18 ft), which represents the wall shared with the director's office, to find its other dimension, representing the wall shared with the reception/front office room: 414 ft$^2 \div 18$ ft $= 23$ ft. The other dimension of the reception/front office room is the combined length of both the conference room and the reception/front office room (56 ft) minus the length of the conference room (18 ft): 56 ft – 18 ft = 38 ft. Multiply for the total area of the reception/front office room: 23 ft × 38 ft = 874 ft². The correct answer is (D).

7. (E)

According to the bulleted info, the reception area is 35% of the combined reception/front office room, or 0.35 × 874 ft² = 306 ft². However, the same bulleted info states that the diagram of the offices is not to scale, and thus it is impossible to approximate or otherwise calculate any of the dimensions of the reception area, which is shaded in the diagram. Both answers (A) and (B) would have an area of 306 ft², and there is no way of determining whether one of these is correct, or whether the dimensions are a third option not listed in the answers. For these reasons, the answer is (E).

8. (A)

First, calculate the total area to be carpeted. The combined area of the director's office and conference room is 18 ft × 40 ft = 720 ft². The area of the front office, not including the reception area, is 65% of the combined reception/front office area: 0.65 × 874 ft² = 568.1 ft². Add these for the total area to be carpeted: 720 ft² + 568.1 ft² = 1,288.1 ft². Next, multiply by the cost of carpeting per sq ft for the total cost: 1,288.1 ft² × £2.99/ft² = £3,851.42. The answer is (A).

9. (E)

A quick glance at the table reveals that Joel scored the highest in Science, with a result of 96 out of 100. The correct answer is (E).

10. (C)

On questions like this, try to answer by comparing the data in the table, rather than making any calculations, which could be very time-consuming. The first step is to see if anyone scored the highest in more than one subject. The only student who did so was Emily. She scored the highest mark in English, Maths and French, and the second highest mark in Science. The only student who scored higher than her is Joel, but his result in Maths is the lowest of all six friends, and he is in the bottom half in the results for English. Thus, it is clear from looking at the data that Emily scored the best across all subjects, out of all her friends. The answer is therefore (C).

11. (D)

Percentage change equals difference divided by original. The difference between David's old score and his new score from his resit is 36 – 4 = 32; his old (original) score is 4. Plug these values into the formula and divide to solve: 32 ÷ 4 = 8, or 800%, answer (D).

12. (B)

To solve, add up the Science scores for all 6 friends and divide by 6, the number of friends. The sum of all 6 scores is 84 + 78 + 54 + 47 + 89 + 96 = 450. The mean score of the six friends is 450 ÷ 6 = 75. Answer (B) is correct.

13. (B)

The information needed to answer is found in the graph, which gives a figure of 2.6 for Retail in 2010. The figures on the bars represent millions of pounds, so 2.6 equals a value of £2.6 million. Answer (B) is correct.

14. (C)

Again, find the relevant information in the graph, which gives a figure of 1.7 for Leisure in 2011. This is the equivalent of £1,700,000, so the correct answer is (C).

15. (D)

The Commercial sector made £2.4 million in profit in 2009, which increased to £3.2 million in profit in 2010. The difference is £3,200,000 – £2,400,000 = £800,000. Use the percentage change formula (difference ÷ original) to solve: 800,000 ÷ 2,400,000 = 0.333, or 33.3%. The answer is therefore (D).

16. (C)

To find the total 2010 profits of all the different business sectors, add up the relevant figures from the graph: 1.6 + 2.6 + 3.2 + 2.2 = 9.6 million. The correct answer is (C).

17. (E)

The information in the table and just below it reveals that the module that most students picked as their favourite is pharmacology, which is therefore the most preferred subject based on the survey. The correct answer is (E).

18. (D)

The three most popular modules are pharmacology, genetics and immunology. Add these up for the first figure for the proportion: 81 + 68 + 67 = 216. The information above the table indicates that 336 students completed the survey. Therefore, the proportion of students who picked the three most popular modules is simply 216:336. This simplifies to 9:14, answer (D).

19. (A)

The bulleted information below the table indicates that two students preferred physiology. Since 336 students took part in the survey, the percentage of students who preferred physiology as a module is 2 ÷ 336 = 0.00595, or 0.595%. This rounds up to 1%, so answer (A) is correct.

20. (E)

The bulleted information below the table explains that five modules not listed were chosen as favourite by a single student. Thus, five modules were each selected by the fewest students, but the names of these modules are not given in the data. For this reason, the answer is (E).

21. (D)

The question provides Christos's speed (45 mph) and time (1 hour, 12 minutes), and asks you to find Christos's distance, so use the speed formula: Distance = Speed × Time. Since the speed is in mph, convert the time into hours: 1 hour, 12 minutes = 72 minutes = 72/60 hours = 1.2 hours. Use this figure to calculate his distance: Distance = 45 mph × 1.2 hours = 54 miles. Answer (D) is correct.

22. (C)

Use the speed formula to solve for Vasilis's speed: Speed = Distance ÷ Time. The distance is 16 miles more than Christos's, or 54 + 16 = 70 miles. The time is 75 minutes = 75/60 = 1.25 hours. Calculate using the speed formula: Speed = 70 miles ÷ 1.25 hours = 56 mph. The answer is (C).

23. (A)

The previous question indicates that Vasilis travels 16 miles further than Christos. This question does not mention the top speed of the jet skis, but this speed is given in the information above the set as 60 mph. Since Christos would travel a mile a minute at top speed, he would need 16 minutes to travel the 16 miles needed to catch up to Vasilis. The answer is therefore (A).

24. (B)

This question requires the percentage change formula: Percentage Change = Difference ÷ Original. The original time is 75 minutes, and the new time is 2 hours, or 120 minutes. The difference is therefore 120 – 75 = 45 minutes. Divide to find the percentage change: 45 ÷ 75 = 0.6, or 60%. The correct answer is (B).

25. (C)

To find the cost of lawn turf for the entire circular garden, find the area of the garden and then multiply by the cost of lawn turf. The garden is a circle, so use the equation $A = \pi r^2$. The radius is 5 metres, so $A = \pi(5)^2 = 3.14 \times 25 = 78.5$ m². Lawn turf costs £2 per m², so multiply to find the cost of lawn turf for the circular garden: 78.5 m² × £2/m² = £157. The correct answer is (C).

26. (B)

This question requires the same approach as the previous one, so simply multiply the area of the circular garden by the cost of paving slabs, which is £6 per m²: 78.5 m² × £6/m² = £471. The answer is therefore (B).

27. (C)

Work on the previous questions gave the area of the circular garden (78.5 m²) and the cost of paving slabs for the garden (£471). The labour cost for installing paving slabs is £2 per m², which is the same as the charge for lawn turf, so the labour cost is the same as the answer to the first question: £157. Subtract the cost of the paving slabs and the labour from the budget figure of £750 to find how much Mr Johnston will have left over: £750 – £471 – £157 = £122. The answer is (C).

28. (E)

To solve, subtract the area of the fountain from the area of the entire garden (78.5 m²). The fountain has a diameter of 2 m, which means it has a radius of 1 m. Use the area formula to solve for the fountain's area: $A = \pi(1)^2 = 3.14 \times 1 = 3.14$ m². Subtract the area of the fountain from the area of the entire garden to find the area that is not covered by the fountain: 78.5 m² – 3.14 m² = 75.36 m². The correct answer is (E).

29. (C)

The price of gold in dollars per ounce is indicated by the lines on the left-hand side of the graph. The price of gold in 2007 is just below the line for $900 per ounce, which is equivalent to a value of $890 per ounce. The correct answer is (C).

30. (E)

The scale of the labels for gold and silver prices make this question a lot more straightforward than it might initially seem. Since the labels for the price of gold increase by $100 for each line, those for silver increase by only $2 for each dash, and both start at $0 at the bottom of the graph, the year with the greatest difference in price per ounce between gold and silver will simply be the year with the greatest price per ounce for gold. In 2010, gold was approximately $1150 per ounce—a few hundred dollars above its price per ounce in the next highest year, and well above the price of silver in any year. The answer is therefore (E).

31. (B)

To find the percentage increase in the price of silver per ounce, use the percentage change formula: Percentage Change = Difference ÷ Original. The price of silver was approximately $5 per ounce in 2000 and $17 per ounce in 2010, for a difference of $12. Calculate the percentage change: 12 ÷ 5 = 2.4, or 240%. Answer (B) is correct.

32. (D)

Gold was $1150 per ounce in 2010, so 100 ounces of gold would have a value of 100 × $1150 = $115,000. Silver was $17 per ounce in 2010, so divide to find the ounces of silver you could buy with this value: $115,000 ÷ $17 per ounce = 6,765 ounces, answer (D).

33. (B)

To solve, use the speed formula: Speed = Distance ÷ Time. Mohsin's distance is 42 km and his time is 3 hours, 25 minutes. Divide the minutes by 60 to convert into hours: 25 ÷ 60 = 0.417 hours; his total time is thus 3.417 hours. Plug these values into the speed formula, and divide to solve: Speed = 42 km ÷ 3.417 h = 12.29 km/h. The correct answer is (B).

34. (C)

The previous answer gives Mohsin's average speed for his fastest time as 12.3 km/h. 21 km is half the total distance, and travelling this distance at 13 km/h, which is 0.7 km/h faster than his previous fastest time, means that he could run 0.7 km/h slower than his fastest speed in the second half of the marathon and still match his fastest time. 12.3 km/h – 0.7 km/h = 11.6 km/h, so any speed faster than this would result in a faster time than Mohsin's previous record. The question asks the minimum average speed to achieve a new fastest time, so the minimum is the answer that is only slightly more than 11.6 km/h. Thus, answer (C) is correct.

35. (A)

Use the speed formula to solve for distance: Distance = Speed × Time. Mohsin's speed was 12 km/h and his total time was 3.75 hours, so plug these values in to solve for his new distance: 12 km/h × 3.75 h = 45 km. The correct answer is (A).

36. (D)

Use the speed formula to solve for Mohsin's new speed: Speed = Distance ÷ Time. However, the new speed is based on a time that is 5% less than 3 hours, 15 minutes, or 3.25 hours. The quickest way to find the quicker time is to find 95% of 3.25 hours: 0.95×3.25 h = 3.0875 h. Plug this value, and the distance of the marathon (42 km), into the speed formula to solve: 42 km ÷ 3.0875 h = 13.6 km/h. The answer is (D).

Abstract Reasoning

1. (C)

This pattern involves arrangement. In Set A, the arrows are arranged so they point at the top or bottom of the boxes. In Set B, the arrows are arranged so they point at the left or right of the boxes. The black arrows in this test shape point at the top and bottom, which fits the pattern for Set A. However, the white arrows point at the left and right, which fits the pattern for Set B. Since the test shape fits into both sets, it belongs to neither.

2. (B)

The arrows in this test shape point to the left and right, so the answer is (B).

3. (C)

The arrows here point at all four sides of the box, so it belongs to neither set. The answer is (C).

4. (A)

This test shape's arrows point at the top and bottom of the box, so the test shape fits into Set A.

5. (C)

The double-headed arrow in this test shape points at the lower left and lower right corners of the box. Since the arrows don't point at the left and right sides of the box, and also don't point at the top and bottom sides of the box, the test shape fits into neither set.

6. (A)

All the boxes in Set A and B contain a shape made up of three line segments, so the difference in this shape must be key to both patterns. In Set A, all the angles in the three-segment shapes are obtuse (greater than 90°); in Set B, all the angles in the three-segment shapes are acute (less than 90°). The first test shape contains a three-segment shape with obtuse angles, so it belongs to Set A.

7. (B)

The three-segment line in this test shape contains only acute angles, so it belongs to Set B.

8. (C)

This line shape consists of only two segments, so it fits neither pattern.

9. (C)

This three-segment shape has an acute and an obtuse angle, so it belongs to neither set.

10. (B)

The three-segment line in this test shape has only acute angles, so it fits into Set B.

11. (B)

This pattern involves a feature of the shapes: whether their sides are curved or straight. In Set A, all the shapes have curved sides. In Set B, all the shapes have straight sides. The first test shape includes three stars, with entirely straight sides; this fits the pattern for Set B.

12. (B)

The three triangles in this test shape have straight sides, so it belongs to Set B.

13. (C)

The test shape contains a rainbow shape, consisting of two curved sides and two straight sides. The curved sides fit the pattern for Set A, and the straight sides fit the pattern for Set B. Since the test shape fits the pattern for both sets, it belongs exclusively to neither. The answer is therefore (C).

14. (A)

This test shape includes three crescent moon shapes, consisting entirely of curved sides. As such, the test shape fits the pattern for Set A.

15. (C)

The test shape contains a cross and a crescent moon. The cross has straight sides, so it fits the pattern for Set A. The crescent has curved sides, so it fits the pattern for Set B. Since the test shape fits the pattern for both sets, it belongs exclusively to neither. The answer is (C).

16. (C)

All the shapes in both sets are circles, and all are the same size. The only difference is in the colour—some are white, some are black—and the number. The boxes in Set A contain a total of 6, 8, 12, 14, 16 or 24 circles, with various circles shaded white or black; the total number of circles in Set A is always a multiple of 2. In Set B, the boxes contain a total of 7, 14 or 21 circles; again, the shading varies, but the total number of circles is always a multiple of 7. The first test shape contains 9 circles, so it fits the pattern for neither set.

17. (B)

This test shape looks very similar to the lower left box in Set B, and indeed contains the same number of circles, a total of 21. This is a multiple of 7, so it fits the pattern for Set B.

18. (B)

The test shape contains 7 circles, so it belongs to Set B.

19. (A)

This test shape includes 10 circles; since 10 is a multiple of 2, it fits the pattern for Set A.

20. (C)

The test shape contains 14 circles. Since 14 is a multiple of 2, it fits the pattern for Set A. However, 14 is also a multiple of 7, so it also fits the pattern for Set B. Since the test shape fits the pattern for both sets, it belongs exclusively to neither. The answer is therefore (C).

21. (C)

All the boxes in both sets feature four white shapes of approximately the same size, so the colour and number of the shapes cannot be the key to the patterns. Check each set to see whether any of the same types of shape appear in each box in the set. In Set A, each box includes a pentagon and a crescent, arranged diagonally opposite each other; in Set B, each box contains an octagon and a circle, arranged diagonally opposite each other. The first test shape includes an octagon diagonally opposite a pentagon, and a circle diagonally opposite a crescent. As such, the test shape fits the pattern for neither set. The answer is (C).

22. (C)

This test shape contains a pentagon diagonally opposite a crescent, so it fits the pattern for Set A. However, the test shape also includes an octagon diagonally opposite a circle, so it also fits the pattern for Set B. Since the test shape fits the patterns for both sets, it belongs exclusively to neither.

23. (A)

The test shape contains a pentagon diagonally opposite a crescent, and therefore belongs to Set A.

24. (C)

This test shape includes a triangle diagonally opposite a diamond, and a heart opposite a 'D' shape. As such, the test shape fits the pattern for neither set.

25. (B)

The test shape contains an octagon diagonally opposite a circle, so it fits the pattern for Set B. Since the crescent in the test shape is diagonally opposite a 'D' shape, the test shape does not fit the pattern for Set A. The answer is therefore (B).

26. (C)

This pattern involves type of shape. In Set A, each box contains a 4-pointed star; in Set B, each box contains a 5-pointed star. The other stars in each set are distractor shapes, and not part of the patterns. The first test shape includes a 4-pointed star, so it belongs to Set A. However, it also includes a 5-pointed star, so it also belongs to Set B. Since the test shape belongs to both sets, it fits exclusively into neither. The answer is therefore (C).

27. (A)

This test shape has a 4-pointed star, so it fits into Set A.

28. (A)

The 4-pointed star in this test shape means that it belongs to Set A.

29. (C)

The 4-pointed star in this test shape matches the pattern for Set A; the 5-pointed star matches the pattern for Set B. Because it can belong to both sets, the answer is (C). Hopefully, you weren't caught out by the fact that this test shape is identical to the lower right box in Set B, which includes a 4-pointed star as a distractor shape.

30. (B)

The test shape contains a 5-pointed star, and no 4-pointed star, so it belongs to Set B.

31. (B)

At first glance, the patterns in both sets appear to be very similar, as all boxes in both sets include two shapes, one large and one small, one black and one white. The type of shape does not appear to be relevant to the pattern, as some boxes have the same type of shape, but most have two shapes of different types. When the boxes appear to be very similar, check for an arrangement pattern—these can be subtle, and less obvious than patterns involving size and colour. In both patterns, the arrangement pattern is based on the colour of the shapes, irrespective of their size: in Set A, the white shape is arranged to the left of the black shape; in Set B, the black shape is arranged above the white shape. In the first test shape, the black oval is to the left of the white parallelogram; as a result, the test shape does not fit into Set A. The black shape is above the white shape, so the test shape fits into Set B.

32. (A)

In this test shape, the white arrow is to the left of the black triangle; the test shape fits the pattern for Set A. The arrow is also above the triangle, so the test shape does not fit the pattern for Set B. The answer is therefore (A).

33. (C)

The white shape is to the left of the black shape, so this test shape belongs to Set A. However, the black shape is also above the white shape, so the test shape also belongs to Set B. Since the test shape belongs to both sets, it belongs exclusively to neither. The answer is therefore (C).

34. (B)

This test shape includes a black cross above a white triangle, fitting the pattern for Set B. The black shape is to the left of the white shape, so the test shape does not also belong to Set A. Thus, the answer is (B).

35. (C)

This test shape includes a white parallelogram above, and to the left of, a black oval. However, both shapes are medium-sized, rather than the one large and one small required in both Set A and Set B. As a result, the test shape cannot fit into either set. The answer is (C).

36. (A)

All the boxes in both sets feature the same seven shapes, with the same shading. This is a great hint to look for an arrangement pattern, as the only difference can be in how the identical shapes are arranged. In Set A, the black donut is always positioned directly above the white cross; in Set B, the black square is always positioned directly above the white triangle. There is no other aspect of the pattern involving the arrangement of the other shapes. In the first test shape, the black donut is directly above the white cross; thus, the test shape belongs to Set A.

37. (C)

This test shape includes all seven shapes, and the black donut is directly above the white cross, which fits the pattern for Set A. However, the black square is directly above the white triangle as well, which fits the pattern for Set B. Since the test shape fits into both sets, it belongs exclusively to neither. The answer is therefore (C).

38. (A)

The test shape features the black donut above the white cross, so it belongs to Set A. The black square is not above the white triangle, so it cannot belong to Set B. The answer is (A).

39. (C)

This test shape includes the seven required shapes; however, the black donut is not above the white cross, and the black square is not above the white triangle. Thus, the test shape fits into neither set.

40. (B)

The test shape has its black square positioned above its white triangle, so it fits the pattern for Set B. Since the black donut is not positioned above the white cross, it does not fit the pattern for Set A. The answer is therefore (B).

41. (C)

Each box in Set A contains a triangle as a standalone shape, or as a shape formed by the intersection of other shapes. Each box in Set B contains a rectangle as a standalone shape, or as a shape formed by the intersection of other shapes. The first test shape contains a star, so there aren't any triangles or rectangles. As such, it fits the pattern for neither set.

42. (C)

The intersection of the arrows creates both a triangle and a rectangle. This test shape therefore fits both patterns, and so it belongs exclusively to neither. The answer is (C).

43. (B)

This test shape includes rectangles, so it fits the pattern for Set B.

44. (A)

This test shape contains only triangles, so it fits the pattern for Set A.

45. (B)

The three-dimensional box contains a rectangle as one of its sides, so it belongs to Set B.

46. (B)

All the boxes in both sets include an arrow, a large shape, a small shape and a medium-sized shape; only one of the shapes in each box is white, and the others are black. Since the boxes are so similar, check for an arrangement pattern. In Set A, the arrow points at the largest shape; in Set B, the arrow points at the white shape. In the first test shape, the arrow points at the white shape; since it is not also the largest shape, the answer is (B).

47. (C)

The arrow in this test shape points at the largest shape, which fits the pattern for Set A. However, the largest shape is also the white shape; thus, the test shape also fits the pattern for Set B. Since the test shape can belong to both sets, it fits exclusively into neither. The answer is (C).

48. (A)

The test shape contains an arrow pointing at the largest shape, which fits the pattern for Set A. The largest shape is black, so the test shape does not fit the pattern for Set B. Thus, the answer is (A).

49. (C)

This test shape includes an arrow pointing at the largest shape, which fits the pattern for Set A. However, the largest shape is also the white shape; the test shape thus also fits the pattern for Set B. Because it fits the pattern for both sets, the test shape belongs exclusively to neither set.

50. (C)

The arrow in this test shape is pointing at the medium-sized shape, not the largest, so it does not belong to Set A. The arrow is pointing at a black shape, so the test shape does not belong to Set B. The answer is therefore (C).

51. (D)

In the first progression, the pentagon—the large outer shape—switches places and sizes with the parallelogram—the smaller inner shape—but both retain their original colour; the final parallelogram has also been flipped, but the final pentagon hasn't. In the second progression, then, the large trapezium will become the smaller inner shape and retain its original orientation. Eliminate (A) and (C), which incorrectly flip the final trapezium. It's the final, large arrow that must be flipped from its original orientation, so (D) is correct.

52. (A)

It's quickest to start with the simplest part of the progression. In the first row of boxes, the bottom shapes are simplest. The two trapeziums switch positions from left to right, but retain their original colours. Thus, the white chevron must be on the left in the correct answer; eliminate (C) and (D). In the first boxes, the colour of the stars shifts by one position to the left, with the leftmost colour moving to the rightmost position; thus, the white circle—which is leftmost in the third box—will be in the rightmost position in the answer. (A) is therefore correct.

53. (B)

In the first progression, the circles move from the bottom to the top; there is one fewer circle, and the remaining circles become wider. Thus, the four hexagons in the bottom of the second progression must move to the top, with one fewer, and the remaining hexagons wider; eliminate (A) and (C). In the first progression, the diamonds at the top move to the bottom, there is one more, and they become shorter. Hence, there must be one more triangle in the bottom of the answer. (B) is correct.

54. (D)

In the first progression, each shape is replaced by a shape that has exactly half as many sides as the original. In the second progression, the two shapes at the left in the first box have eight sides each, so they must each be replaced by a shape with exactly four sides. Answer (D) is therefore correct.

55. (C)

In the first progression, the shape originally on the left moves to the right, and the shape that was on the right moves diagonally into the original position of the shape that was on the left. Thus, the heart must move to the right; eliminate (A) and (B). In the first progression, the black arrow—the inner shape that was originally on the left—flips vertically in the second box. Hence, the white chevron must flip vertically in the answer. (C) is therefore correct.

Decision Analysis

1. (E)

The literal translation is *moon(up), human, stop, head(journey)*. The first part of the message could mean night, as night is the time when the moon is up. Answers (A), (B) and (C) do not include a representation of up in combination with moon, so they cannot be correct. The third part of the message, stop, is correctly interpreted in (E). (D) incorrectly interprets this part of the message as 'go', which is the opposite of stop; opposite is F in the table, but is not found in the message, so eliminate (D). The answer is (E).

2. (B)

The literal translation is *opposite(them), air(journey), opposite(moon), big(journey), opposite(moon)*. Three of the answers interpret the first part of the message as 'we' or 'us'; eliminate (A), which omits this part of the message, and also (E), which omits opposite and instead interprets it as 'them'. It's not clear from the message and the code whether the opposite of moon could mean sun, planet or both; however, (D) interprets the final opposite(moon) as distant moon, which omits opposite, so eliminate (D). The remaining answers interpret the second part of the message as 'flew' and 'travel', but travel does not omit the concept of air, which is combined with journey in this part of the message. Eliminate (C); the answer is therefore (B).

3. (D)

The first part of the coded message is either 16, plant, or G16, one(plant). Plant is plural in the message, so one cannot be part of the correct answer; eliminate (A), (C) and (E). The second part of the coded message is either 14, fuel, or B14, negative(fuel). Since the message requires the negative, the correct answer is (D). **NB** This answer encodes 'aliens' as 4(F5), them(opposite(home)). This information could be useful on a later question.

4. (C)

The literal translation is *opposite(them), opposite(stop), home, plant(negative(grow))*. All the answers give the first part of the message as 'we'. The second part of the message is interpreted as 'went' or 'left' in three of the answers; eliminate (A), which omits opposite, and also (E), which omits this part of the message entirely. Two of the remaining answers give the third part of the message as 'house' or 'home'; (D) is very questionable, because 'Earth' would likely require further elements from the table. The final part of the message includes grow, but (B) and (D) omit grow, so they cannot be correct. The answer is (C).

5. (C)

The literal translation is *grow(human), air(tank), opposite(grow)(grow(fast))*. All the answers give possible interpretations of the first two parts of the message, so eliminate based on the final part of the message. The final part does not include negative, B; eliminate (E), which does include a negative. Grow(fast) could mean something like more quickly; eliminate (D), which incorrectly gives the opposite of fast, rather than grow(fast), and also (A) and (B), which omit this element entirely. The answer is therefore (C).

6. (A)

The answers give the first part of the message, new planet, as either K(F2), new(opposite(moon)), or F2, opposite(moon). Eliminate (D) and (E), which omit new. The remaining answers give the second part of the message, with plants, as 16, plant, J16, grow(plant), or JA16, grow(big)(plant). Plant is not modified in the message, so eliminate (B) and (C). The answer is (A).

7. (E)

The literal translation is *ship(big(burn)(fuel), big(fast)(journey(up))), beyond(today)*. All the answers interpret the final part of the message as 'in future' or 'tomorrow', which both logically fit the meaning of beyond today. The first half of the first part of the message, a ship that 'big burns' fuel, seems to mean rocket ship, as a rocket burns a lot of fuel. Eliminate (B), which separates ship and rocket into different parts of the message, and also (D), which does not include a representation of big(burn)(fuel). The second half of the first part of the message fits well with 'launch', which is quite literally a big, fast journey up. Eliminate (A), which omits fast, and also (C), which includes 'past the sun', as this would require further codes that are not in the message. The answer is therefore (E).

8. (A)

The literal translation is *opposite(moon), grow(cold, fast), negative, opposite(them)(human)*. All the answers interpret the first part of the message as planet or sun, and the second part as fast-freezing or quickly cooling. The third part of the message, negative, is omitted from (E), so it cannot be correct. The final part of the message includes opposite(them), which has been interpreted in previous correct answers as 'we', and also human. Eliminate (D), which does not include a representation of 'we' or 'us'. Of the remaining answers, (B) and (C) each include an element—live and stay, respectively—that would require a further code that is not in the message. (A) can be understood logically using only the codes in the message, so it is correct.

9. (C)

The answers give three possible ways to encode the first part of the message: A(AE11), big(big (beyond(today))); E11, beyond(today); or A(F11), big(opposite(today)). A previous answer interpreted beyond(today) as 'tomorrow', so something further is required for the message here; eliminate (B) and (D). The opposite of today could be tomorrow, but it could also be yesterday; eliminate (E). The only difference between the remaining answers is in the final part of the message: (A) gives this as 9(8), stop(burn), while (C) gives it as FJ, JC, opposite(grow), grow(cold). Stop(burn) could imply become cold, but would not suggest anything to do with the sun shrinking. Shrink is the opposite of grow, and grow cold is a good fit for become cold. The answer is therefore (C). **NB** The correct answer here encodes 'sun' as A1, big(star). This could be useful in answering other questions in this section.

10. (B)

The answers encode the first part of the message as 2D, moon(up), or G(2D), one(moon(up)). A previous correct answer interpreted 2D as 'at night', so a further code would be required for the concept of 'one night'; G(2D) is a good logical fit for this concept. Eliminate (A) and (D). There are a number of differences among the remaining answers, so eliminate on the basis of any of these. The final part of the message, us, is given as F4, opposite(them), in (B); this matches the encoding of 'we' and 'us' in the correct answers to previous questions. (C) and (E) only have 4, them, which cannot logically mean 'us'. Eliminate (C) and (E); the answer is (B).

11. (D)

The literal translation is *them(opposite(home)), negative(stop), ship(opposite(them)), burn(negative)*. All of the answers interpret the first part of the message as 'aliens', except for (E), which instead has the singular form, alien; since the message has 'them', aliens must be plural. Eliminate (E). The second part of the message combines negative and stop; eliminate (B), which omits negative, and (C), because 'allowed to escape' is not a good interpretation of negative(stop). The remaining answers both give the third part of the message as 'our ship'. (D) interprets the final part of the message as 'evil laser'; (A) interprets it as 'burned', which omits a representation of negative. Thus, the answer is (D).

12. (A)

The literal translation is *big(star), negative(special), grow(big)(grow(star), grow(big)(star), grow(moon), grow(opposite)(moon))*. All of the answers interpret the first part of the message as 'sun', which a previous correct answer gave as an acceptable meaning for big(star); eliminate (B), which instead has 'stars', as the code does not seem to use big to form a plural noun. The second part of the message combines negative and single into a single element; eliminate (C) and (E), which omit negative, and also (D), which omits single. The answer is therefore (A).

13. (B)

The literal translation is *head(human), stop(ship, journey), fix(journey, new(star))*. All of the answers give the first part of the message as 'captain', except for (E), which omits human and therefore cannot be correct. The second part of the message combines stop, ship and journey into a single element. Eliminate (A), (C) and (D), which omit a representation of journey in this part of the message. The correct answer is (B).

14. (C)

The literal translation is *big(opposite(give)(air), grow, love, stop(opposite(give)(air))), beyond(moon), opposite(easy)*. All of the answers interpret the first part of the message as 'life' or 'live', and the second part of the message as 'in space'. The final part of the message is the opposite of easy. Eliminate (A), as unusual is the opposite of common or normal, not of easy; also, eliminate (B) and (D), as 'not easy' would need to be encoded as negative(easy), B204. The only difference between the remaining answers is that

(E) includes 'your' and 'whole', but there are no codes in the message corresponding to these concepts. (C) includes only the elements in the message, and is a good logical fit for its meaning; thus, (C) is correct.

15. (E)

The first part of the message is encoded as 3(A106), human(big(money)), or 3(106), human(money). A rich man has a lot of money, so the first option is a better fit; eliminate (B) and (D). The second part of the message is the same in the remaining answers, but they give three different options for the third part of the message: A101, big(launch); 7D, journey(up); M101, special(launch). Since launch is now included in the table, the correct answer must include 101; eliminate (C). Special is a better fit for the concept of private, so the correct answer is (E).

16. (B)

The literal translation is *human(sail, ship), (search, negative(find)), orange(moon), fuel(opposite(stop))*. The first part of the message includes human; eliminate (C) and (D), which omit human and interpret it as 'space shuttle'. It is not clear whether the first part of the message can mean 'astronaut', as a human who sails a ship would be something like a captain or pilot. The second part of the message gives a stronger reason to eliminate the remaining wrong answers: (A) and (E) interpret the second part of the message as 'discovered', but this part of the message combines search and negative(find) into a single element. 'Discovered' would mean 'searched and found', and as such omits a representation of negative. Eliminate (A) and (E), and the answer is (B).

17. (A)

The literal translation is *army(beyond(moon)), stop(fight), new(opposite(big(army))), negative(find), army*. The first part of the message is interpreted as 'space army' in all the answers. The second part of the message does not include negative; eliminate (B), which incorrectly interprets it as 'did not stop fighting'. The remaining answers interpret the third part of the message as 'reinforcements' or 'new troops', both of which could fit logically with the coded message. The fourth part of the message includes negative; eliminate (D) and (E), which omit the negative in this part of the message. The final part of the message is army; eliminate (C), which incorrectly gives it as 'them', as them is 4 in the table but is not included in the message. The correct answer is (A).

18. (D)

The literal translation is *human(sail, star), give, grow(head, heart, opposite(one)), beyond(time), send(ship)*. All the answers interpret the first part of the message as astronaut, which makes logical sense, as an astronaut is quite literally a human who sails the stars. The second part of the message, give, is omitted from (A), which cannot be correct. The third part of the message combines head, heart and the opposite of one—perhaps meaning something like all—into a single element. (B) and (D) interpret this element as 'body'; eliminate (C) and (E), which interpret it overly broadly as 'everything', as this is not specific to the codes in the message. Both of the remaining answers interpret the fourth part of the message as 'future'. (B) interprets the final part of the message as 'sent the ship', and (D) interprets it as 'the mission', which could literally be sending of a ship. However, (B) also includes 'self' at the end of the message, and there is no code corresponding to this concept in the message. For this reason, (B) is not a good fit for the message, and the answer is (D).

19. (E)

The literal translation is *big(rock)(sail(beyond(space), special(time)), negative(opposite(launch)), home(opposite(moon))*. The first part of the message is very long, so it might be faster to start with the other parts of the message. The second part of the message is the opposite of launch, modified by negative. (A) and (E) both give this as 'fell', which could have a negative meaning as well as being the opposite of launching. Eliminate (B), (C) and (D), which omit opposite. (A) also includes down, which is the opposite of up, which are codes in the table that have appeared in other messages but not in this one. Thus, (A) cannot be correct; the answer is (E).

20. (C)

The literal translation is *negative(plant)(grow(human)), big(worry)*. This message includes two elements, and it might be easier to start with the second—compare it to the answer choices, and eliminate those that don't represent it as combining big and worry. Answers (A) and (B) omit a representation of big, and (D) and (E) include a negative with big(worry) that is not part of this element in the original message. Thus, (C) must be the correct answer.

21. (A)

The literal translation is *big(orange)(air), grow(different), human(head, hopeful)*. The first element could mean 'orange gas' or 'orange gas cloud', so it does not allow you to eliminate any answers. The second element could mean 'grow differently' or 'expand differently'; eliminate (B) and (E), which omit a representation of different with this element. (D) includes tank, which is 13 in the table but is not included in the message, so (D) must be wrong. The final element of the message is given in the two remaining answers as 'a person would expect' or 'you would hope'; (A) is the better fit for the message, and is therefore correct.

22. (E)

The first part of the message is encoded as G(F4), one(opposite(them)), or F4, opposite(them). Previous correct answers have used F4 to mean 'we' or 'us', and the singular form of 'we' is 'I'; eliminate (B) and (D). The second part of the message is either 109, scratch, or 108, search. Search fits the message, but scratch does not make sense; eliminate (A). The third part of both remaining answers start with AJ, big(grow). (C) combines 'big grow' with panic, love, sorrow and easy; (E) combines 'big grow' with human and them(opposite(home)), which was used correctly to mean 'aliens' in previous questions. Humans and aliens combined with 'big grow' could mean all beings, but the list of emotions and reactions in (C) would not fit logically with the message. The answer is therefore (E).

23. (B)

The literal translation is *time(opposite(up)), launch, give(opposite(them)), grow(worry, negative(panic))*. All the answers interpret the first part of the message as 'countdown'. (C) omits launch, the second part of the message, so it is incorrect. The third part of the message means something like 'give us'; eliminate (A), which mistakenly uses the singular form, and also (D), which includes them rather than the opposite of them. The final part of the message combines worry and negative panic into a single element. Eliminate (E), which separates 'worry' and 'don't panic' into different parts of the message. The correct answer is (B).

24. (C)

The literal translation is *big(journey), fix, grow(big)(opposite(love), sorrow, fight, opposite(hopeful)), opposite(beyond)(heart, opposite(fix))*. The first part of the message combines big and journey into a single element. Eliminate (A), which omits big, and (B), which includes space instead of big; previous questions have encoded space as E2, beyond(moon), but this is not part of the message here. Eliminate (D) as well, since time is 102 in the table but is not included in the message. Comparing the remaining answers, the most obvious difference is that (E) includes 'your' twice; it's not clear how to represent 'you' with the table of codes, but there are no codes in the message that could encode the concept of 'you' or 'your'. Eliminate (E); the answer is therefore (C).

25. (B)

The correct answer to a previous question encoded 'astronaut' as a human who sails the stars, or 3(107, 1); eliminate (D) and (E), which include ship rather than star. The remaining answers give three different ways to encode the concept of 'expand knowledge': J(FE10), grow(opposite(beyond(head))); J(A112), grow(big(learn)); or J10, grow(head). Big(learn) is the best fit for knowledge, and growing the 'big learn' could mean expanding knowledge. The correct answer is (B).

26. (C) and (D)

All of the answers appear in the message, so check to see which can be represented with the existing table of codes. Itch could be represented with scratch, 109, so eliminate (E). Ivy is a plant, 16, so eliminate (B). The opposite of fix, FH, would mean break or hurt; this could be combined with negative, or big negative, to represent the concept of poison. Eliminate (A). There is no way to encode skin or red, so answers (C) and (D) must be correct.

27. (A) and (D)

The message includes all five answers, so check to see which could be represented with the existing codes. Finish could be encoded as stop, 9; eliminate (B). A soldier is a single human in the army, or G3(105); eliminate (C). There is no way to encode change, blood or transfusion with the existing codes. However, if blood were added to the code as, say, 20, you could encode transfusion as L(K20), since a transfusion involves giving someone new blood. Eliminate (E); the answers are (A) and (D).

28. (A) and (B)

All the answers are in the message except command, but the message is a command, so (A) is likely to be correct. Check to see whether the other answers can be represented with the existing codes. Several previous questions have encoded space as beyond(moon), E2; eliminate (E). Rubbish could be encoded as waste, 17, and bin could be encoded as 17(13), waste(tank); eliminate (C) and (D). There is no clear way to encode drop using the table, so the correct answers are (A) and (B).

Situational Judgement

1. (C)

Telling a peer would allow Adam to leave without disrupting the class, so it is not an awful response. However, leaving the classroom without planning to catch up on what will be missed means Adam will miss part of his training. Thus, this response is inappropriate.

2. (C)

Walking out of the classroom is not an appropriate course of action if Adam is beginning to feel sick. He needs to inform someone, before simply leaving for what may appear to be no good reason. However, Adam does feel sick, so this response is not awful.

3. (D)

Whilst Adam clearly needs to ask for help from the medical school to overcome his anxieties, offering to read from books is a very inappropriate response, as anatomy and dissection classes are a compulsory part of the curriculum. This is also not a local solution; he should discuss his concerns with the tutor first.

4. (A)

Whilst this option is good in that it offers Hayley a chance to explain her actions, the wording is somewhat confrontational and may hinder a successful conversation about the problems that she may be having.

5. (D)

Being dishonest is an inappropriate course of action in any context. This option also demonstrates Adam would not be admitting his need for help, which may have further consequences for his training and for becoming a good doctor. This is therefore highly inappropriate.

6. (C)

This response is inappropriate, as Umar should be more sensitive in addressing Darryl's apparent problem with drink. Since Darryl does seem to have a rather serious drinking problem, this response is not awful, but it is also not likely to be effective at addressing the issues in the scenario.

7. (A)

This response is neutral and supportive, and is thus highly appropriate.

8. (A)

This response addresses one of the underlying issues: Darryl is not in a fit state to encounter patients at the hospital. As such, the response is very appropriate.

9. (D)

This is a highly inappropriate response, as it is not a local solution, and also because it is not likely that anonymous complaint that does not specify which doctor has a drinking problem would lead to any help for Darryl.

10. (A)

This is an immediate, discreet and local solution, and would remove the risk of Darryl encountering patients in his current state.

11. (A)

Darryl may require additional support as he gets his professional and personal life in order, so it would be very appropriate to encourage him to discuss matters with his consultant.

12. (D)

This is an extreme response, given that the message is not threatening or harmful in any way; thus, involving the police would be highly inappropriate. The police would only need to be involved if the patient persistently tries to contact Saba.

13. (C)

This is an inappropriate option, as it could come across as rude and might be awkward if the patient were to be re-admitted to her ward. However, it is not awful, since doctors should not socialise with patients. The better response would be to ignore the request, rather than denying it.

14. (D)

This is a very inappropriate response, as it is unprofessional for Saba to socialise with a patient. Accepting the request in order to explain why she cannot socialise would send the patient a mixed message, and would also begin a conversation on the social networking site, which could lead to serious professional consequences for Saba, despite her best intentions.

15. (A)

This would be a highly appropriate response, since it will not escalate the situation further, and it will ensure that Saba does not engage in any inappropriate social contact with a patient.

16. (C)

It is inappropriate for a doctor to speak to nurses in such a manner; however, the nurses are behaving unprofessionally, so this response is not awful.

17. (A)

This response allows Dr Davies to obtain the information required quickly and directly, and is therefore a very appropriate thing to do.

18. (C)

Clearing her throat will not ensure that the nurses notice her presence or stop their gossiping, so it is not an effective or appropriate response. However, there are no negative consequences from doing so, other than potentially having to wait a bit longer for help from the nurses—so it is not an awful response.

19. (A)

This response is quick and direct, and is thus highly appropriate.

20. (D)

Whilst it is right to tell Ben that he should not cheat next time, this does not resolve the issue that Ben has clearly acted highly inappropriately and dishonestly by cheating, which must be raised with the medical school, particularly as these actions impact on others—for example, Ben may have scored higher than students who did not cheat in the examination. Ben could also interpret Ian's comment as implying that it was okay to cheat this time, so this is a highly inappropriate response.

21. (A)

Whilst this would be a difficult action for Ian to pursue, it is a very appropriate response that deals with the situation immediately, discreetly and locally. No student under any circumstances should be allowed to cheat, and this response ensures that Ben must face the consequences of his actions.

22. (C)

This response is inappropriate, as it does not deal with the situation as swiftly as possible. However, it does deal with the situation, so it is not awful.

23. (A)

This response would allow Ian to determine whether Ben needed any help in dealing with his parents' divorce, and would allow him to support his friend appropriately. As such, it is very appropriate.

24. (D)

This may save Ian from a difficult conversation with his best friend; however, this response is neither immediate nor local. By the time the medical school investigates further, it will be hard to prove that Ben cheated. This means it is likely that Ben will not have to face consequences for having cheated, and that he will be able to maintain an unfair advantage over their fellow medical students. Thus, this is a highly inappropriate response.

25. (D)

There are a number of reasons that the patient is not responding to Arissa. Perhaps Arissa is not speaking loudly or clearly enough, or the patient may have trouble hearing, or may not speak English well or at all. The patient's name will not help in addressing the exact cause of the problem, as a patient with a foreign name could speak English well but could also have a hearing problem. Thus, this is a very inappropriate response.

26. (D)

The patient has not given consent for the treatment, so it would be highly unprofessional for Arissa to proceed with the treatment. This would be a highly inappropriate thing to do, and could result in serious professional consequences for Arissa.

27. (A)

It is always very appropriate for a doctor to seek advice from a senior colleague.

28. (D)

This is not a local solution to the problem, and Freddie should talk to Joanna herself first before risking damaging her reputation with their consultant. Thus, it is a highly inappropriate response.

29. (A)

This would be a very appropriate thing to do, since it would give them both equal opportunities to teach and to help complete the paperwork.

30. (D)

This is very inappropriate, since it is not the fault of the medical students that Joanna is not doing her share of the paperwork. The students are there to learn in a clinical setting.

31. (C)

This response is inappropriate, as it focuses on Freddie's preferences, rather than a fair and professional balance of their responsibilities. However, it is not awful, as it would open a discussion of the division of their responsibilities, which has been made based on Joanna's preferences.

32. (D)

Olubayo is right to be concerned that the power may go out again, and patient health and safety could be compromised if this were to happen once Olubayo starts treatment. However, this is a decision that must be taken by the dentist on behalf of the patient; asking whether the patient is comfortable with proceeding is therefore very inappropriate.

33. (A)

This is a very appropriate response, given that Olubayo cannot be assured of being able to complete the treatment without disruption due to the storm, which could place the patient's health at risk.

34. (A)

This is a highly appropriate thing to do, as many treatments at the dental surgery would require the use of electricity. Given that the back-up generator has already failed once today, proceeding with any treatment as another storm approaches would be reckless and unprofessional.

35. (D)

This is not going to help answer the patient's questions. Eoghan should offer to get someone else to come and talk to him instead. It is not the fault of the patient that the consultant is not there, and it would be very inappropriate for Eoghan not to provide a quick, local solution to this problem.

36. (A)

This is an ideal solution as it ensures the patient's questions will be answered, and does not undermine the consultant in any way by disclosing that she is on holiday.

37. (D)

This would be an inappropriate thing to do since Eoghan is only a medical student and is unlikely to be able to answer all of the patient's questions correctly or satisfactorily. Also, the patient has requested to speak to the consultant, so it would be appropriate to arrange for the patient to speak to a doctor.

38. (D)

This is very appropriate, as Eoghan can deal with the questions that he feels he can answer straightaway so that the patient does not have to wait for answers. By getting a doctor to come and talk to the patient as well, Eoghan would maintain confidence in the profession and continuity of care, and ensure that no incorrect information is given to the patient.

39. (A)

This is a highly appropriate response, as it is an open and neutral question, with no possible negative consequences for Alfie.

40. (A)

If Hannah wants to examine Alfie's injuries, then it would be highly appropriate to get consent from his carer before doing so.

41. (A)

This is a very appropriate thing to do, as it will help to calm Alfie and make it easier for Hannah to treat him.

42. (D)

It is not clear that Alfie has been abused, though his injuries are worrying and would justify further investigation by Hannah before making a report to children's services. The next step would be to examine the injuries, ideally after obtaining consent from Alfie's carer. Phoning in a report before checking the injuries would be highly inappropriate.

43. (A)

Whilst the circumstances of Nieve's ill health are not professional, this is an appropriate course of action in the present situation. In this way, the tutorial will go ahead for other students on time and Nieve will catch up on all that has been missed in her absence.

44. (B)

Attending the tutorial only is another appropriate, if not ideal, response, so that Nieve does not miss out on any of her training. It is appropriate for her to tell the team she is not feeling well enough to work with patients as not feeling well may impact on her behaviour and judgement and thus negatively impact on the care of patients who are the priority, though again, this is not ideal.

45. (D)

It is highly inappropriate for Nieve to ask Leila to lie on her behalf.

46. (D)

Asking Leila to lie, missing her teaching session and skipping her work on the ward are all highly inappropriate things for Nieve to do.

47. (D)

If Nieve is feeling nauseous, it is unlikely she will be able to concentrate fully during the tutorial or perform at her best on the ward, which could have a potentially very serious impact on patient care. Furthermore, not having cleaned is unprofessional and could negatively impact public confidence in students and the profession.

48. (D)

This is a very inappropriate thing to do, as the patient has given consent for his family to be informed of his condition, and it's likely that his niece has come to the hospital for this very purpose. The doctor should make some time to speak with her, even if to briefly explain that she must wait to speak with the consultant.

49. (D)

This response is very inappropriate, and it is also inaccurate, as the patient has given consent for his condition to be explained to his family.

50. (A)

This is a very appropriate thing to do, as it defers to the patient's wish to have the consultant explain his condition to his family. It also allows Dr Miller to guide the woman to a more appropriate place to wait for the consultant.

51. (B)

This response is appropriate, as it confirms the relationship to the patient and supports the patient's family member in the absence of the consultant; however, it is not ideal, as it does not comply entirely with the patient's wishes to have the consultant explain his condition to his family.

52. (D)

This is not at all important, as Jackson should not be stealing the supplies for any reason.

53. (B)

The reason that Jackson is stealing the supplies is irrelevant to how Zakariyah responds to the situation. However, if Jackson has talked about putting up drips on himself and his friends, this is an important factor to consider, as the fact that Jackson is taking drips and bags of intravenous fluids makes it more likely that Jackson is actually engaging in an illegal and potentially dangerous misuse of medical equipment, and Zakariyah should take this into account when dealing with the situation.

54. (D)

Jackson should not be stealing medical supplies from the hospital. The fact that the medical supplies are not safe to use at the hospital is not at all important in responding to Jackson's behaviour.

55. (D)

Whilst it may be tempting for Zakariyah to 'let this one go' in support of his friend, stealing hospital supplies is completely against all regulations and also calls into question a doctor's probity; therefore, it is important that Zakariyah raises this through the appropriate channels without placing any importance at all on the consequences for Jackson's medical career.

56. (D)

This factor is not at all important, as it does not mitigate Liam's unprofessional comments about this patient in any way.

57. (C)

This factor is of minor importance, as it could lead Conor to be more sensitive to Liam's remarks. It could also serve as a constructive point about not prejudging foreigners in Conor's response to Liam.

58. (A)

This is a very important factor to consider, as Conor will need to decide whether to respond to Liam immediately, or to move the conversation to a more private space where they can speak freely.

59. (D)

This is not at all important, as Liam's comments are so extreme that Conor must address them with Liam immediately, directly and discreetly, even if this is the first time that Liam has made them.

60. (A)

This is a very important factor, as it means that it will be simple and direct for Conor to get support in addressing Liam's behaviour effectively. Given the nature of Liam's remarks about not being able to deal with 'another one of these people', it is likely that there are serious issues that need to be addressed, and Conor may need help from a senior member of staff to do so effectively. This factor makes it more likely that Conor could get such help, so it is very important.

61. (C)

This factor is of minor importance. It makes it more likely that Conor would want to be sensitive yet effective in responding to Liam's remarks, but it does not mitigate the need to address Liam's behaviour in any way.

62. (A)

This is a very important factor, since the consultant obviously had a good reason for requesting the X-ray, and patient health and the professionalism of the team may be compromised if it is not completed on time.

63. (A)

This is very important to consider, since the safety of patients has to come first. If there was a very sick patient on the ward who urgently needed medical care, then they should have taken priority over other non-urgent jobs, such as organising this X-ray.

64. (B)

This is an important factor, as it means that there is sufficient time remaining to organise this non-urgent X-ray before the patient leaves the hospital.

65. (D)

Patients must always come first, so this factor is not at all important. The fact that Dr O'Keefe had this news a few days ago means that she had time to organise someone to cover for her if she needed to take a few days off.

66. (A)

This is a very important factor, as it would allow for Maisie to ring Catriona and encourage her to make every effort to come to the meeting before it starts. If Catriona will be delayed, then the group could delay the start of the meeting. This is something best explained directly, rather than in a text message, so a private spot for this conversation would be very important.

67. (B)

This is an important consideration, as it would give Catriona a likelihood of arriving relatively soon, although she would be likely to arrive late. This would be preferable to Catriona skipping the meeting due to car trouble, so Maisie would be right to encourage Catriona to consider other transport options.

68. (A)

This factor is of utmost importance. If they have been clearly assigned a project that must be completed as a group, then it is inappropriate for Catriona to ask Maisie to cover for her.

69. (A)

This factor is extremely important, as it is fundamental to the matter at hand, and Addison must disclose what he observed to the hospital administrator.

70. (D)

This is not at all important, as Addison remembers noticing an error during the procedure and thus has a professional obligation to disclose it to the hospital, even if he is not directly asked about it.

71. (C)

This factor is of minor importance. It does not mitigate Addison's responsibility to disclose Petra's error to the hospital, though it makes it more urgent that he do so, as the other staff may have lacked the training to understand that it was an error, or to comprehend its implications.